W0259412

Cram101 Textbook Outlines to accompany:

Basic Histology: Text and Atlas

Junqueira, Carneiro, 11th Edition

An Academic Internet Publishers (AIPI) publication (c) 2007.

You have a discounted membership at www.Cram101.com with this book.

Get all of the practice tests for the chapters of this textbook, and access in-depth reference material for writing essays and papers. Here is an example from a Cram101 Biology text:

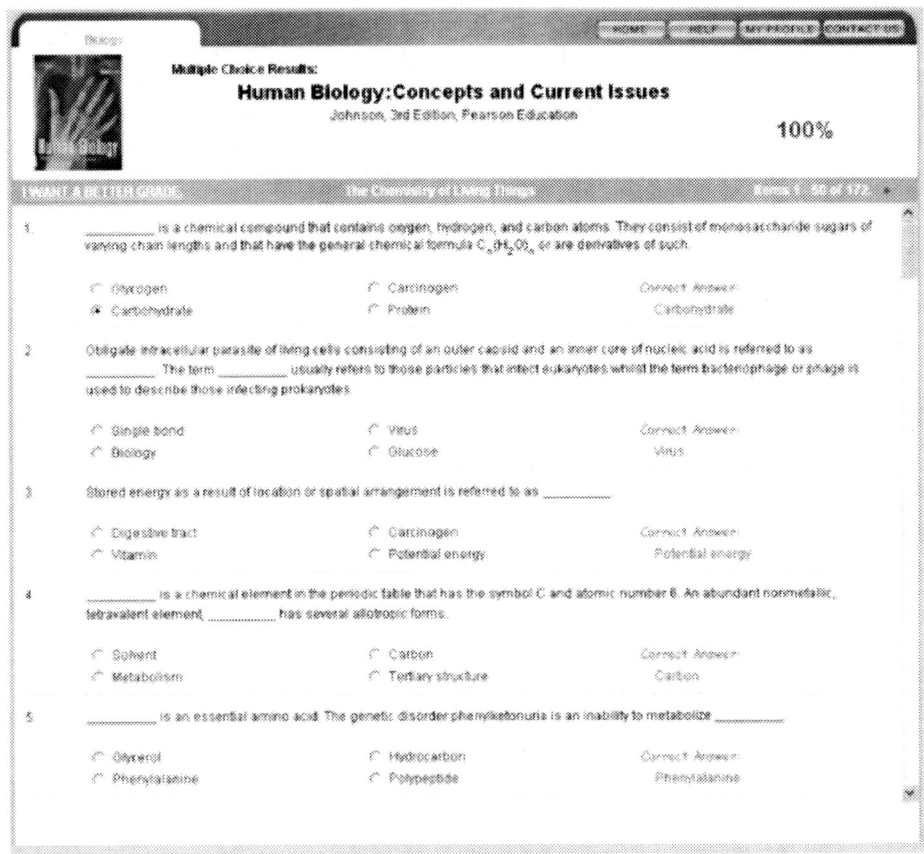

When you need problem solving help with math, stats, and other disciplines, www.Cram101.com will walk through the formulas and solutions step by step.

With Cram101.com online, you also have access to extensive reference material.

You will nail those essays and papers. Here is an example from a Cram101 Biology text:

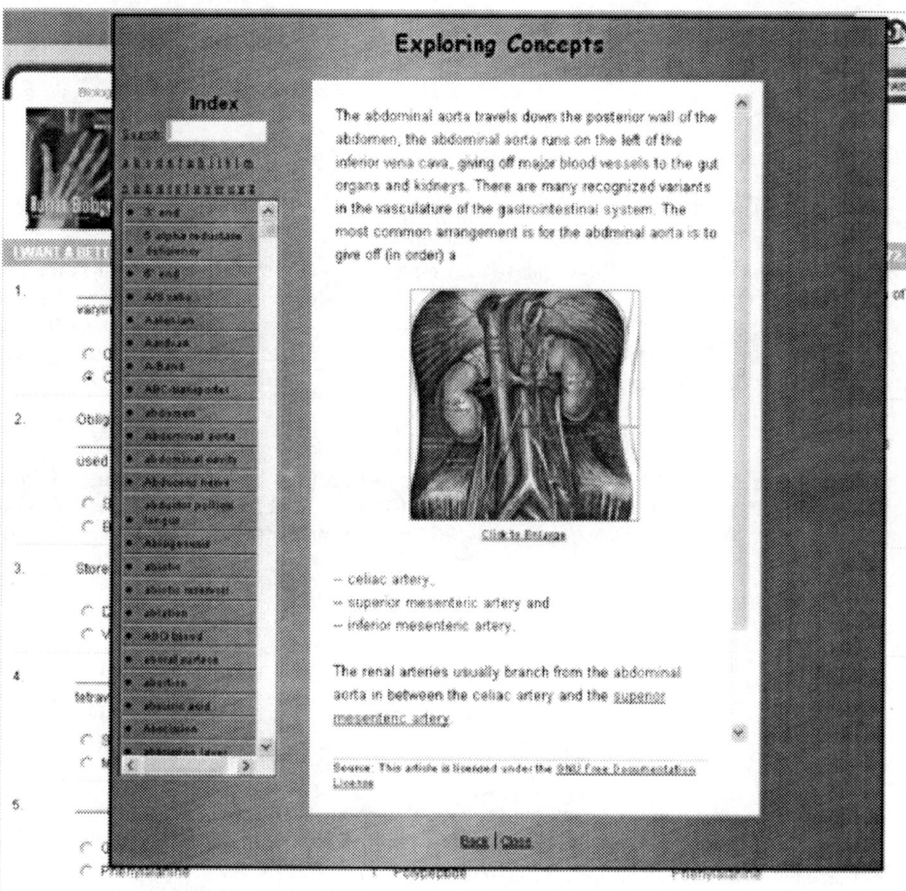

Visit **www.Cram101.com**, click Sign Up at the top of the screen, and enter DK73DW3596 in the promo code box on the registration screen. Access to www.Cram101.com is normally $9.95, but because you have purchased this book, your access fee is only $4.95. Sign up and stop highlighting textbooks forever.

Learning System

Cram101 Textbook Outlines is a learning system. The notes in this book are the highlights of your textbook, you will never have to highlight a book again.

How to use this book. Take this book to class, it is your notebook for the lecture. The notes and highlights on the left hand side of the pages follow the outline and order of the textbook. All you have to do is follow along while your intructor presents the lecture. Circle the items emphasized in class and add other important information on the right side. With Cram101 Textbook Outlines you'll spend less time writing and more time listening. Learning becomes more efficient.

Cram101.com Online

Increase your studying efficiency by using Cram101.com's practice tests and online reference material. It is the perfect complement to Cram101 Textbook Outlines. Use self-teaching matching tests or simulate in-class testing with comprehensive multiple choice tests, or simply use Cram's true and false tests for quick review. Cram101.com even allows you to enter your in-class notes for an integrated studying format combining the textbook notes with your class notes.

Visit **www.Cram101.com**, click Sign Up at the top of the screen, and enter **DK73DW3596** in the promo code box on the registration screen. Access to www.Cram101.com is normally $9.95, but because you have purchased this book, your access fee is only $4.95. Sign up and stop highlighting textbooks forever.

 ISBN: 1-4288-1931-2

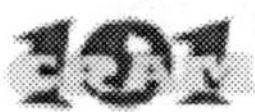

Basic Histology: Text and Atlas
Junqueira, Carneiro, 11th

CONTENTS

Tissue	A collection of interconnected cells that perform a similar function within an organism is called tissue.
Organ	Organ refers to a structure consisting of several tissues adapted as a group to perform specific functions.
Connective tissue	Connective tissue is any type of biological tissue with an extensive extracellular matrix and often serves to support, bind together, and protect organs.
Nervous tissue	Tissue made up of neurons and supportive cells is referred to as nervous tissue. It forms a rapid communication network for the body.
Extracellular	Outside the cell is called extracellular.
Collagen	Collagen is the main protein of connective tissue in animals and the most abundant protein in mammals, making up about 1/4 of the total. It is one of the long, fibrous structural proteins whose functions are quite different from those of globular proteins such as enzymes.
Collagen fibril	Collagen fibril refers to extracellular structure formed by self-assembly of secreted fibrillar collagen subunits. An abundant constituent of the extracellular matrix in many animal tissues.
Cytoplasm	Cytoplasm refers to the contents of a cell excluding the nucleus and cell membrane. Cytoplasm is a homogeneous, generally clear jelly-like material that fills cells.
Receptor	A receptor is a protein on the cell membrane or within the cytoplasm or cell nucleus that binds to a specific molecule (a ligand), such as a neurotransmitter, hormone, or other substance, and initiates the cellular response to the ligand. Receptor, in immunology, the region of an antibody which shows recognition of an antigen.
Central nervous system	The central nervous system comprized of the brain and spinal cord, represents the largest part of the nervous system. Together with the peripheral nervous system, it has a fundamental role in the control of behavior.
Nervous system	The nervous system of an animal coordinates the activity of the muscles, monitors the organs, constructs and processes input from the senses, and initiates actions.
Microscope	A microscope is an instrument for viewing objects that are too small to be seen by the naked or unaided
Histology	Histology is the study of tissue sectioned as a thin slice, using a microscope. It can be described as microscopic anatomy.
Immunology	Immunology refers to the branch of science that deals with the immune system and attempts to understand the many phenomena that are responsible for both acquired and innate immunity. It also includes the use of antibodyantigen reactions in other laboratory work .
Physiology	The study of the function of cells, tissues, and organs is referred to as physiology.
Pathology	Pathology is the study of the processes underlying disease and other forms of illness, harmful abnormality, or dysfunction.
Light microscope	An optical instrument with lenses that refract visible light to magnify images and project them into a viewer's eye or onto photographic film is referred to as light microscope.
Digestion	Digestion refers to the mechanical and chemical breakdown of food into molecules small enough for the body to absorb; the second main stage of food processing, following ingestion.
Bacteria	The domain that contains procaryotic cells with primarily diacyl glycerol diesters in their membranes and with bacterial rRNA. Bacteria also is a general term for organisms that are composed of procaryotic cells and are not multicellular.
Enzyme	An enzyme is a protein that catalyzes, or speeds up, a chemical reaction. They are essential to sustain life because most chemical reactions in biological cells would occur too slowly, or would lead to

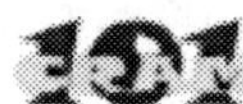

	different products, without them.
Fixative	In biology, a fixative is a solution used to preserve or harden fresh tissue or cell specimens for microscopic examination. Usually they stabilise and firm tissues by denaturing or cross-linking constituent proteins. Formaldehyde solution is an example of a fixative.
Solution	Solution refers to homogenous mixture formed when a solute is dissolved in a solvent.
Agent	Agent refers to an epidemiological term referring to the organism or object that transmits a disease from the environment to the host.
Intravascular	Within the arteries, vessels, veins, or capillaries is intravascular.
Blood vessel	A blood vessel is a part of the circulatory system and function to transport blood throughout the body. The most important types, arteries and veins, are so termed because they carry blood away from or towards the heart, respectively.
Blood	Blood is a circulating tissue composed of fluid plasma and cells. The main function of blood is to supply nutrients (oxygen, glucose) and constitutional elements to tissues and to remove waste products.
Microscopy	Microscopy is any technique for producing visible images of structures or details too small to otherwise be seen by the human eye, using a microscope or other magnification tool.
Isotonic solution	An isotonic solution has an equal amount of dissolved solute in it compared to the things around it. Typically in humans and most other mammals, the isotonic solution is 0.9 weight percent.
Protein	A protein is a complex, high-molecular-weight organic compound that consists of amino acids joined by peptide bonds. They are essential to the structure and function of all living cells and viruses. Many are enzymes or subunits of enzymes.
Amine	An organic compound with one or more amino groups is called amine. They contain nitrogen as the key atom. Structurally amines resemble ammonia, wherein one or more hydrogen atoms are replaced by organic substituents such as alkyl and aryl groups.
Glutaraldehyde	Glutaraldehyde is a colorless liquid with a pungent odor used to sterilize medical and dental equipment. It is also used for industrial water treatment and as a chemical preservative. But it is toxic, causing severe eye, nose, throat and lung irritation, along with headaches, drowsiness and dizziness.
Osmium	Osmium is a chemical element in the periodic table that has the symbol Os and atomic number 76. A hard brittle blue-gray or blue-black transition metal in the platinum family, osmium is the densest natural element and is used in some alloys with platinum and iridium. The extraordinary density of osmium is a consequence of the lanthanide contraction.
Lipid	Lipid is one class of aliphatic hydrocarbon-containing organic compounds essential for the structure and function of living cells. They are characterized by being water-insoluble but soluble in nonpolar organic solvents.
Consistency	The extent to which an individual responds to a given stimulus or situation in the same way on different occasions is a consistency.
Dehydration	Dehydration is the removal of water from an object. Medically, dehydration is a serious and potentially life-threatening condition in which the body contains an insufficient volume of water for normal functioning.
Solvent	A solvent is a liquid that dissolves a solid, liquid, or gaseous solute, resulting in a solution. The most common solvent in everyday life is water.
Ethanol	Ethanol is a flammable, colorless chemical compound, one of the alcohols that is most often found in alcoholic beverages. In common parlance, it is often referred to simply as alcohol. Its chemical formula is C_2H_5OH, also written as C_2H_6O.

Freezing | Freezing is the process in which blood is frozen and all of the plasma and 99% of the WBCs are eliminated when thawing takes place and the nontransferable cryoprotectant is removed.

Staining | Staining is a biochemical technique of adding a class-specific (DNA, proteins, lipids, carbohydrates) dye to a substrate to qualify or quantify the presence of a specific compound. They are frequently used to highlight structures in tissues for viewing, often with the aid of different microscopes.

Salt | Salt is a term used for ionic compounds composed of positively charged cations and negatively charged anions, so that the product is neutral and without a net charge.

Affinity | Chemical affinity results from electronic properties by which dissimilar substances are capable of forming chemical compounds. Specifically, the term refers to the tendency of an atom or compound to combine by chemical reaction with atoms or compounds of unlike composition.

Acid | An acid is a water-soluble, sour-tasting chemical compound that when dissolved in water, gives a solution with a pH of less than 7.

Base | The common definition of a base is a chemical compound that absorbs hydronium ions when dissolved in water (a proton acceptor). An alkali is a special example of a base, where in an aqueous environment, hydroxide ions are donated.

Mitochondria | Cytoplasmic organelles responsible for ATP generation for cellular activities are referred to as mitochondria.

Nucleic acid | A nucleic acid is a complex, high-molecular-weight biochemical macromolecule composed of nucleotide chains that convey genetic information.

Glycosaminoglycan | Glycosaminoglycan is a long unbranched polysaccharide, made up of repeating disaccharides that may be sulphated (e.g. glucuronic acid, iduronic acid, galactose, galactosamine, glucosamine).

Cartilage | Cartilage is a type of dense connective tissue. Cartilage is composed of cells called chondrocytes which are dispersed in a firm gel-like ground substance, called the matrix. Cartilage is avascular (contains no blood vessels) and nutrients are diffused through the matrix.

Hyaline cartilage | Hyaline cartilage is the most abundant type of cartilage. Hyaline cartilage is a translucent matrix or ground substance found lining bones in joints. It is also present inside bones, serving as a center of ossification or bone growth

Muscle | Muscle is a contractile form of tissue. It is one of the four major tissue types, the other three being epithelium, connective tissue and nervous tissue. Muscle contraction is used to move parts of the body, as well as to move substances within the body.

Smooth muscle | Smooth muscle is a type of non-striated muscle, found within the "walls" of hollow organs; such as blood vessels, the bladder, the uterus, and the gastrointestinal tract. Smooth muscle is used to move matter within the body, via contraction; it generally operates "involuntarily", without nerve stimulation.

Rotation | Movement turning a body part on its longitudinal axis is rotation.

Insight | Insight refers to a sudden awareness of the relationships among various elements that had previously appeared to be independent of one another.

Silver | Silver is a chemical element with the symbol Ag. A soft white lustrous transition metal, it has the highest electrical and thermal conductivity of any metal and occurs in minerals and in free form.

Gold | Gold is a chemical element in the periodic table that has the symbol Au and atomic number 79. A soft, shiny, yellow, dense, malleable, ductile (trivalent and univalent) transition metal, gold does not react with most chemicals but is attacked by chlorine, fluorine and aqua regia.

Fluorescence | Fluorescence is a luminescence that is mostly found as an optical phenomenon in cold bodies, in which the molecular absorption of a photon triggers the emission of a lower-energy photon with a longer

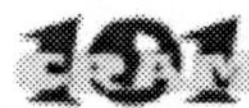

	wavelength. The energy difference between the absorbed and emitted photons ends up as molecular vibrations or heat.
Retina	The retina is a thin layer of cells at the back of the eyeball of vertebrates and some cephalopods; it is the part of the eye which converts light into nervous signals.
Eye	An eye is an organ that detects light. Different kinds of light-sensitive organs are found in a variety of creatures. The simplest eyes do nothing but detect whether the surroundings are light or dark, while more complex eyes can distinguish shapes and colors.
Digital image	A digital image is a representation of a two-dimensional image as a finite set of digital values, called picture elements or pixels.
Actin	A protein in a muscle fiber that, together with myosin, is responsible for contraction and relaxation is actin.
Value	Value is worth in general, and it is thought to be connected to reasons for certain practices, policies, actions, beliefs or emotions. Value is "that which one acts to gain and/or keep."
Lens	The lens or crystalline lens is a transparent, biconvex structure in the eye that, along with the cornea, helps to refract light to focus on the retina. Its function is thus similar to a man-made optical lens.
Microtubule	A hollow rod of the protein tubulin in the cytoplasm is referred to as the microtubule.
Mesentery	A mesentery is a part of the peritoneum that connects an internal organ, such as the small intestine, to the abdominal wall.
Fiber	Fibers used by man come from a wide variety of sources: Natural fiber include those made out of plants, animal and mineral sources. Natural fibers can be classified according to their origin.
Collagen fiber	White fiber in the matrix of connective tissue, giving flexibility and strength is called collagen fiber.
DNA	Deoxyribonucleic acid (DNA) is a nucleic acid —usually in the form of a double helix— that contains the genetic instructions specifying the biological development of all cellular forms of life, and most viruses.
Fluorescence microscope	A Fluorescence Microscope is a light microscope used to study properties of organic or inorganic substances using the phenomena of fluorescence and phosphorescence instead of, or in addition to, reflection and absorption.
Scanning electron microscope	A microscope that uses an electron beam to study the surface architecture of a cell or other specimen is called scanning electron microscope.
Transmission electron microscope	Transmission electron microscope refers to a microscope that uses an electron beam to study the internal structure of thinly sectioned specimens.
Tungsten	Tungsten is a chemical element that has the symbol W (L. wolframium) and atomic number 74. A very hard, heavy, steel-gray to white transition metal, tungsten is found in several ores including wolframite and scheelite and is remarkable for its robust physical properties, especially the fact that it has a higher melting point than any other non-alloy in existence.
Cathode	A cathode is the electrode at which electrons go into a cell, tube or diode, whether driven externally or internally.
Micrograph	A micrograph is a photograph or similar image taken through a microscope or similar device to show a magnified image of an item.
Radiation	The emission of electromagnetic waves by all objects warmer than absolute zero is referred to as

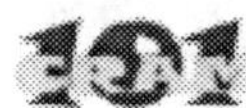

radiation.

Crystal
Crystal is a solid in which the constituent atoms, molecules, or ions are packed in a regularly ordered, repeating pattern extending in all three spatial dimensions.

Amino acid
An amino acid is any molecule that contains both amino and carboxylic acid functional groups. They are the basic structural building units of proteins. They form short polymer chains called peptides or polypeptides which in turn form structures called proteins.

Nucleotide
A building block of a nucleic acid molecule, consisting of a sugar, a nitrogenous base, and a phosphate group is called a nucleotide.

Sugar
A sugar is the simplest molecule that can be identified as a carbohydrate. These include monosaccharides and disaccharides, trisaccharides and the oligosaccharides. The term "glyco-" indicates the presence of a sugar in an otherwise non-carbohydrate substance.

Fucose
Fucose is a hexose sugar with the chemical formula $C_6H_{12}O_5$. It is found on N-linked glycans on the mammalian and plant cell surface. Alpha1□¨3 linked core fucose is a suspected carbohydrate antigen for IgE-mediated allergy.

Gland
A gland is an organ in an animal's body that synthesizes a substance for release such as hormones, often into the bloodstream or into cavities inside the body or its outer surface.

Submandibular gland
The submandibular gland is one of the salivary glands, responsible for producing saliva. It lies inferior to the mylohyoid muscles and superior to the digastric muscle.

Injection
A method of rapid drug delivery that puts the substance directly in the bloodstream, in a muscle, or under the skin is called injection.

Culture
Culture, generally refers to patterns of human activity and the symbolic structures that give such activity significance.

Direct observation
Direct observation refers to assessing behavior through direct surveillance.

In vitro
In vitro is an experimental technique where the experiment is performed in a test tube, or generally outside a living organism or cell.

Vitamin
An organic compound other than a carbohydrate, lipid, or protein that is needed for normal metabolism but that the body cannot synthesize in adequate amounts is called a vitamin.

Serum
Serum is the same as blood plasma except that clotting factors (such as fibrin) have been removed. Blood plasma contains fibrinogen.

Petri dish
Petri dish refers to a shallow dish consisting of two round, overlapping halves that is used to grow microorganisms on solid culture medium; the top is larger than the bottom of the dish to prevent contamination of the culture.

Life span
Life span refers to the upper boundary of life, the maximum number of years an individual can live. The maximum life span of human beings is about 120 years of age.

Cancer
Cancer is a class of diseases or disorders characterized by uncontrolled division of cells and the ability of these cells to invade other tissues, either by direct growth into adjacent tissue through invasion or by implantation into distant sites by metastasis.

Metabolism
Metabolism is the biochemical modification of chemical compounds in living organisms and cells. This includes the biosynthesis of complex organic molecules (anabolism) and their breakdown (catabolism).

Chromosomes
Physical structures in the cell's nucleus that house the genes. Each human cell has 23 pairs of chromosomes.

Morphology
The scientific study of organic form, including both its development and function is morphology.

Genetic disorder	A genetic disorder is a disease caused by abnormal expression of one or more genes in a person causing a clinical phenotype.
Organelle	Organelle refers to any structure within a cell that carries out one of its metabolic roles, such as mitochondria, centrioles, endoplasmic reticulum, and the nucleus.
Trypanosome	Parasitic zooflagellate that causes severe disease in human beings and domestic animals, including a condition called sleeping sickness is a trypanosome. All members are exclusively parasitic, found primarily in insects.
Chemical reaction	Chemical reaction refers to a process leading to chemical changes in matter; involves the making and/or breaking of chemical bonds.
Macromolecule	A macromolecule is a molecule with a large molecular mass, but generally the use of the term is restricted to polymers and molecules which structurally include polymers.
Phosphate	A phosphate is a polyatomic ion or radical consisting of one phosphorus atom and four oxygen. In the ionic form, it carries a -3 formal charge, and is denoted PO_4^{3-}.
Calcium	Calcium is the chemical element in the periodic table that has the symbol Ca and atomic number 20. Calcium is a soft grey alkaline earth metal that is used as a reducing agent in the extraction of thorium, zirconium and uranium. Calcium is also the fifth most abundant element in the Earth's crust.
Iron	Iron is essential to all organisms, except for a few bacteria. It is mostly stably incorporated in the inside of metalloproteins, because in exposed or in free form it causes production of free radicals that are generally toxic to cells.
Ion	Ion refers to an atom or molecule that has gained or lost one or more electrons, thus acquiring an electrical charge.
Phosphatase	A phosphatase is an enzyme that hydrolyses phosphoric acid monoesters into a phosphate ion and a molecule with a free hydroxyl group.
Sulfide	One of the minerals that is abundant in the hot water that seeps through hydrothermal vents is sulfide.
Lead	Lead is a chemical element in the periodic table that has the symbol Pb and atomic number 82. A soft, heavy, toxic and malleable poor metal, lead is bluish white when freshly cut but tarnishes to dull gray when exposed to air. Lead is used in building construction, lead-acid batteries, bullets and shot, and is part of solder, pewter, and fusible alloys.
Substrate	A substrate is a molecule which is acted upon by an enzyme. Each enzyme recognizes only the specific substrate of the reaction it catalyzes. A surface in or on which an organism lives.
Hydrogen	Hydrogen is a chemical element in the periodic table that has the symbol H and atomic number 1. At standard temperature and pressure it is a colorless, odorless, nonmetallic, univalent, tasteless, highly flammable diatomic gas.
Lysosome	Organelle that contains enzymes that degrade worn cell parts is called a lysosome.
Alkaline phosphatase	Alkaline phosphatase (ALP) (EC 3.1.3.1) is a hydrolase enzyme responsible for removing phosphate groups in the 5- and 3- positions from many types of molecules, including nucleotides, proteins, and alkaloids.
Hydrogen ion	A single proton with a charge of + 1. The dissociation of a water molecule leads to the generation of a hydroxide ion and a hydrogen ion. The hydrogen ion is hydrated in aqueous solutions and is usually written as H_3O^+.
Oxidation	Oxidation refers to the loss of electrons from a substance involved in a redox reaction; always accompanies reduction.
Hydrogen peroxide	Hydrogen peroxide is a clear liquid, slightly more viscous than water, that has strong oxidizing properties and is therefore a powerful bleaching agent that has found use as a disinfectant, as an

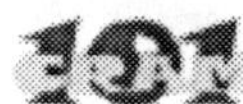

	oxidizer, and in rocketry (particularly in high concentrations as high-test peroxide (HTP) as a monopropellant, and in bipropellant systems.
Diagnosis	In medicine, diagnosis is the process of identifying a medical condition or disease by its signs, symptoms, and from the results of various diagnostic procedures.
Leukemia	Leukemia refers to a type of cancer of the bloodforming tissues, characterized by an excessive production of white blood cells and an abnormally high number of them in the blood; cancer of the bone marrow cells that produce leukocytes.
Oligosaccharide	An oligosaccharide is a saccharide polymer containing a small number (typically three to six) of component sugars, also known as simple sugars. They are generally found either O- or N-linked to compatible amino acid side chains in proteins or to lipid moieties.
Polysaccharide	A carbohydrate composed of many joined monosaccharides is called a polysaccharide.
Isolation	Isolation refers to the degree to which groups do not live in the same communities.
Sodium	Sodium is the chemical element in the periodic table that has the symbol Na (Natrium in Latin) and atomic number 11. Sodium is a soft, waxy, silvery reactive metal belonging to the alkali metals that is abundant in natural compounds (especially halite). It is highly reactive.
Aldehyde	An aldehyde is either a functional group consisting of a terminal carbonyl group or a compound containing a terminal carbonyl group.
Glycogen	Glycogen refers to a complex, extensively branched polysaccharide of many glucose monomers; serves as an energy-storage molecule in liver and muscle cells.
Liver	The liver is an organ in vertebrates, including humans. It plays a major role in metabolism and has a number of functions in the body including drug detoxification, glycogen storage, and plasma protein synthesis. It also produces bile, which is important for digestion.
Striated muscle	Striated muscle refers to contractile tissue characterized by multinucleated cells containing highly ordered arrangements of actin and myosin microfilaments. Also known as skeletal muscle.
Specificity	A medical diagnostic test for a certain disease, specificity is the proportion of true negatives of all the negative samples tested.
Amylase	Amylase is a digestive enzyme classified as a saccharidase. It is mainly a constituent of pancreatic juice and saliva, needed for the breakdown of long-chain carbohydrates (such as starch) into smaller units.
Saliva	Saliva is the moist, clear, and usually somewhat frothy substance produced in the mouths of some animals, including humans.
Proteoglycan	Molecule consisting of one or more glycosaminoglycan chains attached to a core protein is referred to as proteoglycan.
Attachment	Attachment refers to the psychological tendency to seek closeness to another person, to feel secure when that person is present, and to feel anxious when that person is absent.
Monosaccharide	A monosaccharide is simplest form of a carbohydrate. They consist of one sugar and are usually colorless, water-soluble, crystalline solids. Some monosaccharides have a sweet taste. They are the building blocks of disaccharides like sucrose and polysaccharides.
Kidney	The kidney is a bean-shaped excretory organ in vertebrates. Part of the urinary system, the kidneys filter wastes (especially urea) from the blood and excrete them, along with water, as urine.
Carboxyl	A carboxyl is the univalent radical -COOH; present in and characteristic of organic acids.
Alcohol	Alcohol is a general term, applied to any organic compound in which a hydroxyl group (-OH) is bound to a carbon atom, which in turn is bound to other hydrogen and/or carbon atoms. The general formula for a

	simple acyclic alcohol is $C_nH_{2n+1}OH$.
Phospholipid	Phospholipid is a class of lipids formed from four components: fatty acids, a negatively-charged phosphate group, an alcohol and a backbone. Phospholipids with a glycerol backbone are known as glycerophospholipids or phosphoglycerides.
Cholesterol	Cholesterol is a steroid, a lipid, and an alcohol, found in the cell membranes of all body tissues, and transported in the blood plasma of all animals. It is an important component of the membranes of cells, providing stability; it makes the membrane's fluidity stable over a bigger temperature interval.
Glycolipid	Glycolipid refers to lipid in plasma membranes that bears a carbohydrate chain attached to a hydrophobic tail.
Esters	Esters are organic compounds in which an organic group replaces a hydrogen atom in an oxygen acid. An oxygen acid is an acid whose molecule has an -OH group from which the hydrogen (H) can dissociate as an H^+ ion.
Intracellular	Intracellular refers to having to do with the interior of a cell.
Brush border	Brush border refers to dense covering of microvilli on the apical surface of epithelial cells in the intestine and kidney. The microvilli aid absorption by increasing the surface area of the cell.
Goblet cell	A goblet cell is a glandular simple columnar epithelial cell that is specifically designed to secrete mucus.
Villus	Villus refers to a fingerlike projection of the inner surface of the small intestine. A fingerlike projection of the chorion of the mammalian placenta. Large numbers of villus increase the surface areas of these organs.
Atom	An atom is the smallest possible particle of a chemical element that retains its chemical properties.
Actin filament	An actin filament is a helical protein filament formed by the polymerization of globular actin molecules. They provide mechanical support for the cell, determine the cell shape, enable cell movements; and participate in certain cell junctions.
Antibody	An antibody is a protein used by the immune system to identify and neutralize foreign objects like bacteria and viruses. Each antibody recognizes a specific antigen unique to its target.
Staphylococcus aureus	Staphylococcus aureus (which is occasionally given the nickname golden staph) is a bacterium, frequently living on the skin or in the nose of a healthy person, that can cause illnesses ranging from minor skin infections (such as pimples, boils, and cellulitis) and abscesses, to life-threatening diseases such as pneumonia, meningitis, endocarditis and septicemia.
Staphylococcus	Staphylococcus is a genus of gram-positive bacteria. Under the microscope they appear round (cocci), and form in grape-like clusters.
Carbohydrate	Carbohydrate is a chemical compound that contains oxygen, hydrogen, and carbon atoms. They consist of monosaccharide sugars of varying chain lengths and that have the general chemical formula $C_n(H_2O)_n$ or are derivatives of such.
Lectin	Lectin is a protein of non-immune origin that specifically interacts with sugar molecules (carbohydrates) without modifying them.
Antigen	An antigen is a substance that stimulates an immune response, especially the production of antibodies. They are usually proteins or polysaccharides, but can be any type of molecule, including small molecules (haptens) coupled to a protein (carrier).
Lymphocyte	A lymphocyte is a type of white blood cell involved in the human body's immune system. There are two broad categories, namely T cells and B cells.
Tumor	An abnormal mass of cells that forms within otherwise normal tissue is a tumor. This growth can be either malignant or benign

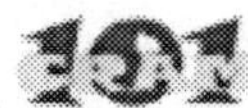

Biotin	Biotin is a low-molecular-weight compound used as a coenzyme. Useful technically as a covalent label for proteins, allowing them to be detected by the egg protein avidin, which binds extremely tightly to biotin.
In situ hybridization	In situ hybridization refers to the use of a DNA or RNA probe to detect the presence of the complementary DNA sequence in cloned bacterial or cultured eukaryotic cells.
Polypeptide	Polypeptide refers to polymer of many amino acids linked by peptide bonds.
Infection	The invasion and multiplication of microorganisms in body tissues is called an infection.
Hormone	A hormone is a chemical messenger from one cell to another. All multicellular organisms produce hormones. The best known hormones are those produced by endocrine glands of vertebrate animals, but hormones are produced by nearly every organ system and tissue type in a human or animal body. Hormone molecules are secreted directly into the bloodstream, they move by circulation or diffusion to their target cells, which may be nearby cells in the same tissue or cells of a distant organ of the body.
Virus	Obligate intracellular parasite of living cells consisting of an outer capsid and an inner core of nucleic acid is referred to as virus. The term virus usually refers to those particles that infect eukaryotes whilst the term bacteriophage or phage is used to describe those infecting prokaryotes.
Gel electrophoresis	Gel electrophoresis is a group of techniques used by scientists to separate molecules based on physical characteristics such as size, shape, or isoelectric point.
Digestive tract	The digestive tract is the system of organs within multicellular animals which takes in food, digests it to extract energy and nutrients, and expels the remaining waste.
Nitrocellulose	Nitrocellulose is a highly flammable compound formed by nitrating cellulose (e.g. through exposure to nitric acid or powerful nitrating agent). This compound, when used as a propellant or low order explosive, was known as guncotton.
Isotope	An isotope is a form of an element whose nuclei have the same atomic number - the number of protons in the nucleus - but different mass numbers because they contain different numbers of neutrons.
Buffer	A chemical substance that resists changes in pH by accepting H^+ ions from or donating H^+ ions to solutions is called a buffer.
Blotting	Biochemical technique in which macromolecules separated on an agarose or polyacrylamide gel are transferred to a nylon membrane or sheet of paper, thereby immobilizing them for further analysis is called blotting.
Northern blotting	Northern blotting refers to technique used in molecular biology research to study gene expression in which RNA fragments separated by electrophoresis are immobilized on a paper sheet. A specific RNA is then detected by hybridization with a labeled nucleic acid probe.
Medicine	Medicine is the branch of health science and the sector of public life concerned with maintaining or restoring human health through the study, diagnosis and treatment of disease and injury.
Immunofluore-cence	Immunofluorescence is the labeling of antibodies or antigens with fluorescent dyes. This technique is sometimes used to make viral plaques more readily visible to the human eye. Immunofluorescently labelled tissue sections are studied using a fluorescence microscope or by confocal microscopy.
Intestine	The intestine is the portion of the alimentary canal extending from the stomach to the anus and, in humans and mammals, consists of two segments, the small intestine and the large intestine. The intestine is the part of the body responsible for extracting nutrition from food.
Lysozyme	Lysozyme is an enzyme (EC 3.2.1.17), commonly referred to as the "body's own antibiotic" since it kills bacteria. It is abundantly present in a number of secretions, such as tears (except bovine tears).
Small intestine	The small intestine is the part of the gastrointestinal tract between the stomach and the large intestine (colon). In humans over 5 years old it is about 7m long. It is divided into three structural

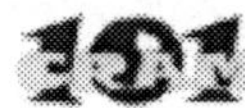

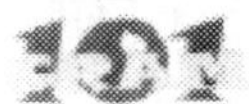

	parts: duodenum, jejunum and ileum.
Human papillomavirus	Human papillomavirus is a member of a group of viruses in the genus Papillomavirus that can infect humans and cause changes in cells leading to abnormal tissue growth.
Theory	Theory refers to an explanatory statement, or set of statements, that concisely summarizes the state of knowledge on a phenomenon and provides direction for further study.

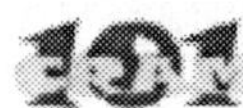

Bacteria	The domain that contains procaryotic cells with primarily diacyl glycerol diesters in their membranes and with bacterial rRNA. Bacteria also is a general term for organisms that are composed of procaryotic cells and are not multicellular.
Prokaryotes	Prokaryotes are organisms without a cell nucleus, or indeed any other membrane-bound organelles, in most cases unicellular.
Organelle	Organelle refers to any structure within a cell that carries out one of its metabolic roles, such as mitochondria, centrioles, endoplasmic reticulum, and the nucleus.
Protein	A protein is a complex, high-molecular-weight organic compound that consists of amino acids joined by peptide bonds. They are essential to the structure and function of all living cells and viruses. Many are enzymes or subunits of enzymes.
DNA	Deoxyribonucleic acid (DNA) is a nucleic acid —usually in the form of a double helix— that contains the genetic instructions specifying the biological development of all cellular forms of life, and most viruses.
Cytoplasm	Cytoplasm refers to the contents of a cell excluding the nucleus and cell membrane. Cytoplasm is a homogeneous, generally clear jelly-like material that fills cells.
Spermatozoon	Spermatozoon is the haploid cell that is the male gamete. It is carried in fluid called semen, and is capable of fertilizing an egg cell to form a zygote.
Zygote	A zygote is a cell that is the result of fertilization. That is, two haploid cells—usually (but not always) an ovum from a female and a sperm cell from a male—merge into a single diploid cell called the zygote.
Fertilization	Fertilization is fusion of gametes to form a new organism. In animals, the process involves a sperm fusing with an ovum, which eventually leads to the development of an embryo.
Receptor	A receptor is a protein on the cell membrane or within the cytoplasm or cell nucleus that binds to a specific molecule (a ligand), such as a neurotransmitter, hormone, or other substance, and initiates the cellular response to the ligand. Receptor, in immunology, the region of an antibody which shows recognition of an antigen.
Hormone	A hormone is a chemical messenger from one cell to another. All multicellular organisms produce hormones. The best known hormones are those produced by endocrine glands of vertebrate animals, but hormones are produced by nearly every organ system and tissue type in a human or animal body. Hormone molecules are secreted directly into the bloodstream, they move by circulation or diffusion to their target cells, which may be nearby cells in the same tissue or cells of a distant organ of the body.
Muscle	Muscle is a contractile form of tissue. It is one of the four major tissue types, the other three being epithelium, connective tissue and nervous tissue. Muscle contraction is used to move parts of the body, as well as to move substances within the body.
Macromolecule	A macromolecule is a molecule with a large molecular mass, but generally the use of the term is restricted to polymers and molecules which structurally include polymers.
Smooth muscle	Smooth muscle is a type of non-striated muscle, found within the "walls" of hollow organs; such as blood vessels, the bladder, the uterus, and the gastrointestinal tract. Smooth muscle is used to move matter within the body, via contraction; it generally operates "involuntarily", without nerve stimulation.
Plasma	Fluid portion of circulating blood is called plasma.
Phospholipid	Phospholipid is a class of lipids formed from four components: fatty acids, a negatively-charged phosphate group, an alcohol and a backbone. Phospholipids with a glycerol backbone are known as glycerophospholipids or phosphoglycerides.

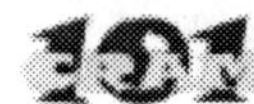

Hydrophobic	Hydrophobic refers to being electrically neutral and nonpolar, and thus prefering other neutral and nonpolar solvents or molecular environments. Hydrophobic is often used interchangeably with "oily" or "lipophilic."
Cholesterol	Cholesterol is a steroid, a lipid, and an alcohol, found in the cell membranes of all body tissues, and transported in the blood plasma of all animals. It is an important component of the membranes of cells, providing stability; it makes the membrane's fluidity stable over a bigger temperature interval.
Fatty acid	A fatty acid is a carboxylic acid (or organic acid), often with a long aliphatic tail (long chains), either saturated or unsaturated.
Phosphate	A phosphate is a polyatomic ion or radical consisting of one phosphorus atom and four oxygen. In the ionic form, it carries a -3 formal charge, and is denoted PO_4^{3-}.
Acid	An acid is a water-soluble, sour-tasting chemical compound that when dissolved in water, gives a solution with a pH of less than 7.
Plasma membrane	The unit membrane that encloses a cell and controls the traffic of molecules in and out of the cell is the plasma membrane.
Phosphate group	The functional group $-0P0_3H_2$; the transfer of energy from one compound to another is often accomplished by the transfer of a phosphate group.
Extracellular	Outside the cell is called extracellular.
Hydrophilic	Pertaining to molecules that attract water or dissolve in it because of their polar nature is hydrophilic.
Microscope	A microscope is an instrument for viewing objects that are too small to be seen by the naked or unaided eye.
Osmium	Osmium is a chemical element in the periodic table that has the symbol Os and atomic number 76. A hard brittle blue-gray or blue-black transition metal in the platinum family, osmium is the densest natural element and is used in some alloys with platinum and iridium. The extraordinary density of osmium is a consequence of the lanthanide contraction.
Intestine	The intestine is the portion of the alimentary canal extending from the stomach to the anus and, in humans and mammals, consists of two segments, the small intestine and the large intestine. The intestine is the part of the body responsible for extracting nutrition from food.
Adrenal	In mammals, the adrenal glands are the triangle-shaped endocrine glands that sit atop the kidneys. They are chiefly responsible for regulating the stress response through the synthesis of corticosteroids and catecholamines, including cortisol and adrenaline.
Enzyme	An enzyme is a protein that catalyzes, or speeds up, a chemical reaction. They are essential to sustain life because most chemical reactions in biological cells would occur too slowly, or would lead to different products, without them.
Kidney	The kidney is a bean-shaped excretory organ in vertebrates. Part of the urinary system, the kidneys filter wastes (especially urea) from the blood and excrete them, along with water, as urine.
Gland	A gland is an organ in an animal's body that synthesizes a substance for release such as hormones, often into the bloodstream or into cavities inside the body or its outer surface.
Ion	Ion refers to an atom or molecule that has gained or lost one or more electrons, thus acquiring an electrical charge.
Adrenal gland	In mammals, the adrenal gland (also known as suprarenal glands or colloquially as kidney

	hats) are the triangle-shaped endocrine glands that sit atop the kidneys; their name indicates that position.
Integrin	An integrin is an integral membrane protein in the plasma membrane of cells. It plays a role in the attachment of a cell to the extracellular matrix (ECM) and in signal transduction from the ECM to the cell.
Constant	A behavior or characteristic that does not vary from one observation to another is referred to as a constant.
Carbohydrate	Carbohydrate is a chemical compound that contains oxygen, hydrogen, and carbon atoms. They consist of monosaccharide sugars of varying chain lengths and that have the general chemical formula $C_n(H_2O)_n$ or are derivatives of such.
Lipid	Lipid is one class of aliphatic hydrocarbon-containing organic compounds essential for the structure and function of living cells. They are characterized by being water-insoluble but soluble in nonpolar organic solvents.
Eukaryotic	Eukaryotic cells are generally much larger than prokaryotes, typically a thousand times by volume. They have a variety of internal membranes and structures, called organelles, and a cytoskeleton composed of microtubules and microfilaments, which play an important role in defining the cell's organization.
Intracellular	Intracellular refers to having to do with the interior of a cell.
Oligosaccharide	An oligosaccharide is a saccharide polymer containing a small number (typically three to six) of component sugars, also known as simple sugars. They are generally found either O- or N-linked to compatible amino acid side chains in proteins or to lipid moieties.
Extracellular fluid	Body fluids outside the individual cells are called extracellular fluid.
Light microscope	An optical instrument with lenses that refract visible light to magnify images and project them into a viewer's eye or onto photographic film is referred to as light microscope.
Lipid bilayer	A lipid bilayer is a membrane or zone of a membrane composed of lipid molecules (usually phospholipids). The lipid bilayer is a critical component of all biological membranes, including cell membranes, and is a prerequisite for cell-based organisms.
Hydrocarbon	A chemical compound composed only of the elements carbon and hydrogen is called hydrocarbon.
Lecithin	Lecithin refers to a group of phospholipids containing two fatty acids, a phosphate group, and a choline molecule. They are a group of compounds, since they can differ based on the types of fatty acids found on each lecithin molecule.
Nonpolar	Lacking any asymmetric accumulation of positive and negative charge. Nonpolar molecules are generally insoluble in water.
Glycolipid	Glycolipid refers to lipid in plasma membranes that bears a carbohydrate chain attached to a hydrophobic tail.
Solution	Solution refers to homogenous mixture formed when a solute is dissolved in a solvent.
Salt	Salt is a term used for ionic compounds composed of positively charged cations and negatively charged anions, so that the product is neutral and without a net charge.
Glycocalyx	A network of polysaccharides extending from the surface of bacteria and other cells is referred to as glycocalyx. It allows the bacterium to attach itself to inert surfaces (like teeth or rocks), prokaryotes or other bacteria.
Membrane protein	A membrane protein is a protein molecule that is attached to, or associated with the membrane of a cell or an organelle. Membrane proteins can be classified into two groups, based on

	their attachment to the membrane.
Amino acid	An amino acid is any molecule that contains both amino and carboxylic acid functional groups. They are the basic structural building units of proteins. They form short polymer chains called peptides or polypeptides which in turn form structures called proteins.
Hydrophobic interaction	The tendency for hydrophobic molecules to cluster together when immersed in water is called hydrophobic interaction.
Distribution	Distribution in pharmacology is a branch of pharmacokinetics describing reversible transfer of drug from one location to another within the body.
Attachment	Attachment refers to the psychological tendency to seek closeness to another person, to feel secure when that person is present, and to feel anxious when that person is absent.
Diffusion	Random movement of molecules from a region of higher concentration toward one of lower concentration is referred to as diffusion.
Sugar	A sugar is the simplest molecule that can be identified as a carbohydrate. These include monosaccharides and disaccharides, trisaccharides and the oligosaccharides. The term "glyco-" indicates the presence of a sugar in an otherwise non-carbohydrate substance.
Proteoglycan	Molecule consisting of one or more glycosaminoglycan chains attached to a core protein is referred to as proteoglycan.
Vesicle	Membranous, cytoplasmic sac formed by an infolding of the cell membrane is called a vesicle.
Golgi apparatus	Golgi apparatus refers to an organelle in eukaryotic cells consisting of stacks of membranous sacs that modify, store, and ship products of the endoplasmic reticulum.
Adenosine	Adenosine is a nucleoside comprized of adenine attached to a ribose (ribofuranose) moiety via a β-N_9-glycosidic bond. Adenosine plays an important role in biochemical processes, such as energy transfer - as adenosine triphosphate (ATP) and adenosine diphosphate (ADP) - as well as in signal transduction as cyclic adenosine monophosphate, cAMP.
Adenosine triphosphate	Organic molecule that stores energy and releases energy for use in cellular processes is adenosine triphosphate.
Exocytosis	Exocytosis is the process by which a cell is able to get rid of large molecules or materials including wastes through its membrane. The process involves a [vacuole], containing the material, fusing with the membrane.
Fusion	Fusion refers to the combination of two atoms into a single atom as a result of a collision, usually accompanied by the release of energy.
Invagination	Infolding of one part of a structure into another is invagination.
Pinocytosis	Process by which a cell engulfs droplets of fluid from its surroundings is referred to as pinocytosis.
Lipoprotein	A lipoprotein is a biochemical assembly that contains both proteins and lipids and may be structural or catalytic in function. They may be enzymes, proton pumps, ion pumps, or some combination of these functions.
Endocytosis	Endocytosis is a process where cells absorb material (molecules or other cells) from outside by engulfing it with their cell membranes.
Polypeptide	Polypeptide refers to polymer of many amino acids linked by peptide bonds.
Affinity	Chemical affinity results from electronic properties by which dissimilar substances are capable of forming chemical compounds. Specifically, the term refers to the tendency of an atom or compound to combine by chemical reaction with atoms or compounds of unlike

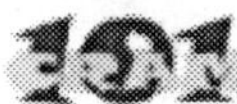

	composition.
Digestion	Digestion refers to the mechanical and chemical breakdown of food into molecules small enough for the body to absorb; the second main stage of food processing, following ingestion.
Lysosome	Organelle that contains enzymes that degrade worn cell parts is called a lysosome.
Motor protein	Protein that uses energy derived from nucleoside triphosphate hydrolysis to propel itself along a protein filament or another polymeric molecule is called motor protein.
Phagocytosis	Phagocytosis (literally, "cell eating") is a form of endocytosis where large particles are enveloped by the cell membrane of a (usually larger) cell and internalized to form a phagosome, or "food vacuole."
Polymorphonu-lear leukocyte	Polymorphonuclear leukocyte refers to a leukocyte that has a variety of nuclear forms.
Leukocyte	A white blood cell is a leukocyte. They help to defend the body against infectious disease and foreign materials as part of the immune system.
Fungi	Fungi refers to simple parasitic life forms, including molds, mildews, yeasts, and mushrooms. They live on dead or decaying organic matter. Fungi can grow as single cells, like yeast, or as multicellular colonies, as seen with molds.
Polymorphonu-lear	Cells with nuclei having several parts or lobes are called polymorphonuclear.
Pancreas	The pancreas is a retroperitoneal organ that serves two functions: exocrine - it produces pancreatic juice containing digestive enzymes, and endocrine - it produces several important hormones, namely insulin.
Salivary gland	The salivary gland produces saliva, which keeps the mouth and other parts of the digestive system moist. It also helps break down carbohydrates and lubricates the passage of food down from the oro-pharynx to the esophagus to the stomach.
Tissue	A collection of interconnected cells that perform a similar function within an organism is called tissue.
Channel	Channel, in communications (sometimes called communications channel), refers to the medium used to convey information from a sender (or transmitter) to a receiver.
Paracrine signaling	Paracrine signaling is a form of signalling in which the target cell is close to the signal releasing cell, and the signal chemical is broken down too quickly to be carried to other parts of the body.
Target cell	Specific cell on which a hormone exerts its effect is a target cell.
Nerve cell	A cell specialized to originate or transmit nerve impulses is referred to as nerve cell.
Synapse	A junction, or relay point, between two neurons, or between a neuron and an effector cell. Electrical and chemical signals are relayed from one cell to another at a synapse.
Nerve	A nerve is an enclosed, cable-like bundle of nerve fibers or axons, which includes the glia that ensheath the axons in myelin.
Blood	Blood is a circulating tissue composed of fluid plasma and cells. The main function of blood is to supply nutrients (oxygen, glucose) and constitutional elements to tissues and to remove waste products.
Synaptic signaling	Synaptic signaling refers to type of cell to cell communication that occurs across chemical synapses in the nervous system.
Neurotransmitter	A neurotransmitter is a chemical that is used to relay, amplify and modulate electrical

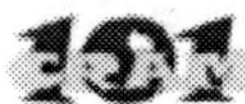

	signals between a neuron and another cell.
Solubility	A solution at equilibrium that cannot hold any more solute is said to be saturated. The equilibrium of a solution is mainly dependent on temperature. The maximum equilibrium amount of solute which can normally dissolve per amount of solvent is the solubility of that solute in that solvent.
Steroid	A steroid is a lipid characterized by a carbon skeleton with four fused rings. Different steroids vary in the functional groups attached to these rings. Hundreds of distinct steroids have been identified in plants and animals. Their most important role in most living systems is as hormones.
Thyroid	The thyroid is one of the larger endocrine glands in the body. It is located in the neck and produces hormones, principally thyroxine and triiodothyronine, that regulate the rate of metabolism and affect the growth and rate of function of many other systems in the body.
Thyroid **hormones**	The thyroid hormones, thyroxine (T4) and triiodothyronine (T3), are tyrosine-based hormones produced by the thyroid gland. An important component in the synthesis is iodine. They act on the body to increase the basal metabolic rate, affect protein synthesis and increase the body's sensitivity to catecholamines.
Nucleotide	A building block of a nucleic acid molecule, consisting of a sugar, a nitrogenous base, and a phosphate group is called a nucleotide.
G **protein**	G protein, short for guanine nucleotide binding proteins, are a family of proteins involved in second messenger cascades. They are so called because of their signaling mechanism, which uses the exchange of guanosine diphosphate (GDP) for guanosine triphosphate (GTP) as a molecular "switch" to allow or inhibit biochemical reactions inside the cell.
Second **messenger**	An intermediary compound that couples extracellular signals to intracellular processes and also amplifies a hormonal signal is referred to as second messenger.
Carrier	Person in apparent health whose chromosomes contain a pathologic mutant gene that may be transmitted to his or her children is a carrier.
Steroid **hormones**	Steroid hormones are steroids which act as hormones. They can be grouped into five groups by the receptors to which they bind: glucocorticoids, mineralocorticoids, androgens, estrogens, and progestagens.
Genes	Genes are the units of heredity in living organisms. They are encoded in the organism's genetic material (usually DNA or RNA), and control the development and behavior of the organism.
Homo**logous**	Homologous refers to structures that have the same embryonic or evolutionary origin but not necessarily the same function, such as the scrotum and labia majora. Also refers to two chromosomes with identical structures and gene loci but not necessarily identical alleles.
Sperm**atozoa**	A sperm cell, spermatozooa (pl. spermatozoa), or spermatozoan, is the haploid cell that is the male gamete. It is carried in fluid called semen, and is capable of fertilising an egg cell to form a zygote.
Metabolite	The term metabolite is usually restricted to small molecules. They are the intermediates and products of metabolism. A primary metabolite is directly involved in the normal growth, development, and reproduction. A secondary metabolite is not directly involved in those processes, but usually has important ecological function.
Base	The common definition of a base is a chemical compound that absorbs hydronium ions when dissolved in water (a proton acceptor). An alkali is a special example of a base, where in an aqueous environment, hydroxide ions are donated.

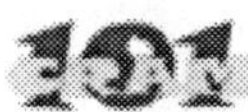

Chemical energy	Chemical energy refers to energy stored in the chemical bonds of molecules; a form of potential energy.
ATPase	ATPase is a class of enzymes that catalyze the decomposition of adenosine triphosphate into adenosine diphosphate and a free phosphate ion. This dephosphorylation reaction releases energy, which the enzyme harnesses to drive other chemical reactions that would not otherwise occur. This process is widely used in all known forms of life.
Mitochondria	Cytoplasmic organelles responsible for ATP generation for cellular activities are referred to as mitochondria.
Mitochondrion	Organelle housing enzymes that catalyze reactions of aerobic respiration is mitochondrion.
Oxidative phosphorylation	Oxidative phosphorylation is a biochemical process in cells. It is the final metabolic pathway of cellular respiration, after glycolysis and the citric acid cycle.
Phosphorylation	Phosphorylation refers to reaction in which a phosphate group becomes covalently coupled to another molecule.
Blood vessel	A blood vessel is a part of the circulatory system and function to transport blood throughout the body. The most important types, arteries and veins, are so termed because they carry blood away from or towards the heart, respectively.
Progesterone	Progesterone is a C-21 steroid hormone involved in the female menstrual cycle, pregnancy (supports gestation) and embryogenesis of humans and other species.
Epinephrine	Epinephrine is a hormone and a neurotransmitter. Epinephrine plays a central role in the short-term stress reaction—the physiological response to threatening or exciting conditions (fight-or-flight response). It is secreted by the adrenal medulla.
Enkephalins	Opiate-like brain chemicals that regulate reactions to pain and stress are enkephalins.
Endorphins	Endorphins refer to neurotransmitters that are composed of amino acids and that are functionally similar to morphine.
Heart rate	Heart rate is a term used to describe the frequency of the cardiac cycle. It is considered one of the four vital signs. Usually it is calculated as the number of contractions of the heart in one minute and expressed as "beats per minute".
Endorphin	Endorphin is an endogenous opioid biochemical compound. They are peptides produced by the pituitary gland and the hypothalamus in vertebrates, and they resemble the opiates in their abilities to produce analgesia and a sense of well-being.
Cone cell	The cone cell is a photoreceptor in the retina of the eye which functions only in relatively bright light. There are about 6 million in the human eye, concentrated at the fovea. They gradually become more sparse towards the outside of the retina. They are less sensitive to light than the rod cells, but allow the perception of color and detail.
Glycogen	Glycogen refers to a complex, extensively branched polysaccharide of many glucose monomers; serves as an energy-storage molecule in liver and muscle cells.
Neuron	The neuron is a major class of cells in the nervous system. In vertebrates, they are found in the brain, the spinal cord and in the nerves and ganglia of the peripheral nervous system, and their primary role is to process and transmit neural information.
Brain	The part of the central nervous system involved in regulating and controlling body activity and interpreting information from the senses transmitted through the nervous system is referred to as the brain.
Blood pressure	Blood pressure is the pressure exerted by the blood on the walls of the blood vessels.
Theory	Theory refers to an explanatory statement, or set of statements, that concisely summarizes

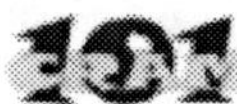

	the state of knowledge on a phenomenon and provides direction for further study.
Proton	Positive subatomic particle, located in the nucleus and having a weight of approximately one atomic mass unit is referred to as a proton.
Chromosomes	Physical structures in the cell's nucleus that house the genes. Each human cell has 23 pairs of chromosomes.
Transfer RNA	Transfer RNA is a small RNA chain (74-93 nucleotides) that transfers a specific amino acid to a growing polypeptide chain at the ribosomal site of protein synthesis during translation. It has sites for amino-acid attachment and codon (a particular sequence of 3 bases) recognition.
Mitochondrial DNA	Mitochondrial DNA is DNA that is located in mitochondria. This is in contrast to most DNA of eukaryotic organisms, which is found the nucleus.
Acetyl	The acetyl radical contains a methyl group single-bonded to a carbonyl. The carbon of the carbonyl has an lone electron available, with which it forms a chemical bond to the remainder of the molecule.
Citric acid cycle	In aerobic organisms, the citric acid cycle is a metabolic pathway that forms part of the break down of carbohydrates, fats and proteins into carbon dioxide and water in order to generate energy. It is the second of three metabolic pathways that are involved in fuel molecule catabolism and ATP production, the other two being glycolysis and oxidative phosphorylation.
Coenzyme Q	Coenzyme Q is a biologically active quinone with an isoprenoid side chain, related in structure to vitamin K and vitamin E. It is found in the membranes of endoplasmic reticulum, peroxisomes, lysosomes, vesicles and notably the inner membrane of the mitochondrion where it is an important part of the electron transport chain.
Oxygen	Oxygen is a chemical element in the periodic table. It has the symbol O and atomic number 8. Oxygen is the second most common element on Earth, composing around 46% of the mass of Earth's crust and 28% of the mass of Earth as a whole, and is the third most common element in the universe.
Aerobic	An aerobic organism is an organism that has an oxygen based metabolism. Aerobes, in a process known as cellular respiration, use oxygen to oxidize substrates (for example sugars and fats) in order to obtain energy.
Glycolysis	Glycolysis refers to the multistep chemical breakdown of a molecule of glucose into two molecules of pyruvic acid; the first stage of cellular respiration in all organisms; occurs in the cytoplasmic fluid.
Glucose	Glucose, a simple monosaccharide sugar, is one of the most important carbohydrates and is used as a source of energy in animals and plants. Glucose is one of the main products of photosynthesis and starts respiration.
Hypothesis	A specific statement about behavior or mental processes that is testable through research is a hypothesis.
Host	Host is an organism that harbors a parasite, mutual partner, or commensal partner; or a cell infected by a virus.
Muscle fiber	Cell with myofibrils containing actin and myosin filaments arranged within sarcomeres is a muscle fiber.
Metabolism	Metabolism is the biochemical modification of chemical compounds in living organisms and cells. This includes the biosynthesis of complex organic molecules (anabolism) and their breakdown (catabolism).
Fiber	Fibers used by man come from a wide variety of sources: Natural fiber include those made out

	of plants, animal and mineral sources. Natural fibers can be classified according to their origin.
Skeletal muscle	Skeletal muscle is a type of striated muscle, attached to the skeleton. They are used to facilitate movement, by applying force to bones and joints; via contraction. They generally contract voluntarily (via nerve stimulation), although they can contract involuntarily.
Mutation	A change in the structure of a gene is called a mutation.
Sperm	Sperm refers to the male sex cell with three distinct parts at maturity: head, middle piece, and tail.
Stomach	The stomach is an organ in the alimentary canal used to digest food. It's primary function is not the absorption of nutrients from digested food; rather, the main job of the stomach is to break down large food molecules into smaller ones, so that they can be absorbed into the blood more easily.
Chloroplasts	Chloroplasts are organelles found in plant cells and eukaryotic algae that conduct photosynthesis.
Erythrocyte	Red blood cells are the most common type of blood cell and are the vertebrate body's principal means of delivering oxygen from the lungs or gills to body tissues via the blood. Red blood cells are also known as erythrocyte.
Hemoglobin	Hemoglobin is the iron-containing oxygen-transport metalloprotein in the red cells of the blood in mammals and other animals. Hemoglobin transports oxygen from the lungs to the rest of the body, such as to the muscles, where it releases the oxygen load.
White blood cell	The white blood cell is a a component of blood. They help to defend the body against infectious disease and foreign materials as part of the immune system.
Micrograph	A micrograph is a photograph or similar image taken through a microscope or similar device to show a magnified image of an item.
Striated muscle	Striated muscle refers to contractile tissue characterized by multinucleated cells containing highly ordered arrangements of actin and myosin microfilaments. Also known as skeletal muscle.
Transduction	In physiology, transduction is transportation of a stimuli to the nervous system. In genetics, transduction is the transfer of viral, bacterial, or both bacterial and viral DNA from one cell to another via bacteriophage.
Shunt	In medicine, a shunt is a hole or passage which moves, or allows movement of, fluid from one part of the body to another. The term may describe either congenital or acquired shunts; and acquired shunts may be either biological or mechanical.
Adipose tissue	Adipose tissue is an anatomical term for loose connective tissue composed of adipocytes. Its main role is to store energy in the form of fat, although it also cushions and insulates the body. It has an important endocrine function in producing recently-discovered hormones such as leptin, resistin and TNFalpha.
Microscopy	Microscopy is any technique for producing visible images of structures or details too small to otherwise be seen by the human eye, using a microscope or other magnification tool.
Collagen	Collagen is the main protein of connective tissue in animals and the most abundant protein in mammals, making up about 1/4 of the total. It is one of the long, fibrous structural proteins whose functions are quite different from those of globular proteins such as enzymes.
Staining	Staining is a biochemical technique of adding a class-specific (DNA, proteins, lipids, carbohydrates) dye to a substrate to qualify or quantify the presence of a specific compound. They are frequently used to highlight structures in tissues for viewing, often with the aid

	of different microscopes.
Glycosylation	Glycosylation refers to the process of adding one or more sugars to a protein or lipid molecule.
Posttranslat-onal modification	Posttranslational modification means the chemical modification of a protein after its translation. It is one of the later steps in protein biosynthesis for many proteins.
Posttranslat-onal	Posttranslational refers to any process involving a protein that occurs after protein synthesis is completed.
Methylation	In biochemistry, methylation refers to the replacement of a hydrogen atom (H) with a methyl group (CH_3), regardless of the substrate.
Barbiturate	A barbiturate is a drug that acts as a central nervous system (CNS) depressant, and by virtue of this produces a wide spectrum of effects, from mild sedation to anesthesia.
Oxidation	Oxidation refers to the loss of electrons from a substance involved in a redox reaction; always accompanies reduction.
Cortex	In anatomy and zoology the cortex is the outermost or superficial layer of an organ or the outer portion of the stem or root of a plant.
Liver	The liver is an organ in vertebrates, including humans. It plays a major role in metabolism and has a number of functions in the body including drug detoxification, glycogen storage, and plasma protein synthesis. It also produces bile, which is important for digestion.
Adrenal cortex	Situated along the perimeter of the adrenal gland, the adrenal cortex mediates the stress response through the production of mineralocorticoids and glucocorticoids, including aldosterone and cortisol respectively. It is also a secondary site of androgen synthesis.
Calcium	Calcium is the chemical element in the periodic table that has the symbol Ca and atomic number 20. Calcium is a soft grey alkaline earth metal that is used as a reducing agent in the extraction of thorium, zirconium and uranium. Calcium is also the fifth most abundant element in the Earth's crust.
Amphipathic	An amphipathic molecule contains both hydrophobic and hydrophilic groups. The hydrophobic group can be a long carbon chain, with the form: $CH_3(CH_2)_n$, with $4 < n < 16$.
Trans face	Trans face refers to face of a Golgi stack at which material leaves the organelle for the cell surface or another cell compartment. It is adjacent to the trans Golgi network.
Cis	A double bond in which the greater radical on both ends is on the same side of the bond is called a cis.
Vacuole	Vacuole refers to a space or cavity within the cytoplasm of a cell.
Proteolysis	Degradation of a protein by cellular enzymes called proteases or by intramolecular digestion at one or more of its peptide bonds is referred to as proteolysis.
Intracellular digestion	Intracellular digestion refers to a form of digestion in which food is taken into cells by phagocytosis. It is found in sponges and most protozoa and coelenterates.
Cellular component	The cellular component involves the movement of white blood cells from blood vessels into the inflamed tissue. The white blood cells, or leukocytes, take on an important role in inflammation; they extravasate (filter out) from the capillaries into tissue, and act as phagocytes, picking up bacteria and cellular debris. They may also aid by walling off an infection and preventing its spread.
Phosphatase	A phosphatase is an enzyme that hydrolyses phosphoric acid monoesters into a phosphate ion

and a molecule with a free hydroxyl group.

Protease | Protease refers to an enzyme that breaks peptide bonds between amino acids of proteins.

Lipase | A lipase is a water-soluble enzyme that catalyzes the hydrolysis of ester bonds in water–insoluble, lipid substrates. Most lipases act at a specific position on the glycerol backbone of a lipid substrate (A1, A2 or A3).

Soma | The soma is the bulbous end of a neuron, containing the nucleus. The cell nucleus is a key feature of the soma. The nucleus is the source of most of the RNA that is produced in neurons and most proteins are produced from mRNAs that do not travel far from the nucleus.

Hydrolytic enzyme | A hydrolytic enzyme breaks down proteins, carbohydrates, and fat molecules into their simplest units. The hydrolysis of polymers by hydrolytic enzymes results in free monomers.

Epididymis | The epididymis is part of the human male reproductive system and is present in all male mammals. It is a narrow, tightly-coiled tube connecting the efferent ducts from the rear of each testicle to its vas deferens.

Silver | Silver is a chemical element with the symbol Ag. A soft white lustrous transition metal, it has the highest electrical and thermal conductivity of any metal and occurs in minerals and in free form.

Glucosamine | Glucosamine ($C_6H_{14}NO_5$) is an amino sugar that is a important precursor in the biochemical synthesis of glycosylated proteins and lipids. Glucosamine is commonly used as a treatment for osteoarthritis, although its acceptance as a medical therapy varies.

Mannose | Mannose is a sugar monomer of the hexose series of carbohydrates. Mannose enters the carbohydrate metabolism stream by phosphorylation and conversion to fructose-6-phosphate.

Trans golgi network | Network of interconnected cisternae and tubules at the trans face of the Golgi apparatus, through which material is transferred out of the Golgi is a trans golgi network.

Nucleolus | A small structure within the nucleus of a cell that contains RNA and protein is referred to as nucleolus. It is where ribonucleoprotein is formed.

Heterogeneous | A heterogeneous compound, mixture, or other such object is one that consists of many different items, which are often not easily sorted or separated, though they are clearly distinct.

Hydrolysis | Hydrolysis is a chemical process in which a molecule is cleaved into two parts by the addition of a molecule of water.

Ganglioside | Ganglioside refers to any glycolipid having one or more sialic acid residues in its structure. Found in the plasma membrane of eucaryotic cells and especially abundant in nerve cells.

Glycosaminog-ycan | Glycosaminoglycan is a long unbranched polysaccharide, made up of repeating disaccharides that may be sulphated (e.g. glucuronic acid, iduronic acid, galactose, galactosamine, glucosamine).

Organ | Organ refers to a structure consisting of several tissues adapted as a group to perform specific functions.

Mental retardation | Mental retardation refers to having significantly below-average intellectual functioning and limitations in at least two areas of adaptive functioning. Many categorize retardation as mild, moderate, severe, or profound.

Spleen | The spleen is a ductless, vertebrate gland that is not necessary for life but is closely associated with the circulatory system, where it functions in the destruction of old red blood cells and removal of other debris from the bloodstream, and also in holding a reservoir

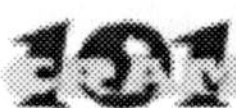

	of blood.
Virus	Obligate intracellular parasite of living cells consisting of an outer capsid and an inner core of nucleic acid is referred to as virus. The term virus usually refers to those particles that infect eukaryotes whilst the term bacteriophage or phage is used to describe those infecting prokaryotes.
Ubiquitin	Ubiquitin is a small protein that occurs in all eukaryotic cells. Its main function is to mark other proteins for destruction, known as proteolysis. Several ubiquitin molecules attach to the condemned protein, and it then moves to a proteasome, a barrel-shaped structure where the proteolysis occurs.
Residue	A residue refers to a portion of a larger molecule, a specific monomer of a polysaccharide, protein or nucleic acid.
Lysine	Lysine is one of the 20 amino acids normally found in proteins. With its 4-aminobutyl side-chain, it is classified as a basic amino acid, along with arginine and histidine.
Peptide	Peptide is the family of molecules formed from the linking, in a defined order, of various amino acids. The link between one amino acid residue and the next is an amide bond, and is sometimes referred to as a peptide bond.
Immune response	The body's defensive reaction to invasion by bacteria, viral agents, or other foreign substances is called immune response.
Substrate	A substrate is a molecule which is acted upon by an enzyme. Each enzyme recognizes only the specific substrate of the reaction it catalyzes. A surface in or on which an organism lives.
Hydrogen	Hydrogen is a chemical element in the periodic table that has the symbol H and atomic number 1. At standard temperature and pressure it is a colorless, odorless, nonmetallic, univalent, tasteless, highly flammable diatomic gas.
Atom	An atom is the smallest possible particle of a chemical element that retains its chemical properties.
Hydrogen peroxide	Hydrogen peroxide is a clear liquid, slightly more viscous than water, that has strong oxidizing properties and is therefore a powerful bleaching agent that has found use as a disinfectant, as an oxidizer, and in rocketry (particularly in high concentrations as high-test peroxide (HTP) as a monopropellant, and in bipropellant systems.
Complement	Complement is a group of proteins of the complement system, found in blood serum which act in concert with antibodies to achieve the destruction of non-self particles such as foreign blood cells or bacteria.
Bile acid	A bile acid is a steroid acid found predominantly in bile of mammals. They are produced in liver by oxidation of cholesterol, in the form of their salts are stored in gallbladder and secreted into the intestine. They act as surfactants, emulsifying lipids and assisting with their digestion and absorption.
Bile	Bile is a bitter, greenish-yellow alkaline fluid secreted by the liver of most vertebrates. In many species, it is stored in the gallbladder between meals and upon eating is discharged into the duodenum where it aids the process of digestion.
Carboxyl	A carboxyl is the univalent radical -COOH; present in and characteristic of organic acids.
Carboxyl terminus	End of a polypeptide that contains a free carboxyl group is called carboxyl terminus.
Nerve tissue	Nerve tissue refers the specialized tissue making up the central and peripheral nervous systems; consists of neurons and glial cells.

Myelin	Myelin is an electrically insulating fatty layer that surrounds the axons of many neurons, especially those in the peripheral nervous system. It is an outgrowth of glial cells: Schwann cells supply the myelin for peripheral neurons while oligodendrocytes supply it to those of the central nervous system.
Peripheral nervous system	The peripheral nervous system consists of the nerves and neurons that reside or extend outside the central nervous system--to serve the limbs and organs. The peripheral nervous system is divided into the somatic nervous system and the autonomic nervous system.
Syndrome	Syndrome is the association of several clinically recognizable features, signs, symptoms, phenomena or characteristics which often occur together, so that the presence of one feature alerts the physician to the presence of the others
Lesion	A lesion is a non-specific term referring to abnormal tissue in the body. It can be caused by any disease process including trauma (physical, chemical, electrical), infection, neoplasm, metabolic and autoimmune.
Nervous system	The nervous system of an animal coordinates the activity of the muscles, monitors the organs, constructs and processes input from the senses, and initiates actions.
Concept	A mental category used to class together objects, relations, events, abstractions, or qualities that have common properties is called concept.
Actin	A protein in a muscle fiber that, together with myosin, is responsible for contraction and relaxation is actin.
Actin filament	An actin filament is a helical protein filament formed by the polymerization of globular actin molecules. They provide mechanical support for the cell, determine the cell shape, enable cell movements; and participate in certain cell junctions.
Microtubule	A hollow rod of the protein tubulin in the cytoplasm is referred to as the microtubule.
Cilia	Microscopic, hairlike processes on the exposed surfaces of certain epithelial cells are cilia.
Variable	A characteristic or aspect in which people, objects, events, or conditions vary is called variable.
Tubulin	Tubulin is the protein which makes up microtubules.
In vitro	In vitro is an experimental technique where the experiment is performed in a test tube, or generally outside a living organism or cell.
In vivo	In vivo is used to indicate the presence of a whole/living organism, in distinction to a partial or dead organism, or a computer model. Animal testing and clinical trials are forms of in vivo research.
Polymerization	Polymerization is a process of reacting monomer molecules together in a chemical reaction to form linear chains or a three-dimensional network of polymer chains.
Colchicine	Colchicine is a highly poisonous alkaloid, originally extracted from plants of the genus Colchicum. Originally used to treat rheumatic complaints and especially gout, it was also prescribed for its cathartic and emetic effects. Its present use is mainly in the treatment of gout.
Alkaloid	Alkaloid refers to small but chemically complex nitrogen-containing metabolite produced by plants as a defense against herbivores. Examples include caffeine, morphine, and colchicine.
Chemotherapy	Chemotherapy is the use of chemical substances to treat disease. In its modern-day use, it refers almost exclusively to cytostatic drugs used to treat cancer.In its non-oncological use, the term may also refer to antibiotics.

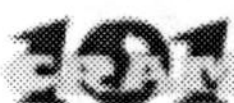

Karyotype	A set of chromosomes characteristic of a species arranged in homologous pairs is referred to as a karyotype. The human karyotype has 23 chromosome pairs.
Cancer	Cancer is a class of diseases or disorders characterized by uncontrolled division of cells and the ability of these cells to invade other tissues, either by direct growth into adjacent tissue through invasion or by implantation into distant sites by metastasis.
Tumor	An abnormal mass of cells that forms within otherwise normal tissue is a tumor. This growth can be either malignant or benign
Centriole	A cellular structure built of microtubules that organizes the mitotic spindle is called a centriole.
Centrosome	Cellular organelle consisting of two centrioles is called a centrosome.
Cell division	Cell division (or local doubling) is the process by which a cell, called the parent cell divides into two cells, called daughter cells. Cell division is usually a small segment of a larger cell cycle.
Axon	An axon is a long slender projection of a nerve cell, or neuron, which conducts electrical impulses away from the neuron's cell body or soma. They are in effect the primary transmission lines of the nervous system, and as bundles they help make up nerves.
Epithelium	Epithelium is a tissue composed of a layer of cells. Epithelium can be found lining internal (e.g. endothelium, which lines the inside of blood vessels) or external (e.g. skin) free surfaces of the body. Functions include secretion, absorption and protection.
Mucus	Mucus is a slippery secretion of the lining of various membranes in the body (mucous membranes). Mucus aids in the protection of the lungs by trapping foreign particles that enter the nose during normal breathing. Additionally, it prevents tissues from drying out.
Helix	A helix is a twisted shape like a spring, screw or a spiral staircase. Helixes are important in biology, as DNA is helical and many proteins have helical substructures, known as alpha helices.
Cleavage	Cleavage refers to the early successive divisions of the blastocyst cells into smaller and smaller cells.
Glutaraldehyde	Glutaraldehyde is a colorless liquid with a pungent odor used to sterilize medical and dental equipment. It is also used for industrial water treatment and as a chemical preservative. But it is toxic, causing severe eye, nose, throat and lung irritation, along with headaches, drowsiness and dizziness.
Epidermis	Epidermis is the outermost layer of the skin. It forms the waterproof, protective wrap over the body's surface and is made up of stratified squamous epithelium with an underlying basement membrane. It contains no blood vessels, and is nourished by diffusion from the dermis. In plants, the outermost layer of cells covering the leaves and young parts of a plant is the epidermis.
Keratin	Keratin is a family of fibrous structural proteins; tough and insoluble, they form the hard but nonmineralized structures found in reptiles, birds and mammals.
Astrocyte	An astrocyte is a characteristic star-shaped cell in the brain. They are the biggest cells found in brain tissue and outnumber the neurons ten to one. A commonly accepted function is to structure physically the brain. A second function is to provide neurons with nutrients such as glucose. They regulate the flow of nutrients provided by capillaries by forming the blood-brain barrier.
Cardiac muscle	Cardiac muscle is a type of striated muscle found within the heart. Its function is to "pump" blood through the circulatory system. Unlike skeletal muscle, which contracts in response to

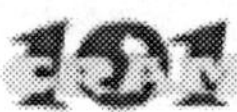

	nerve stimulation, and like smooth muscle, cardiac muscle is myogenic, meaning that it stimulates its own contraction without a requisite electrical impulse.
Lead	Lead is a chemical element in the periodic table that has the symbol Pb and atomic number 82. A soft, heavy, toxic and malleable poor metal, lead is bluish white when freshly cut but tarnishes to dull gray when exposed to air. Lead is used in building construction, lead-acid batteries, bullets and shot, and is part of solder, pewter, and fusible alloys.
Melanocyte	Melanocyte cells are located in the bottom layer of the skin's epidermis. With a process called melanogenesis, they produce melanin, a pigment in the skin, eyes, and hair.
Carotene	Carotene is an orange photosynthetic pigment important for photosynthesis. It is responsible for the orange color of the carrot and many other fruits and vegetables. It contributes to photosynthesis by transmitting the light energy it absorbs to chlorophyll.
Skin	Skin is an organ of the integumentary system composed of a layer of tissues that protect underlying muscles and organs.
Melanin	Broadly, melanin is any of the polyacetylene, polyaniline, and polypyrrole "blacks" or their mixed copolymers. The most common form of biological melanin is a polymer of either or both of two monomer molecules: indolequinone, and dihydroxyindole carboxylic acid.
Retina	The retina is a thin layer of cells at the back of the eyeball of vertebrates and some cephalopods; it is the part of the eye which converts light into nervous signals.
Hepatocyte	Hepatocyte cells make up 60-80% of the cytoplasmic mass of the liver. They are involved in protein synthesis, protein storage and transformation of carbohydrates, synthesis of cholesterol, bile salts and phospholipids, and detoxification, modification and excretion of exogenous and endogenous substances.
Neutrophil	Neutrophil refers to a type of phagocytic leukocyte.
Infection	The invasion and multiplication of microorganisms in body tissues is called an infection.
Diabetes	Diabetes is a medical disorder characterized by varying or persistent elevated blood sugar levels, especially after eating. All types of diabetes share similar symptoms and complications at advanced stages: dehydration and ketoacidosis, cardiovascular disease, chronic renal failure, retinal damage which can lead to blindness, nerve damage which can lead to erectile dysfunction, gangrene with risk of amputation of toes, feet, and even legs.
Basal metabolism	Basal metabolism refers to the minimal energy the body requires to support itself in a fasting state when resting and awake in a warm, quiet environment.
Hyperthyroidism	Hyperthyroidism is the clinical syndrome caused by an excess of circulating free thyroxine (T4) or free triiodothyronine (T3), or both.
Motility	Motility is the ability to move spontaneously and independently. The term can apply to single cells, or to multicellular organisms.
Pathology	Pathology is the study of the processes underlying disease and other forms of illness, harmful abnormality, or dysfunction.

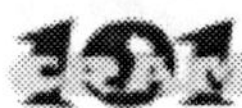

Mitochondria	Cytoplasmic organelles responsible for ATP generation for cellular activities are referred to as mitochondria.
Organelle	Organelle refers to any structure within a cell that carries out one of its metabolic roles, such as mitochondria, centrioles, endoplasmic reticulum, and the nucleus.
Genome	In biology the genome of an organism is the whole hereditary information of an organism that is encoded in the DNA (or, for some viruses, RNA). This includes both the genes and the non-coding sequences.
DNA	Deoxyribonucleic acid (DNA) is a nucleic acid —usually in the form of a double helix— that contains the genetic instructions specifying the biological development of all cellular forms of life, and most viruses.
Mitochondrion	Organelle housing enzymes that catalyze reactions of aerobic respiration is mitochondrion.
Nucleolus	A small structure within the nucleus of a cell that contains RNA and protein is referred to as nucleolus. It is where ribonucleoprotein is formed.
Tissue	A collection of interconnected cells that perform a similar function within an organism is called tissue.
Variable	A characteristic or aspect in which people, objects, events, or conditions vary is called variable.
Cancer	Cancer is a class of diseases or disorders characterized by uncontrolled division of cells and the ability of these cells to invade other tissues, either by direct growth into adjacent tissue through invasion or by implantation into distant sites by metastasis.
Microscopy	Microscopy is any technique for producing visible images of structures or details too small to otherwise be seen by the human eye, using a microscope or other magnification tool.
Protein structure	A protein structure are amino acid chains, made up from 20 different L-α-amino acids, also referred to as residues, that fold into unique three-dimensional structures.
Protein	A protein is a complex, high-molecular-weight organic compound that consists of amino acids joined by peptide bonds. They are essential to the structure and function of all living cells and viruses. Many are enzymes or subunits of enzymes.
Lamina	A thin layer, such as the lamina of a vertebra or the lamina propria of a mucous membrane is referred to as lamina.
Chromosomes	Physical structures in the cell's nucleus that house the genes. Each human cell has 23 pairs of chromosomes.
Cytoplasm	Cytoplasm refers to the contents of a cell excluding the nucleus and cell membrane. Cytoplasm is a homogeneous, generally clear jelly-like material that fills cells.
Hepatocyte	Hepatocyte cells make up 60-80% of the cytoplasmic mass of the liver. They are involved in protein synthesis, protein storage and transformation of carbohydrates, synthesis of cholesterol, bile salts and phospholipids, and detoxification, modification and excretion of exogenous and endogenous substances.
Liver	The liver is an organ in vertebrates, including humans. It plays a major role in metabolism and has a number of functions in the body including drug detoxification, glycogen storage, and plasma protein synthesis. It also produces bile, which is important for digestion.
Ion	Ion refers to an atom or molecule that has gained or lost one or more electrons, thus acquiring an electrical charge.
Euchromatin	Euchromatin is a type of chromatin that is rich in gene concentration (contrast this to heterochromatin). This type of chromatin generally appears as light-colored bands when

stained in GTG banding and observed under an optical microscope.

Distribution Distribution in pharmacology is a branch of pharmacokinetics describing reversible transfer of drug from one location to another within the body.

Microscope A microscope is an instrument for viewing objects that are too small to be seen by the naked or unaided eye.

Light microscope An optical instrument with lenses that refract visible light to magnify images and project them into a viewer's eye or onto photographic film is referred to as light microscope.

Intestine The intestine is the portion of the alimentary canal extending from the stomach to the anus and, in humans and mammals, consists of two segments, the small intestine and the large intestine. The intestine is the part of the body responsible for extracting nutrition from food.

Condensation Combining several people, objects, or events into a single dream image is referred to as condensation.

Staining Staining is a biochemical technique of adding a class-specific (DNA, proteins, lipids, carbohydrates) dye to a substrate to qualify or quantify the presence of a specific compound. They are frequently used to highlight structures in tissues for viewing, often with the aid of different microscopes.

Base The common definition of a base is a chemical compound that absorbs hydronium ions when dissolved in water (a proton acceptor). An alkali is a special example of a base, where in an aqueous environment, hydroxide ions are donated.

Fiber Fibers used by man come from a wide variety of sources: Natural fiber include those made out of plants, animal and mineral sources. Natural fibers can be classified according to their origin.

Meiosis In biology, meiosis is the process that transforms one diploid cell into four haploid cells in eukaryotes in order to redistribute the diploid's cell's genome.

Y chromosome Male sex chromosome that carries genes involved in sex determination is referred to as the Y chromosome. It contains the genes that cause testis development, thus determining maleness.

Leukocyte A white blood cell is a leukocyte. They help to defend the body against infectious disease and foreign materials as part of the immune system.

Organ Organ refers to a structure consisting of several tissues adapted as a group to perform specific functions.

Blood Blood is a circulating tissue composed of fluid plasma and cells. The main function of blood is to supply nutrients (oxygen, glucose) and constitutional elements to tissues and to remove waste products.

Hermaphroditism The coexistence of both female and male sex organs in the same organism is called hermaphroditism.

Spermatozoa A sperm cell, spermatozooa (pl. spermatozoa), or spermatozoan, is the haploid cell that is the male gamete. It is carried in fluid called semen, and is capable of fertilising an egg cell to form a zygote.

Colchicine Colchicine is a highly poisonous alkaloid, originally extracted from plants of the genus Colchicum. Originally used to treat rheumatic complaints and especially gout, it was also prescribed for its cathartic and emetic effects. Its present use is mainly in the treatment of gout.

Culture Culture, generally refers to patterns of human activity and the symbolic structures that give

	such activity significance.
Hypotonic	Condition in which a solution contains a lesser concentration of dissolved particles than the solution to which it is compared is called hypotonic.
Solution	Solution refers to homogenous mixture formed when a solute is dissolved in a solvent.
Hypotonic solution	A hypotonic solution contains a higher concentration compared to the cell.
Helix	A helix is a twisted shape like a spring, screw or a spiral staircase. Helixes are important in biology, as DNA is helical and many proteins have helical substructures, known as alpha helices.
Segmentation	Segmentation in biology refers to the division of some metazoan bodies and plant body plans into a series of semi-repetitive segments, and the question of the benefits and costs of doing so.
Transverse	A transverse (also known as axial or horizontal) plane is an X-Y plane, parallel to the ground, which (in humans) separates the superior from the inferior, or put another way, the head from the feet.
Genes	Genes are the units of heredity in living organisms. They are encoded in the organism's genetic material (usually DNA or RNA), and control the development and behavior of the organism.
In situ hybridization	In situ hybridization refers to the use of a DNA or RNA probe to detect the presence of the complementary DNA sequence in cloned bacterial or cultured eukaryotic cells.
Polymorphonu-lear leukocyte	Polymorphonuclear leukocyte refers to a leukocyte that has a variety of nuclear forms.
Epithelium	Epithelium is a tissue composed of a layer of cells. Epithelium can be found lining internal (e.g. endothelium, which lines the inside of blood vessels) or external (e.g. skin) free surfaces of the body. Functions include secretion, absorption and protection.
Polymorphonu-lear	Cells with nuclei having several parts or lobes are called polymorphonuclear.
Tumor	An abnormal mass of cells that forms within otherwise normal tissue is a tumor. This growth can be either malignant or benign
Cell division	Cell division (or local doubling) is the process by which a cell, called the parent cell divides into two cells, called daughter cells. Cell division is usually a small segment of a larger cell cycle.
Ovulation	Ovulation is the process in the menstrual cycle by which a mature ovarian follicle ruptures and discharges an ovum (also known as an oocyte, female gamete, or casually, an egg) that participates in reproduction.
Ovary	The primary reproductive organ of a female is called an ovary.
Metabolite	The term metabolite is usually restricted to small molecules. They are the intermediates and products of metabolism. A primary metabolite is directly involved in the normal growth, development, and reproduction. A secondary metabolite is not directly involved in those processes, but usually has important ecological function.
Nucleic acid	A nucleic acid is a complex, high-molecular-weight biochemical macromolecule composed of nucleotide chains that convey genetic information.
Acid	An acid is a water-soluble, sour-tasting chemical compound that when dissolved in water, gives a solution with a pH of less than 7.

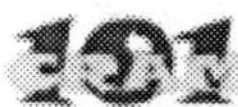

Vesicle	Membranous, cytoplasmic sac formed by an infolding of the cell membrane is called a vesicle.
Phosphorylation	Phosphorylation refers to reaction in which a phosphate group becomes covalently coupled to another molecule.
Centrosome	Cellular organelle consisting of two centrioles is called a centrosome.
Centriole	A cellular structure built of microtubules that organizes the mitotic spindle is called a centriole.
Microtubule	A hollow rod of the protein tubulin in the cytoplasm is referred to as the microtubule.
Micrograph	A micrograph is a photograph or similar image taken through a microscope or similar device to show a magnified image of an item.
Constant	A behavior or characteristic that does not vary from one observation to another is referred to as a constant.
Nerve tissue	Nerve tissue refers the specialized tissue making up the central and peripheral nervous systems; consists of neurons and glial cells.
Muscle	Muscle is a contractile form of tissue. It is one of the four major tissue types, the other three being epithelium, connective tissue and nervous tissue. Muscle contraction is used to move parts of the body, as well as to move substances within the body.
Nerve	A nerve is an enclosed, cable-like bundle of nerve fibers or axons, which includes the glia that ensheath the axons in myelin.
Cardiac muscle	Cardiac muscle is a type of striated muscle found within the heart. Its function is to "pump" blood through the circulatory system. Unlike skeletal muscle, which contracts in response to nerve stimulation, and like smooth muscle, cardiac muscle is myogenic, meaning that it stimulates its own contraction without a requisite electrical impulse.
Epidermis	Epidermis is the outermost layer of the skin. It forms the waterproof, protective wrap over the body's surface and is made up of stratified squamous epithelium with an underlying basement membrane. It contains no blood vessels, and is nourished by diffusion from the dermis. In plants, the outermost layer of cells covering the leaves and young parts of a plant is the epidermis.
Pancreas	The pancreas is a retroperitoneal organ that serves two functions: exocrine - it produces pancreatic juice containing digestive enzymes, and endocrine - it produces several important hormones, namely insulin.
Thyroid	The thyroid is one of the larger endocrine glands in the body. It is located in the neck and produces hormones, principally thyroxine and triiodothyronine, that regulate the rate of metabolism and affect the growth and rate of function of many other systems in the body.
Gland	A gland is an organ in an animal's body that synthesizes a substance for release such as hormones, often into the bloodstream or into cavities inside the body or its outer surface.
Digestive tract	The digestive tract is the system of organs within multicellular animals which takes in food, digests it to extract energy and nutrients, and expels the remaining waste.
Serum	Serum is the same as blood plasma except that clotting factors (such as fibrin) have been removed. Blood plasma contains fibrinogen.
Medicine	Medicine is the branch of health science and the sector of public life concerned with maintaining or restoring human health through the study, diagnosis and treatment of disease and injury.
Mutation	A change in the structure of a gene is called a mutation.

Tubulin	Tubulin is the protein which makes up microtubules.
Benign tumor	A benign tumor does not invade neighboring tissues and do not seed metastases, but may locally grow to great size. They usually do not return after surgical removal.
Reproduction	Biological reproduction is the biological process by which new individual organisms are produced. Reproduction is a fundamental feature of all known life; each individual organism exists as the result of reproduction by an antecedent.
Neoplasia	Neoplasia refers to abnormal, disorganized growth in a tissue or organ; often used to mean formation of cancer.
Erythrocyte	Red blood cells are the most common type of blood cell and are the vertebrate body's principal means of delivering oxygen from the lungs or gills to body tissues via the blood. Red blood cells are also known as erythrocyte.
Erythropoietin	Erythropoietin is a glycoprotein hormone that is a growth factor for erythrocyte (red blood cell) precursors in the bone marrow. It increases the number of red blood cells in the blood.
Squamous cell carcinoma	In medicine, squamous cell carcinoma is a form of cancer of the carcinoma type that may occur in many different organs, including the skin, the esophagus, the lungs, and the cervix.
Morphology	The scientific study of organic form, including both its development and function is morphology.
Carcinoma	Cancer that originates in the coverings of the body, such as the skin or the lining of the intestinal tract is a carcinoma.
Skin	Skin is an organ of the integumentary system composed of a layer of tissues that protect underlying muscles and organs.
Radiation	The emission of electromagnetic waves by all objects warmer than absolute zero is referred to as radiation.
Infection	The invasion and multiplication of microorganisms in body tissues is called an infection.
Bypass	In medicine, a bypass generally means an alternate or additional route for blood flow, which is created in bypass surgery, e.g. coronary artery bypass surgery by moving blood vessels or implanting synthetic tubing.
Viral	Viral phenomena are objects or patterns able to replicate themselves or convert other objects into copies of themselves when these objects are exposed to them.
Neoplasm	Neoplasm refers to abnormal growth of cells; often used to mean a tumor.
Plasma	Fluid portion of circulating blood is called plasma.
Apoptosis	In biology, apoptosis is one of the main types of programmed cell death (PCD). As such, it is a process of deliberate life relinquishment by an unwanted cell in a multicellular organism.
Health	Health is a term that refers to a combination of the absence of illness, the ability to cope with everyday activities, physical fitness, and high quality of life.
Lymphocyte	A lymphocyte is a type of white blood cell involved in the human body's immune system. There are two broad categories, namely T cells and B cells.
Thymus	The thymus is a ductless gland located in the upper anterior portion of the chest cavity. It is most active during puberty, after which it shrinks in size and activity in most individuals and is replaced with fat. The thymus plays an important role in the development of the immune system.
Embryo	A prenatal stage of development after germ layers form but before the rudiments of all organs are present is referred to as an embryo.

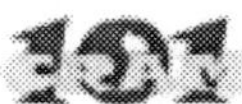

Plasma membrane | The unit membrane that encloses a cell and controls the traffic of molecules in and out of the cell is the plasma membrane.

Necrosis | Necrosis is the name given to unprogrammed death of cells/living tissue. There are many causes of necrosis including injury, infection, cancer, infarction, and inflammation. Necrosis is caused by special enzymes that are released by lysosomes.

Agent | Agent refers to an epidemiological term referring to the organism or object that transmits a disease from the environment to the host.

Microorganism | A microorganism or microbe is an organism that is so small that it is microscopic (invisible to the naked eye).

Extracellular | Outside the cell is called extracellular.

Inflammation | Inflammation is the first response of the immune system to infection or irritation and may be referred to as the innate cascade.

Phagocytosis | Phagocytosis (literally, "cell eating") is a form of endocytosis where large particles are enveloped by the cell membrane of a (usually larger) cell and internalized to form a phagosome, or "food vacuole."

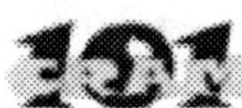

Nerve tissue	Nerve tissue refers the specialized tissue making up the central and peripheral nervous systems; consists of neurons and glial cells.
Tissue	A collection of interconnected cells that perform a similar function within an organism is called tissue.
Muscle	Muscle is a contractile form of tissue. It is one of the four major tissue types, the other three being epithelium, connective tissue and nervous tissue. Muscle contraction is used to move parts of the body, as well as to move substances within the body.
Nerve	A nerve is an enclosed, cable-like bundle of nerve fibers or axons, which includes the glia that ensheath the axons in myelin.
Connective tissue	Connective tissue is any type of biological tissue with an extensive extracellular matrix and often serves to support, bind together, and protect organs.
Extracellular	Outside the cell is called extracellular.
Parenchyma	The parenchyma are the functional parts of an organ in the body (i.e. the nephrons of the kidney, the alveoli of the lungs). In plants parenchyma cells are thin-walled cells of the ground tissue that make up the bulk of most nonwoody structures, although sometimes their cell walls can be lignified.
Organ	Organ refers to a structure consisting of several tissues adapted as a group to perform specific functions.
Spinal cord	The spinal cord is a part of the vertebrate nervous system that is enclosed in and protected by the vertebral column (it passes through the spinal canal). It consists of nerve cells. The spinal cord carries sensory signals and motor innervation to most of the skeletal muscles in the body.
Brain	The part of the central nervous system involved in regulating and controlling body activity and interpreting information from the senses transmitted through the nervous system is referred to as the brain.
Absorption	Absorption is a physical or chemical phenomenon or a process in which atoms, molecules, or ions enter some bulk phase - gas, liquid or solid material. In nutrition, amino acids are broken down through digestion, which begins in the stomach.
Olfactory	Pertaining to the sense of smell is referred to as olfactory.
Intestine	The intestine is the portion of the alimentary canal extending from the stomach to the anus and, in humans and mammals, consists of two segments, the small intestine and the large intestine. The intestine is the part of the body responsible for extracting nutrition from food.
Gland	A gland is an organ in an animal's body that synthesizes a substance for release such as hormones, often into the bloodstream or into cavities inside the body or its outer surface.
Skin	Skin is an organ of the integumentary system composed of a layer of tissues that protect underlying muscles and organs.
Myoepithelial cell	Myoepithelial cell refers to type of unstriated muscle cell found in epithelia, e.g. In the iris of the eye and in glandular tissue.
Microscope	A microscope is an instrument for viewing objects that are too small to be seen by the naked or unaided eye.
Light microscope	An optical instrument with lenses that refract visible light to magnify images and project them into a viewer's eye or onto photographic film is referred to as light microscope.
Criterion	Criterion refers to a standard of comparison. For performance appraisal, it is the definition

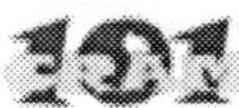

of good performance.

Value Value is worth in general, and it is thought to be connected to reasons for certain practices, policies, actions, beliefs or emotions. Value is "that which one acts to gain and/or keep."

Lamina A thin layer, such as the lamina of a vertebra or the lamina propria of a mucous membrane is referred to as lamina.

Urinary system The urinary system is the organ system that produces, stores, and carries urine. In humans it includes two kidneys, two ureters, the urinary bladder, two sphincter muscles, and the urethra.

Epithelium Epithelium is a tissue composed of a layer of cells. Epithelium can be found lining internal (e.g. endothelium, which lines the inside of blood vessels) or external (e.g. skin) free surfaces of the body. Functions include secretion, absorption and protection.

Papilla A papilla can be a small projection, such as a nipplelike projection on the skin, at the base of a hair or the root of a feather; the base of a new tooth.

Stress Stress refers to a condition that is a response to factors that change the human systems normal state.

Glomerulus A glomerulus is a capillary tuft surrounded by Bowman's capsule in nephrons of the vertebrate kidney. It receives its blood supply from an afferent arteriole of the renal circulation, and empties into an efferent arteriole.

Alveoli Alveoli are anatomical structures that have the form of a hollow cavity. In the lung, the pulmonary alveoli are spherical outcroppings of the respiratory bronchioles and are the primary sites of gas exchange with the blood.

Fusion Fusion refers to the combination of two atoms into a single atom as a result of a collision, usually accompanied by the release of energy.

Renal Pertaining to the kidney is referred to as renal.

Nervous tissue Tissue made up of neurons and supportive cells is referred to as nervous tissue. It forms a rapid communication network for the body.

Proteoglycan Molecule consisting of one or more glycosaminoglycan chains attached to a core protein is referred to as proteoglycan.

Collagen Collagen is the main protein of connective tissue in animals and the most abundant protein in mammals, making up about 1/4 of the total. It is one of the long, fibrous structural proteins whose functions are quite different from those of globular proteins such as enzymes.

Laminin Laminin is a family of heterotrimeric glycoproteins found in the basal lamina underlying epithelia. Their binding to type IV collagen contributes to the self-assembly of the basal lamina from components secreted by cells, and their recognition by growth cone integrins is important to the function of the basal lamina.

Fiber Fibers used by man come from a wide variety of sources: Natural fiber include those made out of plants, animal and mineral sources. Natural fibers can be classified according to their origin.

Micrograph A micrograph is a photograph or similar image taken through a microscope or similar device to show a magnified image of an item.

Collagen fibril Collagen fibril refers to extracellular structure formed by self-assembly of secreted fibrillar collagen subunits. An abundant constituent of the extracellular matrix in many animal tissues.

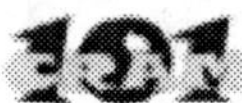

Traction	Traction refers to the set of mechanisms for straightening broken bones or relieving pressure on the skeletal system. It is largely replaced now by more modern techniques, but certain approaches are still used today for hip fractures.
Glomeruli	Glomeruli are important waystations in the pathway from the nose to the olfactory cortex. Each receives input from olfactory receptor neurons expressing only one type of olfactory receptor. There are tens of millions of olfactory receptor cells, but only about two thousand glomeruli. By combining so much input, the olfactory system is able to detect even very faint odors.
Kidney	The kidney is a bean-shaped excretory organ in vertebrates. Part of the urinary system, the kidneys filter wastes (especially urea) from the blood and excrete them, along with water, as urine.
Macromolecule	A macromolecule is a molecule with a large molecular mass, but generally the use of the term is restricted to polymers and molecules which structurally include polymers.
Metabolism	Metabolism is the biochemical modification of chemical compounds in living organisms and cells. This includes the biosynthesis of complex organic molecules (anabolism) and their breakdown (catabolism).
Neuromuscular junction	A neuromuscular junction is the junction of the axon terminal of a motoneuron with the motor end plate, the highly-excitable region of muscle fiber plasma membrane responsible for initiation of action potentials across the muscle's surface.
Acid	An acid is a water-soluble, sour-tasting chemical compound that when dissolved in water, gives a solution with a pH of less than 7.
Desmosome	A desmosome (also known as macula adherens) is a cell structure specialized for cell-to-cell adhesion. It is a type of junctional complex.
Base	The common definition of a base is a chemical compound that absorbs hydronium ions when dissolved in water (a proton acceptor). An alkali is a special example of a base, where in an aqueous environment, hydroxide ions are donated.
A band	A band is a dark band corresponding to an area where actin and myosin filaments overlap in cardiac or skeletal muscle.
Correlation	A statistical technique for determining the degree of association between two or more variables is referred to as correlation.
Bladder	A hollow muscular storage organ for storing urine is a bladder.
Solute	Substance that is dissolved in a solvent, forming a solution is referred to as a solute.
Urinary bladder	In the anatomy of mammals, the urinary bladder is the organ that collects urine excreted by the kidneys prior to disposal by urination. Urine enters the bladder via the ureters and exits via the urethra.
Actin	A protein in a muscle fiber that, together with myosin, is responsible for contraction and relaxation is actin.
Actin filament	An actin filament is a helical protein filament formed by the polymerization of globular actin molecules. They provide mechanical support for the cell, determine the cell shape, enable cell movements; and participate in certain cell junctions.
Hydrophilic	Pertaining to molecules that attract water or dissolve in it because of their polar nature is hydrophilic.
Protein	A protein is a complex, high-molecular-weight organic compound that consists of amino acids joined by peptide bonds. They are essential to the structure and function of all living cells

and viruses. Many are enzymes or subunits of enzymes.

Channel — Channel, in communications (sometimes called communications channel), refers to the medium used to convey information from a sender (or transmitter) to a receiver.

Large intestine — In anatomy of the digestive system, the colon, also called the large intestine or large bowel, is the part of the intestine from the cecum ('caecum' in British English) to the rectum. Its primary purpose is to extract water from feces.

Hormone — A hormone is a chemical messenger from one cell to another. All multicellular organisms produce hormones. The best known hormones are those produced by endocrine glands of vertebrate animals, but hormones are produced by nearly every organ system and tissue type in a human or animal body. Hormone molecules are secreted directly into the bloodstream, they move by circulation or diffusion to their target cells, which may be nearby cells in the same tissue or cells of a distant organ of the body.

Ion — Ion refers to an atom or molecule that has gained or lost one or more electrons, thus acquiring an electrical charge.

Macula — The macula is an oval yellow spot near the center of the retina of the human eye. Near its center is the fovea, a small pit that contains the largest concentration of cone cells in the eye and is responsible for central vision.

Soma — The soma is the bulbous end of a neuron, containing the nucleus. The cell nucleus is a key feature of the soma. The nucleus is the source of most of the RNA that is produced in neurons and most proteins are produced from mRNAs that do not travel far from the nucleus.

Attachment — Attachment refers to the psychological tendency to seek closeness to another person, to feel secure when that person is present, and to feel anxious when that person is absent.

Cytoplasm — Cytoplasm refers to the contents of a cell excluding the nucleus and cell membrane. Cytoplasm is a homogeneous, generally clear jelly-like material that fills cells.

In vitro — In vitro is an experimental technique where the experiment is performed in a test tube, or generally outside a living organism or cell.

Lipid — Lipid is one class of aliphatic hydrocarbon-containing organic compounds essential for the structure and function of living cells. They are characterized by being water-insoluble but soluble in nonpolar organic solvents.

Receptor — A receptor is a protein on the cell membrane or within the cytoplasm or cell nucleus that binds to a specific molecule (a ligand), such as a neurotransmitter, hormone, or other substance, and initiates the cellular response to the ligand. Receptor, in immunology, the region of an antibody which shows recognition of an antigen.

Projection — Attributing one's own undesirable thoughts, impulses, traits, or behaviors to others is referred to as projection.

Course — Pattern of development and change of a disorder over time is a course.

Extension — Movement increasing the angle between parts at a joint is referred to as extension.

Villus — Villus refers to a fingerlike projection of the inner surface of the small intestine. A fingerlike projection of the chorion of the mammalian placenta. Large numbers of villus increase the surface areas of these organs.

Glycocalyx — A network of polysaccharides extending from the surface of bacteria and other cells is referred to as glycocalyx. It allows the bacterium to attach itself to inert surfaces (like teeth or rocks), prokaryotes or other bacteria.

Small intestine — The small intestine is the part of the gastrointestinal tract between the stomach and the

	large intestine (colon). In humans over 5 years old it is about 7m long. It is divided into three structural parts: duodenum, jejunum and ileum.
Plasma	Fluid portion of circulating blood is called plasma.
Plasma membrane	The unit membrane that encloses a cell and controls the traffic of molecules in and out of the cell is the plasma membrane.
Stereocilia	Stereocilia are mechanosensing organelles of hair cells, which respond to fluid motion or fluid pressure changes in numerous types of animals for numerous functions. As acoustic sensors in mammals, they are lined up in the Organ of Corti in the cochlea of the inner ear.
Epididymis	The epididymis is part of the human male reproductive system and is present in all male mammals. It is a narrow, tightly-coiled tube connecting the efferent ducts from the rear of each testicle to its vas deferens.
Cilia	Microscopic, hairlike processes on the exposed surfaces of certain epithelial cells are cilia.
Ductus deferens	The ductus deferens is part of the human male anatomy. There are two of them; they are muscular tubes (surrounded by smooth muscle) connecting the left and right epididymis to the ejaculatory ducts in order to move sperm.
Lipid bilayer	A lipid bilayer is a membrane or zone of a membrane composed of lipid molecules (usually phospholipids). The lipid bilayer is a critical component of all biological membranes, including cell membranes, and is a prerequisite for cell-based organisms.
Microscopy	Microscopy is any technique for producing visible images of structures or details too small to otherwise be seen by the human eye, using a microscope or other magnification tool.
Liver	The liver is an organ in vertebrates, including humans. It plays a major role in metabolism and has a number of functions in the body including drug detoxification, glycogen storage, and plasma protein synthesis. It also produces bile, which is important for digestion.
Microtubule	A hollow rod of the protein tubulin in the cytoplasm is referred to as the microtubule.
Centriole	A cellular structure built of microtubules that organizes the mitotic spindle is called a centriole.
Adenosine	Adenosine is a nucleoside comprized of adenine attached to a ribose (ribofuranose) moiety via a β-N_9-glycosidic bond. Adenosine plays an important role in biochemical processes, such as energy transfer - as adenosine triphosphate (ATP) and adenosine diphosphate (ADP) - as well as in signal transduction as cyclic adenosine monophosphate, cAMP.
Adenosine triphosphate	Organic molecule that stores energy and releases energy for use in cellular processes is adenosine triphosphate.
Trachea	Trachea is an airway through which respiratory gas transport takes place in organisms. In terrestrial vertebrates, such as birds and humans, the trachea lets air move from the throat to the lungs. In terrestrial invertebrates, such as onychophorans and beetles, they conduct air from outside the organism directly to all of its internal tissues.
Serous	The term serous fluid is used for various bodily fluids that are typically pale yellow and transparent, and of a benign nature.
Pericardium	The pericardium is a double-walled sac that contains the heart and the roots of the great vessels. There are two layers to this sac: the fibrous pericardium, serous pericardium.
Endothelium	The endothelium is the layer of thin, flat cells that lines the interior surface of blood vessels, forming an interface between circulating blood in the lumen and the rest of the vessel wall.

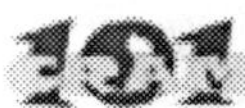

Peritoneum	In higher vertebrates, the peritoneum is the serous membrane that forms the lining of the abdominal cavity - it covers most of the intra-abdominal organs. The peritoneum both supports the abdominal organs and serves as a conduit for their blood and lymph vessels and nerves.
Active transport	Process that requires an expenditure of energy to move a substance across a cell membrane is referred to as active transport.
Mucus	Mucus is a slippery secretion of the lining of various membranes in the body (mucous membranes). Mucus aids in the protection of the lungs by trapping foreign particles that enter the nose during normal breathing. Additionally, it prevents tissues from drying out.
Anal canal	The anal canal is the terminal part of the large intestine. It is situated between the rectum and anus, below the level of the pelvic diaphram.
Esophagus	The esophagus, or gullet is the muscular tube in vertebrates through which ingested food passes from the mouth area to the stomach. Food is passed through the esophagus by using the process of peristalsis.
Vagina	The vagina is the tubular tract leading from the uterus to the exterior of the body in female placental mammals and marsupials, or to the cloaca in female birds, monotremes, and some reptiles. Female insects and other invertebrates also have a vagina, which is the terminal part of the oviduct.
Larynx	The larynx is an organ in the neck of mammals involved in protection of the trachea and sound production. The larynx houses the vocal cords, and is situated at the point where the upper tract splits into the trachea and the esophagus.
Ureter	A ureter is a duct that carries urine from the kidneys to the urinary bladder. They are muscular tubes that can propel urine along by the motions of peristalsis.
Goblet cell	A goblet cell is a glandular simple columnar epithelial cell that is specifically designed to secrete mucus.
Blood vessel	A blood vessel is a part of the circulatory system and function to transport blood throughout the body. The most important types, arteries and veins, are so termed because they carry blood away from or towards the heart, respectively.
Blood	Blood is a circulating tissue composed of fluid plasma and cells. The main function of blood is to supply nutrients (oxygen, glucose) and constitutional elements to tissues and to remove waste products.
Squamous epithelium	The squamous epithelium is epithelium consisting of one or more cell layers, the most superficial of which is composed of flat, scalelike or platelike cells.
Spermatozoa	A sperm cell, spermatozooa (pl. spermatozoa), or spermatozoan, is the haploid cell that is the male gamete. It is carried in fluid called semen, and is capable of fertilising an egg cell to form a zygote.
Body cavity	A fluid-containing space between the digestive tract and the body wall is referred to as body cavity.
Loose connective tissue	Loose connective tissue or Areolar connective tissue holds organs and epithelia in place, and has a variety of proteinaceous fibers, including collagen and elastin. It is also important in inflammation.
Lymphocyte	A lymphocyte is a type of white blood cell involved in the human body's immune system. There are two broad categories, namely T cells and B cells.
Urethra	In anatomy, the urethra is a tube which connects the urinary bladder to the outside of the body. The urethra has an excretory function in both sexes, to pass urine to the outside, and

also a reproductive function in the male, as a passage for sperm.

Taste bud A taste bud is a small structure on the upper surface of the tongue, soft palate, and epiglottis that provides information about the taste of food being eaten. The majority on the tongue sit on raized protrusions of the tongue surface called papillae.

Mucosa The mucosa is a lining of ectodermic origin, covered in epithelium, and involved in absorption and secretion. They line various body cavities that are exposed to the external environment and internal organs.

Olfactory mucosa The olfactory mucosa is an organ made up of the olfactory epithelium and the mucosa, or mucus secreting glands, behind the epithelium. The mucus protects the olfactory epithelium and allows odors to dissolve so that they can be detected by olfactory receptor neurons.

Vesicle Membranous, cytoplasmic sac formed by an infolding of the cell membrane is called a vesicle.

Carbohydrate Carbohydrate is a chemical compound that contains oxygen, hydrogen, and carbon atoms. They consist of monosaccharide sugars of varying chain lengths and that have the general chemical formula $C_n(H_2O)_n$ or are derivatives of such.

Sebaceous The sebaceous glands are glands found in the skin of mammals. They secrete an oily substance called sebum that is made of fat (lipids) and the debris of dead fat-producing cells.

Pancreas The pancreas is a retroperitoneal organ that serves two functions: exocrine - it produces pancreatic juice containing digestive enzymes, and endocrine - it produces several important hormones, namely insulin.

Adrenal In mammals, the adrenal glands are the triangle-shaped endocrine glands that sit atop the kidneys. They are chiefly responsible for regulating the stress response through the synthesis of corticosteroids and catecholamines, including cortisol and adrenaline.

Sebaceous gland The sebaceous gland is found in the skin of mammals. They secrete an oily substance called sebum that is made of fat and the debris of dead fat-producing cells. These glands exist in humans througout the skin except in the palms and soles.

Salivary gland The salivary gland produces saliva, which keeps the mouth and other parts of the digestive system moist. It also helps break down carbohydrates and lubricates the passage of food down from the oro-pharynx to the esophagus to the stomach.

Mammary gland The mammary gland is the organ in the female mammal that produces milk for the sustenance of the young. These exocrine glands are enlarged and modified sweat glands and are the characteristic of mammals which gave the class its name.

Sweat gland Gland responsible for the loss of a watery fluid, consisting mainly of sodium chloride (commonly known as salt) and urea in solution, that is secreted through the skin is a sweat gland.

Endocrine gland An endocrine gland is one of a set of internal organs involved in the secretion of hormones into the blood. These glands are known as ductless, which means they do not have tubes inside them.

Exocrine gland Exocrine gland refers to glands that secrete their products via a duct. Typically, they include sweat glands, salivary glands, mammary glands and many glands of the digestive system.

Follicle Follicle refers to a cluster of cells surrounding, protecting, and nourishing a developing egg cell in the ovary; also secretes estrogen. In botany, a follicle is a type of simple dry fruit produced by certain flowering plants. It is regarded as one the most primitive types of fruits, and derives from a simple pistil or carpel.

Histology Histology is the study of tissue sectioned as a thin slice, using a microscope. It can be

described as microscopic anatomy.

Unicellular | Microorganisms are often illustrated using single-celled, or unicellular organisms; however, some unicellular protists are visible to the naked eye, and some multicellular species are microscopic.

Bile | Bile is a bitter, greenish-yellow alkaline fluid secreted by the liver of most vertebrates. In many species, it is stored in the gallbladder between meals and upon eating is discharged into the duodenum where it aids the process of digestion.

Glucagon | A peptide hormone secreted by islet cells in the pancreas that raises the level of glucose in the blood is referred to as glucagon. Glucagon is a 29 amino acid polypeptide acting as an important hormone in carbohydrate metabolism.

Insulin | Insulin is a polypeptide hormone that regulates carbohydrate metabolism. Apart from being the primary effector in carbohydrate homeostasis, it also has a substantial effect on small vessel muscle tone, controls storage and release of fat (triglycerides) and cellular uptake of both amino acids and some electrolytes.

Enzyme | An enzyme is a protein that catalyzes, or speeds up, a chemical reaction. They are essential to sustain life because most chemical reactions in biological cells would occur too slowly, or would lead to different products, without them.

Exocytosis | Exocytosis is the process by which a cell is able to get rid of large molecules or materials including wastes through its membrane. The process involves a [vacuole], containing the material, fusing with the membrane.

Septa | Septa are thin walls or partitions between the internal chambers (camerae) of the shell of a cephalopod, namely nautiloids or ammonoids.

Distribution | Distribution in pharmacology is a branch of pharmacokinetics describing reversible transfer of drug from one location to another within the body.

Organelle | Organelle refers to any structure within a cell that carries out one of its metabolic roles, such as mitochondria, centrioles, endoplasmic reticulum, and the nucleus.

Membrane protein | A membrane protein is a protein molecule that is attached to, or associated with the membrane of a cell or an organelle. Membrane proteins can be classified into two groups, based on their attachment to the membrane.

Cornea | The cornea is the transparent front part of the eye that covers the iris, pupil, and anterior chamber and provides most of an eye's optical power.

Eye | An eye is an organ that detects light. Different kinds of light-sensitive organs are found in a variety of creatures. The simplest eyes do nothing but detect whether the surroundings are light or dark, while more complex eyes can distinguish shapes and colors.

Anterior surface | The anterior surface of the body presents, in the middle line, a vertical crest, the sphenoidal crest, which articulates with the perpendicular plate of the ethmoid, and forms part of the septum of the nose.

Labile | Easily moved or changed, quickly shifting from one emotion to another, or easily aroused is referred to as labile.

Variable | A characteristic or aspect in which people, objects, events, or conditions vary is called variable.

Capillaries | Capillaries refer to the smallest of the blood vessels and the sites of exchange between the blood and tissue cells.

Capillary | A capillary is the smallest of a body's blood vessels, measuring 5-10 micro meters. They

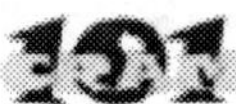

	connect arteries and veins, and most closely interact with tissues. Their walls are composed of a single layer of cells, the endothelium. This layer is so thin that molecules such as oxygen, water and lipids can pass through them by diffusion and enter the tissues.
Neurotransmitter	A neurotransmitter is a chemical that is used to relay, amplify and modulate electrical signals between a neuron and another cell.
Digestion	Digestion refers to the mechanical and chemical breakdown of food into molecules small enough for the body to absorb; the second main stage of food processing, following ingestion.
Vitamin	An organic compound other than a carbohydrate, lipid, or protein that is needed for normal metabolism but that the body cannot synthesize in adequate amounts is called a vitamin.
Sodium	Sodium is the chemical element in the periodic table that has the symbol Na (Natrium in Latin) and atomic number 11. Sodium is a soft, waxy, silvery reactive metal belonging to the alkali metals that is abundant in natural compounds (especially halite). It is highly reactive.
Extracellular fluid	Body fluids outside the individual cells are called extracellular fluid.
Intracellular	Intracellular refers to having to do with the interior of a cell.
Concentration gradient	Gradual change in chemical concentration from one point to another is called concentration gradient.
Gallbladder	The gallbladder is a pear-shaped organ that stores bile until the body needs it for digestion. It is connected to the liver and the duodenum by the biliary tract.
Proximal convoluted tubule	Highly coiled region of a nephron near the glomerular capsule, where tubular reabsorption takes place is called the proximal convoluted tubule.
Ciliary body	The ciliary body is the part of the eye containing the ciliary muscle and ciliary processes. When the ciliary muscle relaxes, it flattens the lens which generally improves the focus for farther objects. When it contracts, the lens becomes more convex which generally improves the focus for closer objects.
Choroid	The choroid is the vascular layer of the eye lying between the retina and the sclera. The choroid provides oxygen and nourishment to the outer layers of the retina.
Plexus	A plexus is also a network of blood vessels, with the choroid plexuses of the brain being the most commonly mentioned example. A choroid plexus is very thin and vascular roof plates of the most anterior and most posterior cavities of the brain which expand into the interiors of the cavities.
Choroid plexus	The choroid plexus is the area on the ventricles of the brain where cerebrospinal fluid (CSF) is produced. Choroid plexus is present in the superior part of the inferior horn of the lateral ventricles.
Invagination	Infolding of one part of a structure into another is invagination.
Mitochondria	Cytoplasmic organelles responsible for ATP generation for cellular activities are referred to as mitochondria.
Pinocytosis	Process by which a cell engulfs droplets of fluid from its surroundings is referred to as pinocytosis.
Zymogen	An inactive precursor of a digestive enzyme secreted into the lumen of the gut, where a protease cleaves it to form the active enzyme is called zymogen.
Lysosome	Organelle that contains enzymes that degrade worn cell parts is called a lysosome.

Go to **Cram101.com** for the Practice Tests for this Chapter.

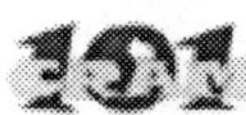

Motor protein	Protein that uses energy derived from nucleoside triphosphate hydrolysis to propel itself along a protein filament or another polymeric molecule is called motor protein.
Staining	Staining is a biochemical technique of adding a class-specific (DNA, proteins, lipids, carbohydrates) dye to a substrate to qualify or quantify the presence of a specific compound. They are frequently used to highlight structures in tissues for viewing, often with the aid of different microscopes.
Golgi apparatus	Golgi apparatus refers to an organelle in eukaryotic cells consisting of stacks of membranous sacs that modify, store, and ship products of the endoplasmic reticulum.
Monosaccharide	A monosaccharide is simplest form of a carbohydrate. They consist of one sugar and are usually colorless, water-soluble, crystalline solids. Some monosaccharides have a sweet taste. They are the building blocks of disaccharides like sucrose and polysaccharides.
Digestive system	The organ system that ingests food, breaks it down into smaller chemical units, and absorbs the nutrient molecules is referred to as the digestive system.
Neuroendocrine system	The network of neurons and glands that make and secrete hormones is referred to as the neuroendocrine system.
Amino acid	An amino acid is any molecule that contains both amino and carboxylic acid functional groups. They are the basic structural building units of proteins. They form short polymer chains called peptides or polypeptides which in turn form structures called proteins.
Polypeptide	Polypeptide refers to polymer of many amino acids linked by peptide bonds.
Epinephrine	Epinephrine is a hormone and a neurotransmitter. Epinephrine plays a central role in the short-term stress reaction—the physiological response to threatening or exciting conditions (fight-or-flight response). It is secreted by the adrenal medulla.
Serotonin	Serotonin is a monoamine neurotransmitter synthesized in serotonergic neurons in the central nervous system and enterochromaffin cells in the gastrointestinal tract. It is believed to play an important part of the biochemistry of depression, migraine, bipolar disorder and anxiety.
Amine	An organic compound with one or more amino groups is called amine. They contain nitrogen as the key atom. Structurally amines resemble ammonia, wherein one or more hydrogen atoms are replaced by organic substituents such as alkyl and aryl groups.
Biogenic amine	A biogenic amine is a biogenic substance involved in chemical signalling. Some prominent examples include neurotransmitters such as acetylcholine, catecholamines, and serotonin.
Silver	Silver is a chemical element with the symbol Ag. A soft white lustrous transition metal, it has the highest electrical and thermal conductivity of any metal and occurs in minerals and in free form.
Salt	Salt is a term used for ionic compounds composed of positively charged cations and negatively charged anions, so that the product is neutral and without a net charge.
Nervous system	The nervous system of an animal coordinates the activity of the muscles, monitors the organs, constructs and processes input from the senses, and initiates actions.
Glycosylation	Glycosylation refers to the process of adding one or more sugars to a protein or lipid molecule.
Transmission electron microscope	Transmission electron microscope refers to a microscope that uses an electron beam to study the internal structure of thinly sectioned specimens.
Tumor	An abnormal mass of cells that forms within otherwise normal tissue is a tumor. This growth

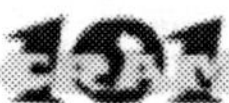

	can be either malignant or benign
Diagnosis	In medicine, diagnosis is the process of identifying a medical condition or disease by its signs, symptoms, and from the results of various diagnostic procedures.
Biopsy	Removal of small tissue sample from the body for microscopic examination is called biopsy.
Conducting portion	The portion of the respiratory system in lung-breathing vertebrates that carries air to the lungs is the conducting portion. It includes the nasal cavity, paranasal sinuses, nasopharynx, larynx, trachea, and bronchi.
Steroid	A steroid is a lipid characterized by a carbon skeleton with four fused rings. Different steroids vary in the functional groups attached to these rings. Hundreds of distinct steroids have been identified in plants and animals. Their most important role in most living systems is as hormones.
Cholesterol	Cholesterol is a steroid, a lipid, and an alcohol, found in the cell membranes of all body tissues, and transported in the blood plasma of all animals. It is an important component of the membranes of cells, providing stability; it makes the membrane's fluidity stable over a bigger temperature interval.
Substrate	A substrate is a molecule which is acted upon by an enzyme. Each enzyme recognizes only the specific substrate of the reaction it catalyzes. A surface in or on which an organism lives.
Androgen	Androgen is the generic term for any natural or synthetic compound, usually a steroid hormone, that stimulates or controls the development and maintenance of masculine characteristics in vertebrates by binding to androgen receptors.
Estrogen	Estrogen is a steroid that functions as the primary female sex hormone. While present in both men and women, they are found in women in significantly higher quantities.
Acetate	Acetate is the anion of a salt or ester of acetic acid.
Steroid hormones	Steroid hormones are steroids which act as hormones. They can be grouped into five groups by the receptors to which they bind: glucocorticoids, mineralocorticoids, androgens, estrogens, and progestagens.
Carcinoma	Cancer that originates in the coverings of the body, such as the skin or the lining of the intestinal tract is a carcinoma.
Brush border	Brush border refers to dense covering of microvilli on the apical surface of epithelial cells in the intestine and kidney. The microvilli aid absorption by increasing the surface area of the cell.

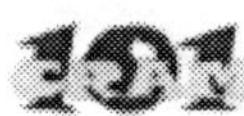

Organ	Organ refers to a structure consisting of several tissues adapted as a group to perform specific functions.
Tissue	A collection of interconnected cells that perform a similar function within an organism is called tissue.
Fiber	Fibers used by man come from a wide variety of sources: Natural fiber include those made out of plants, animal and mineral sources. Natural fibers can be classified according to their origin.
Connective tissue	Connective tissue is any type of biological tissue with an extensive extracellular matrix and often serves to support, bind together, and protect organs.
Epithelium	Epithelium is a tissue composed of a layer of cells. Epithelium can be found lining internal (e.g. endothelium, which lines the inside of blood vessels) or external (e.g. skin) free surfaces of the body. Functions include secretion, absorption and protection.
Muscle	Muscle is a contractile form of tissue. It is one of the four major tissue types, the other three being epithelium, connective tissue and nervous tissue. Muscle contraction is used to move parts of the body, as well as to move substances within the body.
Nerve	A nerve is an enclosed, cable-like bundle of nerve fibers or axons, which includes the glia that ensheath the axons in myelin.
Extracellular	Outside the cell is called extracellular.
Collagen	Collagen is the main protein of connective tissue in animals and the most abundant protein in mammals, making up about 1/4 of the total. It is one of the long, fibrous structural proteins whose functions are quite different from those of globular proteins such as enzymes.
Protein	A protein is a complex, high-molecular-weight organic compound that consists of amino acids joined by peptide bonds. They are essential to the structure and function of all living cells and viruses. Many are enzymes or subunits of enzymes.
Meninges	The meninges are the system of membranes that envelop the central nervous system. The meninges consist of three layers, the dura mater, the arachnoid mater, and the pia mater.
Central nervous system	The central nervous system comprized of the brain and spinal cord, represents the largest part of the nervous system. Together with the peripheral nervous system, it has a fundamental role in the control of behavior.
Nervous system	The nervous system of an animal coordinates the activity of the muscles, monitors the organs, constructs and processes input from the senses, and initiates actions.
Proteoglycan	Molecule consisting of one or more glycosaminoglycan chains attached to a core protein is referred to as proteoglycan.
Hydrophilic	Pertaining to molecules that attract water or dissolve in it because of their polar nature is hydrophilic.
Fibronectin	Fibronectin is a high molecular weight glycoprotein containing about 5% carbohydrate that bind to receptor proteins spanning the cell membrane called integrins. In addition to integrins, they also bind extracellular matrix components such as collagen, fibrin and heparin.
Integrin	An integrin is an integral membrane protein in the plasma membrane of cells. It plays a role in the attachment of a cell to the extracellular matrix (ECM) and in signal transduction from the ECM to the cell.
Receptor	A receptor is a protein on the cell membrane or within the cytoplasm or cell nucleus that binds to a specific molecule (a ligand), such as a neurotransmitter, hormone, or other

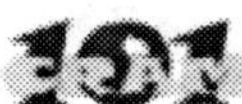

	substance, and initiates the cellular response to the ligand. Receptor, in immunology, the region of an antibody which shows recognition of an antigen.
Laminin	Laminin is a family of heterotrimeric glycoproteins found in the basal lamina underlying epithelia. Their binding to type IV collagen contributes to the self-assembly of the basal lamina from components secreted by cells, and their recognition by growth cone integrins is important to the function of the basal lamina.
Glycosaminog-ycan	Glycosaminoglycan is a long unbranched polysaccharide, made up of repeating disaccharides that may be sulphated (e.g. glucuronic acid, iduronic acid, galactose, galactosamine, glucosamine).
Macromolecule	A macromolecule is a molecule with a large molecular mass, but generally the use of the term is restricted to polymers and molecules which structurally include polymers.
Reservoir	Reservoir is the source of infection. It is the environment in which microorganisms are able to live and grow.
Hormone	A hormone is a chemical messenger from one cell to another. All multicellular organisms produce hormones. The best known hormones are those produced by endocrine glands of vertebrate animals, but hormones are produced by nearly every organ system and tissue type in a human or animal body. Hormone molecules are secreted directly into the bloodstream, they move by circulation or diffusion to their target cells, which may be nearby cells in the same tissue or cells of a distant organ of the body.
Blood	Blood is a circulating tissue composed of fluid plasma and cells. The main function of blood is to supply nutrients (oxygen, glucose) and constitutional elements to tissues and to remove waste products.
Mesenchyme	Mesenchyme is the mass of tissue that develops mainly from the mesoderm of an embryo. It later becomes differentiated into blood vessels and blood-related organs such as the spleen, and into connective tissues.
Mesoderm	Mesoderm forms in the embryos of animals more complex than cnidarians. Some of the cells migrating inward to form the endoderm form an additional layer between the other two. It gives rise to muscles, bones, the dermis of the skin, and most other organs in the adult.
Embryo	A prenatal stage of development after germ layers form but before the rudiments of all organs are present is referred to as an embryo.
Endothelial cell	A endothelial cell also controls the passage of materials — and the transit of white blood cells — into and out of the bloodstream. In some organs, there are highly differentiated endothelial cells to perform specialized 'filtering' functions.
Bone marrow	Bone marrow is the tissue comprising the center of large bones. It is the place where new blood cells are produced. Bone marrow contains two types of stem cells: hemopoietic (which can produce blood cells) and stromal (which can produce fat, cartilage and bone).
Leukocyte	A white blood cell is a leukocyte. They help to defend the body against infectious disease and foreign materials as part of the immune system.
Elastin	Elastin, is a protein in connective tissue that is elastic and allows many tissues in the body to resume their shape after stretching or contracting. Elastin helps skin to return to its original position when it is poked or pinched.
Cytoplasm	Cytoplasm refers to the contents of a cell excluding the nucleus and cell membrane. Cytoplasm is a homogeneous, generally clear jelly-like material that fills cells.
Nucleolus	A small structure within the nucleus of a cell that contains RNA and protein is referred to as nucleolus. It is where ribonucleoprotein is formed.

Staining	Staining is a biochemical technique of adding a class-specific (DNA, proteins, lipids, carbohydrates) dye to a substrate to qualify or quantify the presence of a specific compound. They are frequently used to highlight structures in tissues for viewing, often with the aid of different microscopes.
Elastic fiber	Elastic fiber is a bundles of proteins (elastin) found in connective tissue and produced by fibroblasts and smooth muscle cells in arteries.
Inflammation	Inflammation is the first response of the immune system to infection or irritation and may be referred to as the innate cascade.
Phagocytosis	Phagocytosis (literally, "cell eating") is a form of endocytosis where large particles are enveloped by the cell membrane of a (usually larger) cell and internalized to form a phagosome, or "food vacuole."
Modulation	Modulation is the process of varying a carrier signal, typically a sinusoidal signal, in order to use that signal to convey information.
Osteoblast	An osteoblast is a mononucleate cell that produces a protein that produces osteoid.
Antibody	An antibody is a protein used by the immune system to identify and neutralize foreign objects like bacteria and viruses. Each antibody recognizes a specific antigen unique to its target.
Bacteria	The domain that contains procaryotic cells with primarily diacyl glycerol diesters in their membranes and with bacterial rRNA. Bacteria also is a general term for organisms that are composed of procaryotic cells and are not multicellular.
Antigen	An antigen is a substance that stimulates an immune response, especially the production of antibodies. They are usually proteins or polysaccharides, but can be any type of molecule, including small molecules (haptens) coupled to a protein (carrier).
Scar	A scar results from the biologic process of wound repair in the skin and other tissues of the body. It is a connective tissue that fills the wound.
Wound	A wound is type of physical trauma wherein the skin is torn, cut or punctured, or where blunt force trauma causes a contusion.
Smooth muscle	Smooth muscle is a type of non-striated muscle, found within the "walls" of hollow organs; such as blood vessels, the bladder, the uterus, and the gastrointestinal tract. Smooth muscle is used to move matter within the body, via contraction; it generally operates "involuntarily", without nerve stimulation.
Dermis	The dermis is the layer of skin beneath the epidermis that consists of connective tissue and cushions the body from stress and strain.
Actin	A protein in a muscle fiber that, together with myosin, is responsible for contraction and relaxation is actin.
Microscope	A microscope is an instrument for viewing objects that are too small to be seen by the naked or unaided eye.
Protrusion	Protrusion is the anterior movement of an object. This term is often applied to the jaw.
Vacuole	Vacuole refers to a space or cavity within the cytoplasm of a cell.
Light microscope	An optical instrument with lenses that refract visible light to magnify images and project them into a viewer's eye or onto photographic film is referred to as light microscope.
Capillaries	Capillaries refer to the smallest of the blood vessels and the sites of exchange between the blood and tissue cells.
Capillary	A capillary is the smallest of a body's blood vessels, measuring 5-10 micro meters. They

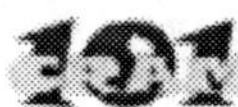

	connect arteries and veins, and most closely interact with tissues. Their walls are composed of a single layer of cells, the endothelium. This layer is so thin that molecules such as oxygen, water and lipids can pass through them by diffusion and enter the tissues.
Venule	A vessel that conveys blood between a capillary bed and a vein is a venule.
Micrograph	A micrograph is a photograph or similar image taken through a microscope or similar device to show a magnified image of an item.
Dense connective tissue	Dense connective tissue has collagen fibers as its main matrix element. Crowded between the collagen fibers are rows of fibroblasts, fiber-forming cells, that manufacture the fibers. Dense connective tissue forms strong, rope-like structures such as tendons and ligaments. Tendons attach skeletal muscles to bones; ligaments connect bones to bones at joints.
Mitochondria	Cytoplasmic organelles responsible for ATP generation for cellular activities are referred to as mitochondria.
Vesicle	Membranous, cytoplasmic sac formed by an infolding of the cell membrane is called a vesicle.
Collagen **fibril**	Collagen fibril refers to extracellular structure formed by self-assembly of secreted fibrillar collagen subunits. An abundant constituent of the extracellular matrix in many animal tissues.
Langer**hans cell**	A Langerhans cell is an immature dendritic cell containing large granules called Birbeck granules. On infection of an area of skin, they will take up and process microbial antigens before travelling to the T-cell areas in the cortex of the draining lymph node and maturing to become fully-functional antigen-presenting cells.
Epidermis	Epidermis is the outermost layer of the skin. It forms the waterproof, protective wrap over the body's surface and is made up of stratified squamous epithelium with an underlying basement membrane. It contains no blood vessels, and is nourished by diffusion from the dermis. In plants, the outermost layer of cells covering the leaves and young parts of a plant is the epidermis.
Digestion	Digestion refers to the mechanical and chemical breakdown of food into molecules small enough for the body to absorb; the second main stage of food processing, following ingestion.
Astrocyte	An astrocyte is a characteristic star-shaped cell in the brain. They are the biggest cells found in brain tissue and outnumber the neurons ten to one. A commonly accepted function is to structure physically the brain. A second function is to provide neurons with nutrients such as glucose. They regulate the flow of nutrients provided by capillaries by forming the blood-brain barrier.
Thyroid	The thyroid is one of the larger endocrine glands in the body. It is located in the neck and produces hormones, principally thyroxine and triiodothyronine, that regulate the rate of metabolism and affect the growth and rate of function of many other systems in the body.
Skin	Skin is an organ of the integumentary system composed of a layer of tissues that protect underlying muscles and organs.
Erythrocyte	Red blood cells are the most common type of blood cell and are the vertebrate body's principal means of delivering oxygen from the lungs or gills to body tissues via the blood. Red blood cells are also known as erythrocyte.
Resistance	Resistance refers to a nonspecific ability to ward off infection or disease regardless of whether the body has been previously exposed to it. A force that opposes the flow of a fluid such as air or blood. Compare with immunity.
Metabolism	Metabolism is the biochemical modification of chemical compounds in living organisms and cells. This includes the biosynthesis of complex organic molecules (anabolism) and their

	breakdown (catabolism).
Infection	The invasion and multiplication of microorganisms in body tissues is called an infection.
Tumor	An abnormal mass of cells that forms within otherwise normal tissue is a tumor. This growth can be either malignant or benign
Fungi	Fungi refers to simple parasitic life forms, including molds, mildews, yeasts, and mushrooms. They live on dead or decaying organic matter. Fungi can grow as single cells, like yeast, or as multicellular colonies, as seen with molds.
Bile	Bile is a bitter, greenish-yellow alkaline fluid secreted by the liver of most vertebrates. In many species, it is stored in the gallbladder between meals and upon eating is discharged into the duodenum where it aids the process of digestion.
Iron	Iron is essential to all organisms, except for a few bacteria. It is mostly stably incorporated in the inside of metalloproteins, because in exposed or in free form it causes production of free radicals that are generally toxic to cells.
Injection	A method of rapid drug delivery that puts the substance directly in the bloodstream, in a muscle, or under the skin is called injection.
Kupffer cell	Kupffer cell is a specialized macrophage located in the liver that forms part of the reticuloendothelial system.
Liver	The liver is an organ in vertebrates, including humans. It plays a major role in metabolism and has a number of functions in the body including drug detoxification, glycogen storage, and plasma protein synthesis. It also produces bile, which is important for digestion.
Monocyte	A monocyte is a leukocyte, part of the human body's immune system that protect against blood-borne pathogens and move quickly to sites of infection in the tissues.
Microtubule	A hollow rod of the protein tubulin in the cytoplasm is referred to as the microtubule.
Lysosome	Organelle that contains enzymes that degrade worn cell parts is called a lysosome.
Kidney	The kidney is a bean-shaped excretory organ in vertebrates. Part of the urinary system, the kidneys filter wastes (especially urea) from the blood and excrete them, along with water, as urine.
Lymph node	A lymph node acts as a filter, with an internal honeycomb of connective tissue filled with lymphocytes that collect and destroy bacteria and viruses. When the body is fighting an infection, these lymphocytes multiply rapidly and produce a characteristic swelling of the lymph node.
Lymph	Lymph originates as blood plasma lost from the circulatory system, which leaks out into the surrounding tissues. The lymphatic system collects this fluid by diffusion into lymph capillaries, and returns it to the circulatory system.
Parturition	Processes that lead to and include birth and the expulsion of the afterbirth are called parturition.
Involution	Shrinkage of a tissue or organ by autolysis, such as involution of the thymus after childhood and of the uterus after pregnancy is referred to as involution.
Uterus	The uterus is the major female reproductive organ of most mammals. One end, the cervix, opens into the vagina; the other is connected on both sides to the fallopian tubes. The main function is to accept a fertilized ovum which becomes implanted into the endometrium, and derives nourishment from blood vessels which develop exclusively for this purpose.
Nerve tissue	Nerve tissue refers the specialized tissue making up the central and peripheral nervous systems; consists of neurons and glial cells.

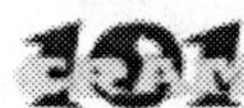

Cytokine	A type of protein secreted by a T lymphocyte that attacks viruses, virally infected cells, and cancer cells is referred to as cytokine.
Fusion	Fusion refers to the combination of two atoms into a single atom as a result of a collision, usually accompanied by the release of energy.
Lungs	Lungs are the essential organs of respiration in air-breathing vertebrates. Their principal function is to transport oxygen from the atmosphere into the bloodstream, and to excrete carbon dioxide from the bloodstream into the atmosphere.
Dendritic cell	The dendritic cell is an immune cell and forms part of the mammal immune system. Once activated, they migrate to the lymphoid tissues where they interact with T cells and B cells to initiate and shape the immune response.
Lymphoid organ	Organ other than a lymphatic vessel that is part of the lymphatic system is referred to as a lymphoid organ.
Inflammatory response	Inflammatory response refers to a complex sequence of events involving chemicals and immune cells that results in the isolation and destruction of antigens and tissues near the antigens.
Heparin	Heparin as a drug is used as an injectable anticoagulant. Heparin is a highly sulfated glycosaminoglycan widely used as an injectable anticoagulant. It is also used to form an inner anticoagulant surface on various experimental and medical devices such as test tubes and renal dialysis machines.
Anaphylaxis	Anaphylaxis refers to an immediate hypersensitivity reaction following exposure of a sensitized individual to the appropriate antigen.
Protease	Protease refers to an enzyme that breaks peptide bonds between amino acids of proteins.
Morphology	The scientific study of organic form, including both its development and function is morphology.
Population	Population refers to all members of a well-defined group of organisms, events, or things.
Anticoagulant	A biochemical that inhibits blood clotting is referred to as an anticoagulant.
Plasma	Fluid portion of circulating blood is called plasma.
Immunoglobulin E	Immunoglobulin E is an antibody subclass (known as "isotypes"), found only in mammals.
Hypersensitivity	Hypersensitivity is an immune response that damages the body's own tissues. Four or five types of hypersensitivity are often described; immediate, antibody-dependent, immune complex, cell-mediated, and stimulatory.
Blood vessel	A blood vessel is a part of the circulatory system and function to transport blood throughout the body. The most important types, arteries and veins, are so termed because they carry blood away from or towards the heart, respectively.
Shock	Circulatory shock, a state of cardiac output that is insufficient to meet the body's physiological needs, with consequences ranging from fainting to death is referred to as shock. Insulin shock, a state of severe hypoglycemia caused by administration of insulin.
Anaphylactic shock	A precipitous drop in blood pressure caused by loss of fluid from capillaries because of an increase in their permeability stimulated by an allergic reaction is called anaphylactic shock.
Blood clotting	A complex process by which platelets, the protein fibrin, and red blood cells block an irregular surface in or on the body, such as a damaged blood vessel, sealing the wound is referred to as blood clotting.

Respiratory tract	In humans the respiratory tract is the part of the anatomy that has to do with the process of respiration or breathing.
Centriole	A cellular structure built of microtubules that organizes the mitotic spindle is called a centriole.
Lymphocyte	A lymphocyte is a type of white blood cell involved in the human body's immune system. There are two broad categories, namely T cells and B cells.
Variable	A characteristic or aspect in which people, objects, events, or conditions vary is called variable.
Epitope	An epitope is the part of a foreign organism or its proteins that is being recognized by the immune system and targeted by antibodies, cytotoxic T cells or both.
Diphtheria	Diphtheria refers to an acute, highly contagious childhood disease that generally affects the membranes of the throat and less frequently the nose. It is caused by Corynehacterium diphtheriae.
Tetanus	Tetanus is a serious and often fatal disease caused by the neurotoxin tetanospasmin which is produced by the Gram-positive, obligate anaerobic bacterium Clostridium tetani. Tetanus also refers to a state of muscle tension.
Toxin	Toxin refers to a microbial product or component that can injure another cell or organism at low concentrations. Often the term refers to a poisonous protein, but toxins may be lipids and other substances.
Exocytosis	Exocytosis is the process by which a cell is able to get rid of large molecules or materials including wastes through its membrane. The process involves a [vacuole], containing the material, fusing with the membrane.
Lead	Lead is a chemical element in the periodic table that has the symbol Pb and atomic number 82. A soft, heavy, toxic and malleable poor metal, lead is bluish white when freshly cut but tarnishes to dull gray when exposed to air. Lead is used in building construction, lead-acid batteries, bullets and shot, and is part of solder, pewter, and fusible alloys.
Intracellular	Intracellular refers to having to do with the interior of a cell.
Phospholipid	Phospholipid is a class of lipids formed from four components: fatty acids, a negatively-charged phosphate group, an alcohol and a backbone. Phospholipids with a glycerol backbone are known as glycerophospholipids or phosphoglycerides.
Glycosylation	Glycosylation refers to the process of adding one or more sugars to a protein or lipid molecule.
Histology	Histology is the study of tissue sectioned as a thin slice, using a microscope. It can be described as microscopic anatomy.
Cardinal sign	Cardinal sign is the body temperature, pulse and respiratory rates, and blood pressure.
Pain	Pain is an unpleasant sensation which may be associated with actual or potential tissue damage and which may have physical and emotional components.
Blood plasma	Blood plasma is the liquid component of blood, in which the blood cells are suspended. Serum is the same as blood plasma except that clotting factors (such as fibrin) have been removed.
Chemotaxis	Chemotaxis is the phenomenon in which bodily cells, bacteria, and other single-celled or multicellular organisms direct their movements according to certain chemicals in their environment.
Lamina	A thin layer, such as the lamina of a vertebra or the lamina propria of a mucous membrane is referred to as lamina.

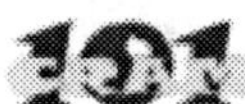

Edema	Edema is swelling of any organ or tissue due to accumulation of excess fluid. Edema has many root causes, but its common mechanism is accumulation of fluid into the tissues.
Taxis	A taxis is an innate behavioral response by an organism (or cell) to a directional stimulus (a stimulus from a particular direction) whereby an organism moves (orientation movement) either towards (positive taxis) or away from (negative taxis) the stimulus.
Filtration	Filtration involved in passive transport is the movement of water and solute molecules across the cell membrane due to hydrostatic pressure by the cardiovascular system.
Placenta	The placenta is an organ present only in female placental mammals during gestation. It is composed of two parts, one genetically and biologically part of the fetus, the other part of the mother. It is implanted in the wall of the uterus, where it receives nutrients and oxygen from the mother's blood and passes out waste.
Tendon	A tendon or sinew is a tough band of fibrous connective tissue that connects muscle to bone. They are similar to ligaments except that ligaments join one bone to another.
Collagen fiber	White fiber in the matrix of connective tissue, giving flexibility and strength is called collagen fiber.
Distribution	Distribution in pharmacology is a branch of pharmacokinetics describing reversible transfer of drug from one location to another within the body.
Pathology	Pathology is the study of the processes underlying disease and other forms of illness, harmful abnormality, or dysfunction.
Dentin	Dentin is the substance between the enamel (substance in the crown) or cementum (substance in the root) of a tooth and the pulp chamber. Dentin is secreted by the odontoblasts of the dental pulp.
Proline	Proline is one of the twenty proteinogenic units which are used in living organisms as the building blocks of proteins. The other nineteen units are all primary amino acids, but due to the (3-carbon) cyclic sidechain binding back to the nitrogen of the backbone, proline lacks a primary amine group ($-NH_2$).
Amino acid	An amino acid is any molecule that contains both amino and carboxylic acid functional groups. They are the basic structural building units of proteins. They form short polymer chains called peptides or polypeptides which in turn form structures called proteins.
Glycine	Glycine (Gly, G) is a nonpolar amino acid. It is the simplest of the 20 standard (proteinogenic) amino acids: its side chain is a hydrogen atom. Because there is a second hydrogen atom at the α carbon, glycine is not optically active.
Acid	An acid is a water-soluble, sour-tasting chemical compound that when dissolved in water, gives a solution with a pH of less than 7.
Hydroxyproline	Hydroxyproline is an uncommon amino acid. Hydroxyproline differs from proline by the presence of a hydroxyl (OH) group attached to the C (gamma) atom.
Hydroxylysine	Hydroxylysine is an amino acid, $C_6H_{14}N_2O_3$. It is most widely known as a component of collagen.
Helix	A helix is a twisted shape like a spring, screw or a spiral staircase. Helixes are important in biology, as DNA is helical and many proteins have helical substructures, known as alpha helices.
Polypeptide	Polypeptide refers to polymer of many amino acids linked by peptide bonds.
Hydrophobic interaction	The tendency for hydrophobic molecules to cluster together when immersed in water is called hydrophobic interaction.

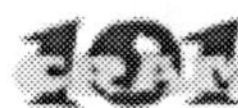

Hydrophobic	Hydrophobic refers to being electrically neutral and nonpolar, and thus prefering other neutral and nonpolar solvents or molecular environments. Hydrophobic is often used interchangeably with "oily" or "lipophilic."
Hydrogen	Hydrogen is a chemical element in the periodic table that has the symbol H and atomic number 1. At standard temperature and pressure it is a colorless, odorless, nonmetallic, univalent, tasteless, highly flammable diatomic gas.
Hydrogen bond	A hydrogen bond is a type of attractive intermolecular force that exists between two partial electric charges of opposite polarity. Although stronger than most other intermolecular forces, the typical hydrogen bond is much weaker than both the ionic bond and the covalent bond.
Enzyme	An enzyme is a protein that catalyzes, or speeds up, a chemical reaction. They are essential to sustain life because most chemical reactions in biological cells would occur too slowly, or would lead to different products, without them.
Transverse	A transverse (also known as axial or horizontal) plane is an X-Y plane, parallel to the ground, which (in humans) separates the superior from the inferior, or put another way, the head from the feet.
Striation	Striation refers to the tiny grooves of muscle across major muscle groups characteristic of a well-developed body.
Solution	Solution refers to homogenous mixture formed when a solute is dissolved in a solvent.
Cartilage	Cartilage is a type of dense connective tissue. Cartilage is composed of cells called chondrocytes which are dispersed in a firm gel-like ground substance, called the matrix. Cartilage is avascular (contains no blood vessels) and nutrients are diffused through the matrix.
Biosynthesis	Biosynthesis is a phenomenon where chemical compounds are produced from simpler reagents. Biosynthesis, unlike chemical synthesis, takes place within living organisms and is generally catalysed by enzymes.
Peptide	Peptide is the family of molecules formed from the linking, in a defined order, of various amino acids. The link between one amino acid residue and the next is an amide bond, and is sometimes referred to as a peptide bond.
Lysine	Lysine is one of the 20 amino acids normally found in proteins. With its 4-aminobutyl side-chain, it is classified as a basic amino acid, along with arginine and histidine.
Carbohydrate	Carbohydrate is a chemical compound that contains oxygen, hydrogen, and carbon atoms. They consist of monosaccharide sugars of varying chain lengths and that have the general chemical formula $C_n(H_2O)_n$ or are derivatives of such.
Galactose	Galactose is a type of sugar found in dairy products, in sugar beets and other gums and mucilages. It is also synthesized by the body, where it forms part of glycolipids and glycoproteins in several tissues.
Carboxyl	A carboxyl is the univalent radical -COOH; present in and characteristic of organic acids.
Precipitation	The crystallization or suspension of particles that occurs due to the mixing of incompatible solutions or adding solutes to incompatible solutions is called precipitation. This results in the occlusion of an intravenous line.
Residue	A residue refers to a portion of a larger molecule, a specific monomer of a polysaccharide, protein or nucleic acid.
Genes	Genes are the units of heredity in living organisms. They are encoded in the organism's genetic material (usually DNA or RNA), and control the development and behavior of the

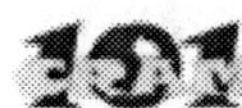

	organism.
Posttranslat-onal	Posttranslational refers to any process involving a protein that occurs after protein synthesis is completed.
Mutation	A change in the structure of a gene is called a mutation.
Fibrosis	Replacement of damaged tissue with fibrous scar tissue rather than by the original tissue type is called fibrosis.
Digestive tract	The digestive tract is the system of organs within multicellular animals which takes in food, digests it to extract energy and nutrients, and expels the remaining waste.
Vitamin	An organic compound other than a carbohydrate, lipid, or protein that is needed for normal metabolism but that the body cannot synthesize in adequate amounts is called a vitamin.
Ascorbic acid	Ascorbic acid is an organic acid with antioxidant properties. Its appearance is white to light yellow crystals or powder. It is water soluble. The L-enantiomer of ascorbic acid is commonly known as vitamin C.
Ligament	A ligament is a short band of tough fibrous connective tissue composed mainly of long, stringy collagen fibres. They connect bones to other bones to form a joint. (They do not connect muscles to bones.)
Cofactor	A cofactor is any substance that needs to be present in addition to an enzyme to catalyze a certain reaction.
Articular	The articular is a bone in the lower jaw of most tetrapods, including reptiles, birds, and amphibians, but has become a middle ear bone (the malleus) in mammals. It is the site of articulation between the lower jaw and the skull, and is connected to two other lower jaw bones, the suprangular and the angular.
Mesentery	A mesentery is a part of the peritoneum that connects an internal organ, such as the small intestine, to the abdominal wall.
Course	Pattern of development and change of a disorder over time is a course.
Squamous epithelium	The squamous epithelium is epithelium consisting of one or more cell layers, the most superficial of which is composed of flat, scalelike or platelike cells.
Affinity	Chemical affinity results from electronic properties by which dissimilar substances are capable of forming chemical compounds. Specifically, the term refers to the tendency of an atom or compound to combine by chemical reaction with atoms or compounds of unlike composition.
Silver	Silver is a chemical element with the symbol Ag. A soft white lustrous transition metal, it has the highest electrical and thermal conductivity of any metal and occurs in minerals and in free form.
Salt	Salt is a term used for ionic compounds composed of positively charged cations and negatively charged anions, so that the product is neutral and without a net charge.
Artery	Vessel that takes blood away from the heart to the tissues and organs of the body is called an artery.
Tunica media	The tunica media is the middle layer of an artery. It is made up of smooth muscle cells and elastic tissue. It lays between the tunica intima on the inside and the tunica adventitia on the outside.
Adventitia	Adventitia is the outermost connective tissue covering of any organ, vessel, or other structure. For example, the connective tissue that surrounds an artery is called the adventitia because it is considered extraneous to the artery.

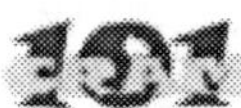

Tunica adventitia	The Tunica Adventitia is the outermost layer of a blood vessel, surrounding the tunica media.
Sugar	A sugar is the simplest molecule that can be identified as a carbohydrate. These include monosaccharides and disaccharides, trisaccharides and the oligosaccharides. The term "glyco-" indicates the presence of a sugar in an otherwise non-carbohydrate substance.
Hexose	A hexose is a monosaccharide with six carbon atoms having the chemical formula $C_6H_{12}O_6$.
Microscopy	Microscopy is any technique for producing visible images of structures or details too small to otherwise be seen by the human eye, using a microscope or other magnification tool.
Histogram	In statistics, a histogram is a graphical display of tabulated frequencies. It is the graphical version of a table which shows what proportion of cases fall into each of several or many specified categories. The categories are usually specified as nonoverlapping intervals of some variable.
Eye	An eye is an organ that detects light. Different kinds of light-sensitive organs are found in a variety of creatures. The simplest eyes do nothing but detect whether the surroundings are light or dark, while more complex eyes can distinguish shapes and colors.
Alkali	In chemistry, an alkali is a specific type of base, formed as a carbonate, hydroxide or other ionic salt of an alkali metal or alkali earth metal element. The word alkali or the adjective alkaline are frequently used to refer to all bases, since most common bases are alkalis, although such use is really a synecdoche.
Syndrome	Syndrome is the association of several clinically recognizable features, signs, symptoms, phenomena or characteristics which often occur together, so that the presence of one feature alerts the physician to the presence of the others
Marfan syndrome	Marfan syndrome is a connective tissue disorder characterized by unusually long limbs. The disease also affects other bodily structures — including the skeleton, lungs, eyes, heart and blood vessels — in less obvious ways.
Aorta	The largest artery in the human body, the aorta originates from the left ventricle of the heart and brings oxygenated blood to all parts of the body in the systemic circulation.
Blood pressure	Blood pressure is the pressure exerted by the blood on the walls of the blood vessels.
Disaccharide	A disaccharide is a sugar (a carbohydrate) composed of two monosaccharides. The two monosaccharides are bonded via a condensation reaction.
Polysaccharide	A carbohydrate composed of many joined monosaccharides is called a polysaccharide.
Glucosamine	Glucosamine ($C_6H_{14}NO_5$) is an amino sugar that is a important precursor in the biochemical synthesis of glycosylated proteins and lipids. Glucosamine is commonly used as a treatment for osteoarthritis, although its acceptance as a medical therapy varies.
Galactosamine	An amino derivative of galactose commonly found in glycolipids is a galactosamine.
Notochord	The notochord is a flexible rod-shaped body found in embryos of all chordates. It is composed of cells derived from the mesoblast and defining the primitive axis of the embryo. In lower vertebrates, it persists throughout life as the main axial support of the body, while in higher vertebrates it is replaced by the vertebral column.
Skeleton	In biology, the skeleton or skeletal system is the biological system providing physical support in living organisms.
Cornea	The cornea is the transparent front part of the eye that covers the iris, pupil, and anterior chamber and provides most of an eye's optical power.
Humor	In traditional medicine practiced before the advent of modern technology, the four humours

	(or four humors) were four fluids that were thought to permeate the body and influence its health. A humor is any fluid substance in the body.
Vitreous humor	Vitreous humor refers to a jellylike substance filling the space behind the lens in the vertebrate eye; helps maintain the shape of the eye.
Amino acid residue	An amino acid residue is what is left of an amino acid once a molecule of water has been lost (an H+ from the nitrogenous side and an OH- from the carboxylic side) in the formation of a peptide bond.
Plasma membrane	The unit membrane that encloses a cell and controls the traffic of molecules in and out of the cell is the plasma membrane.
Extension	Movement increasing the angle between parts at a joint is referred to as extension.
Hydrolase	Hydrolase is a general term for any enzyme that catalyzes a hydrolysis reaction, the chemical breakdown of polymers into smaller molecules through the addition of water molecules.
Microorganism	A microorganism or microbe is an organism that is so small that it is microscopic (invisible to the naked eye).
Hydrolyze	Hydrolyze refers to break a chemical bond, as in a peptide linkage, with the insertion of the components of water, -H and -OH, at the cleaved ends of a chain. The digestion of proteins is hydrolysis.
Hyaluronidase	Hyaluronidase refers to an enzyme that digests proteoglycans. Found in sperm cells, it helps digest the coatings surrounding an egg so the sperm can penetrate the egg cell membrane.
Substrate	A substrate is a molecule which is acted upon by an enzyme. Each enzyme recognizes only the specific substrate of the reaction it catalyzes. A surface in or on which an organism lives.
Cancer	Cancer is a class of diseases or disorders characterized by uncontrolled division of cells and the ability of these cells to invade other tissues, either by direct growth into adjacent tissue through invasion or by implantation into distant sites by metastasis.
Embryogenesis	Embryogenesis is the process by which the embryo is formed and develops. It starts with the fertilization of the ovum, which is then called a zygote.
Trimer	In biochemistry, a trimer is a macromolecular compound formed by three non-covalently bound macromolecules.
Ion	Ion refers to an atom or molecule that has gained or lost one or more electrons, thus acquiring an electrical charge.
Hydrostatic pressure	Hydrostatic pressure refers to pressure exerted by fluids, such as blood pressure.
Molecular weight	The molecular mass of a substance, called molecular weight and abbreviated as MW, is the mass of one molecule of that substance, relative to the unified atomic mass unit u (equal to 1/12 the mass of one atom of carbon-12).
Colloid osmotic pressure	Colloid osmotic pressure refers to a portion of the osmotic pressure of a body fluid that is due to its protein concentration.
Colloid	Colloid refers to a mixture that contains dispersed particles larger than molecules but small enough so that they do not settle out.
Osmotic pressure	Osmotic pressure is the pressure produced by a solution in a space that is enclosed by a differentially permeable membrane.
Striated muscle	Striated muscle refers to contractile tissue characterized by multinucleated cells containing highly ordered arrangements of actin and myosin microfilaments. Also known as skeletal

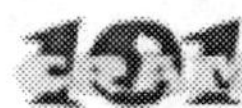

	muscle.
Veins	Blood vessels that return blood toward the heart from the circulation are referred to as veins.
Base	The common definition of a base is a chemical compound that absorbs hydronium ions when dissolved in water (a proton acceptor). An alkali is a special example of a base, where in an aqueous environment, hydroxide ions are donated.
Vein	Vein in animals, is a vessel that returns blood to the heart. In plants, a vascular bundle in a leaf, composed of xylem and phloem.
Congestive heart failure	Congestive heart failure is the inability of the heart to pump a sufficient amount of blood throughout the body, or requiring elevated filling pressures in order to pump effectively.
Venous blood	In the circulatory system, venous blood or peripheral blood is blood returning to the heart. With one exception (the pulmonary vein) this blood is deoxygenated and high in carbon dioxide, having released oxygen and absorbed CO_2 in the tissues.
Depression	In everyday language depression refers to any downturn in mood, which may be relatively transitory and perhaps due to something trivial. This is differentiated from Clinical depression which is marked by symptoms that last two weeks or more and are so severe that they interfere with daily living.
Endothelium	The endothelium is the layer of thin, flat cells that lines the interior surface of blood vessels, forming an interface between circulating blood in the lumen and the rest of the vessel wall.
Endometrium	The endometrium is the inner uterine membrane in mammals which is developed in preparation for the implantation of a fertilized egg upon its arrival into the uterus.
Gland	A gland is an organ in an animal's body that synthesizes a substance for release such as hormones, often into the bloodstream or into cavities inside the body or its outer surface.
Loose connective tissue	Loose connective tissue or Areolar connective tissue holds organs and epithelia in place, and has a variety of proteinaceous fibers, including collagen and elastin. It is also important in inflammation.
Friction	Friction is the force that opposes the relative motion or tendency of such motion of two surfaces in contact. The resulting injury to skin resembles an abrasion and can also damage superficial blood vessels directly under the skin.
Pleural cavity	The lungs are surrounded by two membranes, the pleura. The outer is attached to the chest wall and is known as the parietal pleura; the inner is attached to the lung and other visceral tissues and is known as the visceral pleura. In between the two is a thin space known as the pleural cavity or pleural space. It is filled with pleural fluid, a serous fluid produced by the pleura.
Lesion	A lesion is a non-specific term referring to abnormal tissue in the body. It can be caused by any disease process including trauma (physical, chemical, electrical), infection, neoplasm, metabolic and autoimmune.
Consistency	The extent to which an individual responds to a given stimulus or situation in the same way on different occasions is a consistency.
Stress	Stress refers to a condition that is a response to factors that change the human systems normal state.
Traction	Traction refers to the set of mechanisms for straightening broken bones or relieving pressure on the skeletal system. It is largely replaced now by more modern techniques, but certain approaches are still used today for hip fractures.

Joint	A joint (articulation) is the location at which two bones make contact (articulate). They are constructed to both allow movement and provide mechanical support.
Synovial joint	Synovial joint refers to freely moving joint in which two bones are separated by a cavity.
Penis	The penis is the male reproductive organ and for mammals additionally serves as the external male organ of urination.
Vertebral column	In human anatomy, the vertebral column is a column of vertebrae situated in the dorsal aspect of the abdomen. It houses the spinal cord in its spinal canal.
Spleen	The spleen is a ductless, vertebrate gland that is not necessary for life but is closely associated with the circulatory system, where it functions in the destruction of old red blood cells and removal of other debris from the bloodstream, and also in holding a reservoir of blood.
Umbilical cord	A structure containing arteries and veins that connects a developing embryo to the placenta of the mother is an umbilical cord.
Sinus	A sinus is a pouch or cavity in any organ or tissue, or an abnormal cavity or passage caused by the destruction of tissue.
Activation	As reflected by facial expressions, the degree of arousal a person is experiencing is referred to as activation.
Biochemistry	Biochemistry studies how complex chemical reactions give rise to life. It is a hybrid branch of chemistry which specialises in the chemical processes in living organisms.

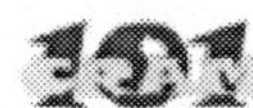

Tissue	A collection of interconnected cells that perform a similar function within an organism is called tissue.
Organ	Organ refers to a structure consisting of several tissues adapted as a group to perform specific functions.
Adipose tissue	Adipose tissue is an anatomical term for loose connective tissue composed of adipocytes. Its main role is to store energy in the form of fat, although it also cushions and insulates the body. It has an important endocrine function in producing recently-discovered hormones such as leptin, resistin and TNFalpha.
Triglyceride	Triglyceride is a glyceride in which the glycerol is esterified with three fatty acids. They are the main constituent of vegetable oil and animal fats and play an important role in metabolism as energy sources. They contain a bit more than twice as much energy as carbohydrates and proteins.
Triglycerides	Triglycerides refer to fats and oils composed of fatty acids and glycerol; are the body's most concentrated source of energy fuel; also known as neutral fats.
Glycogen	Glycogen refers to a complex, extensively branched polysaccharide of many glucose monomers; serves as an energy-storage molecule in liver and muscle cells.
Muscle	Muscle is a contractile form of tissue. It is one of the four major tissue types, the other three being epithelium, connective tissue and nervous tissue. Muscle contraction is used to move parts of the body, as well as to move substances within the body.
Liver	The liver is an organ in vertebrates, including humans. It plays a major role in metabolism and has a number of functions in the body including drug detoxification, glycogen storage, and plasma protein synthesis. It also produces bile, which is important for digestion.
Skeletal muscle	Skeletal muscle is a type of striated muscle, attached to the skeleton. They are used to facilitate movement, by applying force to bones and joints; via contraction. They generally contract voluntarily (via nerve stimulation), although they can contract involuntarily.
Calorie	Calorie refers to a unit used to measure heat energy and the energy contents of foods.
Carbohydrate	Carbohydrate is a chemical compound that contains oxygen, hydrogen, and carbon atoms. They consist of monosaccharide sugars of varying chain lengths and that have the general chemical formula $C_n(H_2O)_n$ or are derivatives of such.
Value	Value is worth in general, and it is thought to be connected to reasons for certain practices, policies, actions, beliefs or emotions. Value is "that which one acts to gain and/or keep."
Subcutaneous	Subcutaneous injections are given by injecting a fluid into the subcutis. It is relatively painless and an effective way to administer particular types of medication.
Shock	Circulatory shock, a state of cardiac output that is insufficient to meet the body's physiological needs, with consequences ranging from fainting to death is referred to as shock. Insulin shock, a state of severe hypoglycemia caused by administration of insulin.
Subcutaneous layer	A sheet that lies just beneath the skin and consists of loose connective and adipose tissue is called the subcutaneous layer.
Insulation	The practice of managing our role performances so that role partners cannot observe our behavior in two or more conflicting roles is referred to as an insulation.
Blood	Blood is a circulating tissue composed of fluid plasma and cells. The main function of blood is to supply nutrients (oxygen, glucose) and constitutional elements to tissues and to remove waste products.

Cytoplasm	Cytoplasm refers to the contents of a cell excluding the nucleus and cell membrane. Cytoplasm is a homogeneous, generally clear jelly-like material that fills cells.
Mitochondria	Cytoplasmic organelles responsible for ATP generation for cellular activities are referred to as mitochondria.
Lipid	Lipid is one class of aliphatic hydrocarbon-containing organic compounds essential for the structure and function of living cells. They are characterized by being water-insoluble but soluble in nonpolar organic solvents.
Scrotum	In some male mammals the scrotum is an external bag of skin and muscle containing the testicles. It is an extension of the abdomen, and is located between the penis and anus.
Penis	The penis is the male reproductive organ and for mammals additionally serves as the external male organ of urination.
Distribution	Distribution in pharmacology is a branch of pharmacokinetics describing reversible transfer of drug from one location to another within the body.
Hormone	A hormone is a chemical messenger from one cell to another. All multicellular organisms produce hormones. The best known hormones are those produced by endocrine glands of vertebrate animals, but hormones are produced by nearly every organ system and tissue type in a human or animal body. Hormone molecules are secreted directly into the bloodstream, they move by circulation or diffusion to their target cells, which may be nearby cells in the same tissue or cells of a distant organ of the body.
Vacuole	Vacuole refers to a space or cavity within the cytoplasm of a cell.
Alcohol	Alcohol is a general term, applied to any organic compound in which a hydroxyl group (-OH) is bound to a carbon atom, which in turn is bound to other hydrogen and/or carbon atoms. The general formula for a simple acyclic alcohol is $C_nH_{2n+1}OH$.
Vesicle	Membranous, cytoplasmic sac formed by an infolding of the cell membrane is called a vesicle.
Microscope	A microscope is an instrument for viewing objects that are too small to be seen by the naked or unaided eye.
Light microscope	An optical instrument with lenses that refract visible light to magnify images and project them into a viewer's eye or onto photographic film is referred to as light microscope.
Lamina	A thin layer, such as the lamina of a vertebra or the lamina propria of a mucous membrane is referred to as lamina.
Nerve	A nerve is an enclosed, cable-like bundle of nerve fibers or axons, which includes the glia that ensheath the axons in myelin.
Connective tissue	Connective tissue is any type of biological tissue with an extensive extracellular matrix and often serves to support, bind together, and protect organs.
Fiber	Fibers used by man come from a wide variety of sources: Natural fiber include those made out of plants, animal and mineral sources. Natural fibers can be classified according to their origin.
Blood vessel	A blood vessel is a part of the circulatory system and function to transport blood throughout the body. The most important types, arteries and veins, are so termed because they carry blood away from or towards the heart, respectively.
Ratio	In number and more generally in algebra, a ratio is the linear relationship between two quantities.
Striated muscle	Striated muscle refers to contractile tissue characterized by multinucleated cells containing highly ordered arrangements of actin and myosin microfilaments. Also known as skeletal

	muscle.
Fatty acid	A fatty acid is a carboxylic acid (or organic acid), often with a long aliphatic tail (long chains), either saturated or unsaturated.
Glycerol	Glycerol is a three-carbon substance that forms the backbone of fatty acids in fats. When the body uses stored fat as a source of energy, glycerol and fatty acids are released into the bloodstream. The glycerol component can be converted to glucose by the liver and provides energy for cellular metabolism.
Esters	Esters are organic compounds in which an organic group replaces a hydrogen atom in an oxygen acid. An oxygen acid is an acid whose molecule has an -OH group from which the hydrogen (H) can dissociate as an H^+ ion.
Acid	An acid is a water-soluble, sour-tasting chemical compound that when dissolved in water, gives a solution with a pH of less than 7.
Lipoprotein	A lipoprotein is a biochemical assembly that contains both proteins and lipids and may be structural or catalytic in function. They may be enzymes, proton pumps, ion pumps, or some combination of these functions.
Glucose	Glucose, a simple monosaccharide sugar, is one of the most important carbohydrates and is used as a source of energy in animals and plants. Glucose is one of the main products of photosynthesis and starts respiration.
Blood plasma	Blood plasma is the liquid component of blood, in which the blood cells are suspended. Serum is the same as blood plasma except that clotting factors (such as fibrin) have been removed.
Plasma	Fluid portion of circulating blood is called plasma.
Lymph	Lymph originates as blood plasma lost from the circulatory system, which leaks out into the surrounding tissues. The lymphatic system collects this fluid by diffusion into lymph capillaries, and returns it to the circulatory system.
Chylomicron	Particles of lipid coated with protein, produced in by the absorptive cells of the small intestine and secreted into the extracellular fluids are referred to as chylomicron.
Cholesterol	Cholesterol is a steroid, a lipid, and an alcohol, found in the cell membranes of all body tissues, and transported in the blood plasma of all animals. It is an important component of the membranes of cells, providing stability; it makes the membrane's fluidity stable over a bigger temperature interval.
Capillaries	Capillaries refer to the smallest of the blood vessels and the sites of exchange between the blood and tissue cells.
Capillary	A capillary is the smallest of a body's blood vessels, measuring 5-10 micro meters. They connect arteries and veins, and most closely interact with tissues. Their walls are composed of a single layer of cells, the endothelium. This layer is so thin that molecules such as oxygen, water and lipids can pass through them by diffusion and enter the tissues.
Enzyme	An enzyme is a protein that catalyzes, or speeds up, a chemical reaction. They are essential to sustain life because most chemical reactions in biological cells would occur too slowly, or would lead to different products, without them.
Lipase	A lipase is a water-soluble enzyme that catalyzes the hydrolysis of ester bonds in water–insoluble, lipid substrates. Most lipases act at a specific position on the glycerol backbone of a lipid substrate (A1, A2 or A3).
Lipoprotein lipase	Lipoprotein lipase is an enzyme which hydrolyzes lipids in lipoproteins like those found in chylomicrons into fatty acids and an alcohol.

Diffusion	Random movement of molecules from a region of higher concentration toward one of lower concentration is referred to as diffusion.
Active transport	Process that requires an expenditure of energy to move a substance across a cell membrane is referred to as active transport.
Metabolism	Metabolism is the biochemical modification of chemical compounds in living organisms and cells. This includes the biosynthesis of complex organic molecules (anabolism) and their breakdown (catabolism).
Phosphate	A phosphate is a polyatomic ion or radical consisting of one phosphorus atom and four oxygen. In the ionic form, it carries a -3 formal charge, and is denoted PO_4^{3-}.
Protein	A protein is a complex, high-molecular-weight organic compound that consists of amino acids joined by peptide bonds. They are essential to the structure and function of all living cells and viruses. Many are enzymes or subunits of enzymes.
Carrier	Person in apparent health whose chromosomes contain a pathologic mutant gene that may be transmitted to his or her children is a carrier.
Organelle	Organelle refers to any structure within a cell that carries out one of its metabolic roles, such as mitochondria, centrioles, endoplasmic reticulum, and the nucleus.
Insulin	Insulin is a polypeptide hormone that regulates carbohydrate metabolism. Apart from being the primary effector in carbohydrate homeostasis, it also has a substantial effect on small vessel muscle tone, controls storage and release of fat (triglycerides) and cellular uptake of both amino acids and some electrolytes.
Norepinephrine	Norepinephrine is a catecholamine and a phenethylamine with chemical formula $C_8H_{11}NO_3$. It is released from the adrenal glands as a hormone into the blood, but it is also a neurotransmitter in the nervous system where it is released from noradrenergic neurons during synaptic transmission.
Sympathetic	The sympathetic nervous system activates what is often termed the "fight or flight response". It is an automatic regulation system, that is, one that operates without the intervention of conscious thought.
Albumin	Albumin refers generally to any protein with water solubility, which is moderately soluble in concentrated salt solutions, and experiences heat coagulation (protein denaturation).
Serum	Serum is the same as blood plasma except that clotting factors (such as fibrin) have been removed. Blood plasma contains fibrinogen.
Prolactin	Prolactin is a hormone synthesised and secreted by lactotrope cells in the anterior pituitary gland. It is made up of 199 amino acids, and has a molecular weight of about 23,000 daltons and has many effects, the most significant of which is to stimulate the mammary glands to produce milk (lactation).
Thyroid	The thyroid is one of the larger endocrine glands in the body. It is located in the neck and produces hormones, principally thyroxine and triiodothyronine, that regulate the rate of metabolism and affect the growth and rate of function of many other systems in the body.
Glucocorticoid	Glucocorticoid is a class of steroid hormones characterized by the ability to bind with the cortisol receptor and trigger similar effects. They are distinguished from mineralocorticoids and sex steroids by the specific receptors, target cells, and effects.
Growth hormone	Growth hormone is a polypeptide hormone synthesised and secreted by the anterior pituitary gland which stimulates growth and cell reproduction in humans and other vertebrate animals.
Endothelium	The endothelium is the layer of thin, flat cells that lines the interior surface of blood vessels, forming an interface between circulating blood in the lumen and the rest of the

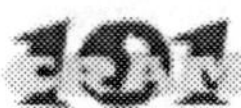

vessel wall.

Amino acid — An amino acid is any molecule that contains both amino and carboxylic acid functional groups. They are the basic structural building units of proteins. They form short polymer chains called peptides or polypeptides which in turn form structures called proteins.

Leptin — Leptin is a 16 kDa protein hormone that plays a key role in metabolism and regulation of adipose tissue. It is released by fat cells in amounts mirroring overall body fat stores. Thus, circulating leptin levels give the brain a reading of energy storage for the purposes of regulating appetite and metabolism.

Receptor — A receptor is a protein on the cell membrane or within the cytoplasm or cell nucleus that binds to a specific molecule (a ligand), such as a neurotransmitter, hormone, or other substance, and initiates the cellular response to the ligand. Receptor, in immunology, the region of an antibody which shows recognition of an antigen.

Brain — The part of the central nervous system involved in regulating and controlling body activity and interpreting information from the senses transmitted through the nervous system is referred to as the brain.

Hypothalamus — Located below the thalamus, the hypothalamus links the nervous system to the endocrine system by synthesizing and secreting neurohormones often called releasing hormones because they function by stimulating the secretion of hormones from the anterior pituitary gland.

Autonomic nervous system — The autonomic nervous system is the part of the nervous system that is not consciously controlled. It is commonly divided into two usually antagonistic subsystems: the sympathetic and parasympathetic nervous system.

Sympathetic division — Sympathetic division refers to one of two sets of neurons in the autonomic nervous system. It generally prepares the body for energy-consuming activities, such as fleeing or fighting. It also is a subdivision of the autonomic nervous system.

Nervous system — The nervous system of an animal coordinates the activity of the muscles, monitors the organs, constructs and processes input from the senses, and initiates actions.

Intestine — The intestine is the portion of the alimentary canal extending from the stomach to the anus and, in humans and mammals, consists of two segments, the small intestine and the large intestine. The intestine is the part of the body responsible for extracting nutrition from food.

Hydrolyze — Hydrolyze refers to break a chemical bond, as in a peptide linkage, with the insertion of the components of water, -H and -OH, at the cleaved ends of a chain. The digestion of proteins is hydrolysis.

Obesity — The state of being more than 20 percent above the average weight for a person of one's height is called obesity.

Gestation — Gestation refers to pregnancy; the state of carrying developing young within the female reproductive tract.

Brown fat — Brown fat refers to fat tissue in mammals that is specialized to produce heat. It has many mitochondria and capillaries, and a protein that uncouples oxidative phosphorylation.

Embryo — A prenatal stage of development after germ layers form but before the rudiments of all organs are present is referred to as an embryo.

Physiology — The study of the function of cells, tissues, and organs is referred to as physiology.

Hibernation — Hibernation is a state of regulated hypothermia, lasting several days or weeks, that allows animals to conserve energy during the winter. During hibernation animals slow their metabolism to a very low level, with body temperature and breathing rates lowered, gradually

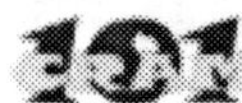

	using up the body fat reserves stored during the warmer months.
Oxygen	Oxygen is a chemical element in the periodic table. It has the symbol O and atomic number 8. Oxygen is the second most common element on Earth, composing around 46% of the mass of Earth's crust and 28% of the mass of Earth as a whole, and is the third most common element in the universe.
Adenosine	Adenosine is a nucleoside comprized of adenine attached to a ribose (ribofuranose) moiety via a β-N_9-glycosidic bond. Adenosine plays an important role in biochemical processes, such as energy transfer - as adenosine triphosphate (ATP) and adenosine diphosphate (ADP) - as well as in signal transduction as cyclic adenosine monophosphate, cAMP.
Proton	Positive subatomic particle, located in the nucleus and having a weight of approximately one atomic mass unit is referred to as a proton.
Adenosine triphosphate	Organic molecule that stores energy and releases energy for use in cellular processes is adenosine triphosphate.
Immune response	The body's defensive reaction to invasion by bacteria, viral agents, or other foreign substances is called immune response.
Immune **system**	The immune system is the system of specialized cells and organs that protect an organism from outside biological influences. When the immune system is functioning properly, it protects the body against bacteria and viral infections, destroying cancer cells and foreign substances.
Diabetes	Diabetes is a medical disorder characterized by varying or persistent elevated blood sugar levels, especially after eating. All types of diabetes share similar symptoms and complications at advanced stages: dehydration and ketoacidosis, cardiovascular disease, chronic renal failure, retinal damage which can lead to blindness, nerve damage which can lead to erectile dysfunction, gangrene with risk of amputation of toes, feet, and even legs.
Health	Health is a term that refers to a combination of the absence of illness, the ability to cope with everyday activities, physical fitness, and high quality of life.
Epithelium	Epithelium is a tissue composed of a layer of cells. Epithelium can be found lining internal (e.g. endothelium, which lines the inside of blood vessels) or external (e.g. skin) free surfaces of the body. Functions include secretion, absorption and protection.
Gland	A gland is an organ in an animal's body that synthesizes a substance for release such as hormones, often into the bloodstream or into cavities inside the body or its outer surface.
Endocrine **gland**	An endocrine gland is one of a set of internal organs involved in the secretion of hormones into the blood. These glands are known as ductless, which means they do not have tubes inside them.
Benign tumor	A benign tumor does not invade neighboring tissues and do not seed metastases, but may locally grow to great size. They usually do not return after surgical removal.
Tumor	An abnormal mass of cells that forms within otherwise normal tissue is a tumor. This growth can be either malignant or benign

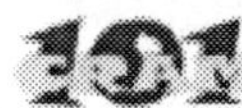

Cartilage	Cartilage is a type of dense connective tissue. Cartilage is composed of cells called chondrocytes which are dispersed in a firm gel-like ground substance, called the matrix. Cartilage is avascular (contains no blood vessels) and nutrients are diffused through the matrix.
Consistency	The extent to which an individual responds to a given stimulus or situation in the same way on different occasions is a consistency.
Tissue	A collection of interconnected cells that perform a similar function within an organism is called tissue.
Connective tissue	Connective tissue is any type of biological tissue with an extensive extracellular matrix and often serves to support, bind together, and protect organs.
Extracellular	Outside the cell is called extracellular.
Shock	Circulatory shock, a state of cardiac output that is insufficient to meet the body's physiological needs, with consequences ranging from fainting to death is referred to as shock. Insulin shock, a state of severe hypoglycemia caused by administration of insulin.
Joint	A joint (articulation) is the location at which two bones make contact (articulate). They are constructed to both allow movement and provide mechanical support.
Chondrocyte	Chondrocyte refers to a living cell of cartilage. With their extracellular secretions of collagen, chondrocytes form cartilage.
Fiber	Fibers used by man come from a wide variety of sources: Natural fiber include those made out of plants, animal and mineral sources. Natural fibers can be classified according to their origin.
Proteoglycan	Molecule consisting of one or more glycosaminoglycan chains attached to a core protein is referred to as proteoglycan.
Collagen	Collagen is the main protein of connective tissue in animals and the most abundant protein in mammals, making up about 1/4 of the total. It is one of the long, fibrous structural proteins whose functions are quite different from those of globular proteins such as enzymes.
Acid	An acid is a water-soluble, sour-tasting chemical compound that when dissolved in water, gives a solution with a pH of less than 7.
Macromolecule	A macromolecule is a molecule with a large molecular mass, but generally the use of the term is restricted to polymers and molecules which structurally include polymers.
Protein	A protein is a complex, high-molecular-weight organic compound that consists of amino acids joined by peptide bonds. They are essential to the structure and function of all living cells and viruses. Many are enzymes or subunits of enzymes.
Elastin	Elastin, is a protein in connective tissue that is elastic and allows many tissues in the body to resume their shape after stretching or contracting. Elastin helps skin to return to its original position when it is poked or pinched.
Elastic cartilage	Elastic cartilage is a stiff yet elastic tissue found in the pinna of the ear and several tubes, such as the walls of the auditory and eustachian canals and larynx.
Glycosaminog-ycan	Glycosaminoglycan is a long unbranched polysaccharide, made up of repeating disaccharides that may be sulphated (e.g. glucuronic acid, iduronic acid, galactose, galactosamine, glucosamine).
Collagen fiber	White fiber in the matrix of connective tissue, giving flexibility and strength is called collagen fiber.
Hyaline	Hyaline cartilage is the most abundant type of cartilage. Hyaline cartilage is a translucent

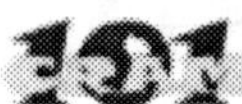

cartilage	matrix or ground substance found lining bones in joints. It is also present inside bones, serving as a center of ossification or bone growth
Elastic fiber	Elastic fiber is a bundles of proteins (elastin) found in connective tissue and produced by fibroblasts and smooth muscle cells in arteries.
Fibrocartilage	Fibrocartilage, as its name implies, is a type of cartilage arranged in a fibrous matrix that is similar to fibrous connective tissues. It is found in areas that require tensile strength, such as intervertebral disks.
Capillaries	Capillaries refer to the smallest of the blood vessels and the sites of exchange between the blood and tissue cells.
Diffusion	Random movement of molecules from a region of higher concentration toward one of lower concentration is referred to as diffusion.
Capillary	A capillary is the smallest of a body's blood vessels, measuring 5-10 micro meters. They connect arteries and veins, and most closely interact with tissues. Their walls are composed of a single layer of cells, the endothelium. This layer is so thin that molecules such as oxygen, water and lipids can pass through them by diffusion and enter the tissues.
Blood vessel	A blood vessel is a part of the circulatory system and function to transport blood throughout the body. The most important types, arteries and veins, are so termed because they carry blood away from or towards the heart, respectively.
Blood	Blood is a circulating tissue composed of fluid plasma and cells. The main function of blood is to supply nutrients (oxygen, glucose) and constitutional elements to tissues and to remove waste products.
Dense connective tissue	Dense connective tissue has collagen fibers as its main matrix element. Crowded between the collagen fibers are rows of fibroblasts, fiber-forming cells, that manufacture the fibers. Dense connective tissue forms strong, rope-like structures such as tendons and ligaments. Tendons attach skeletal muscles to bones; ligaments connect bones to bones at joints.
Nerve	A nerve is an enclosed, cable-like bundle of nerve fibers or axons, which includes the glia that ensheath the axons in myelin.
Articular	The articular is a bone in the lower jaw of most tetrapods, including reptiles, birds, and amphibians, but has become a middle ear bone (the malleus) in mammals. It is the site of articulation between the lower jaw and the skull, and is connected to two other lower jaw bones, the suprangular and the angular.
Oxygen	Oxygen is a chemical element in the periodic table. It has the symbol O and atomic number 8. Oxygen is the second most common element on Earth, composing around 46% of the mass of Earth's crust and 28% of the mass of Earth as a whole, and is the third most common element in the universe.
Skeleton	In biology, the skeleton or skeletal system is the biological system providing physical support in living organisms.
Embryo	A prenatal stage of development after germ layers form but before the rudiments of all organs are present is referred to as an embryo.
Trachea	Trachea is an airway through which respiratory gas transport takes place in organisms. In terrestrial vertebrates, such as birds and humans, the trachea lets air move from the throat to the lungs. In terrestrial invertebrates, such as onychophorans and beetles, they conduct air from outside the organism directly to all of its internal tissues.
Ventral	The surface or side of the body normally oriented upwards, away from the pull of gravity, is the dorsal side; the opposite side, typically the one closest to the ground when walking on

all legs, swimming or flying, is the ventral side.

Sternum Sternum or breastbone is a long, flat bone located in the center of the thorax (chest). It connects to the rib bones via cartilage, forming the rib cage with them, and thus helps to protect the lungs and heart from physical trauma.

Larynx The larynx is an organ in the neck of mammals involved in protection of the trachea and sound production. The larynx houses the vocal cords, and is situated at the point where the upper tract splits into the trachea and the esophagus.

Collagen fibril Collagen fibril refers to extracellular structure formed by self-assembly of secreted fibrillar collagen subunits. An abundant constituent of the extracellular matrix in many animal tissues.

Histology Histology is the study of tissue sectioned as a thin slice, using a microscope. It can be described as microscopic anatomy.

Lactic acid Lactic acid accumulates in skeletal muscles during extensive anaerobic exercise, causing temporary muscle pain. Lactic acid is quickly removed from muscles when they resume aerobic metabolism.

Glycolysis Glycolysis refers to the multistep chemical breakdown of a molecule of glucose into two molecules of pyruvic acid; the first stage of cellular respiration in all organisms; occurs in the cytoplasmic fluid.

Glucose Glucose, a simple monosaccharide sugar, is one of the most important carbohydrates and is used as a source of energy in animals and plants. Glucose is one of the main products of photosynthesis and starts respiration.

Solute Substance that is dissolved in a solvent, forming a solution is referred to as a solute.

Testosterone Testosterone is a steroid hormone from the androgen group. Testosterone is secreted in the testes of men and the ovaries of women. It is the principal male sex hormone and the "original" anabolic steroid. In both males and females, it plays key roles in health and well-being.

Estradiol Estradiol is a sex hormone. Labelled the "female" hormone but also present in males it represents the major estrogen in humans. Critical for sexual functioning estradiol also supports bone growth.

Hormone A hormone is a chemical messenger from one cell to another. All multicellular organisms produce hormones. The best known hormones are those produced by endocrine glands of vertebrate animals, but hormones are produced by nearly every organ system and tissue type in a human or animal body. Hormone molecules are secreted directly into the bloodstream, they move by circulation or diffusion to their target cells, which may be nearby cells in the same tissue or cells of a distant organ of the body.

Growth hormone Growth hormone is a polypeptide hormone synthesised and secreted by the anterior pituitary gland which stimulates growth and cell reproduction in humans and other vertebrate animals.

Tumor An abnormal mass of cells that forms within otherwise normal tissue is a tumor. This growth can be either malignant or benign

Condensation Combining several people, objects, or events into a single dream image is referred to as condensation.

Mesenchyme Mesenchyme is the mass of tissue that develops mainly from the mesoderm of an embryo. It later becomes differentiated into blood vessels and blood-related organs such as the spleen, and into connective tissues.

Extension Movement increasing the angle between parts at a joint is referred to as extension.

Cytoplasm	Cytoplasm refers to the contents of a cell excluding the nucleus and cell membrane. Cytoplasm is a homogeneous, generally clear jelly-like material that fills cells.
Vertebrae	Vertebrae are the individual bones that make up the vertebral column (aka spine) - a flexuous and flexible column.
Ligament	A ligament is a short band of tough fibrous connective tissue composed mainly of long, stringy collagen fibres. They connect bones to other bones to form a joint. (They do not connect muscles to bones.)
Intervertebral disk	Layer of cartilage located between adjacent vertebrae is referred to as intervertebral disk. Each disc forms a cartilaginous joint to allow slight movement of the vertebrae, and acts as a ligament to hold the vertebrae together.
Regeneration	Regeneration is the ability to restore lost or damaged tissues, organs or limbs. It is a common feature in invertebrates, but far more limited in most vertebrates.
Scar	A scar results from the biologic process of wound repair in the skin and other tissues of the body. It is a connective tissue that fills the wound.
Epiglottis	The epiglottis is a thin, lid-like flap of cartilage tissue covered with a mucous membrane, attached to the root of the tongue, that guards the entrance of the glottis, the opening between the vocal cords.
Auditory	Pertaining to the ear or to the sense of hearing is called auditory.
Auditory canal	A canal within the outer ear that conducts sound from the external ear to the tympanic membrane is called the auditory canal.
Attachment	Attachment refers to the psychological tendency to seek closeness to another person, to feel secure when that person is present, and to feel anxious when that person is absent.
Pubis	The pubis, the anterior part of the hip bone, is divisible into a body, a superior and an inferior ramus.
Tendon	A tendon or sinew is a tough band of fibrous connective tissue that connects muscle to bone. They are similar to ligaments except that ligaments join one bone to another.
Notochord	The notochord is a flexible rod-shaped body found in embryos of all chordates. It is composed of cells derived from the mesoblast and defining the primitive axis of the embryo. In lower vertebrates, it persists throughout life as the main axial support of the body, while in higher vertebrates it is replaced by the vertebral column.
Spinal cord	The spinal cord is a part of the vertebrate nervous system that is enclosed in and protected by the vertebral column (it passes through the spinal canal). It consists of nerve cells. The spinal cord carries sensory signals and motor innervation to most of the skeletal muscles in the body.
Pain	Pain is an unpleasant sensation which may be associated with actual or potential tissue damage and which may have physical and emotional components.
Lumbar	In anatomy, lumbar is an adjective that means of or pertaining to the abdominal segment of the torso, between the diaphragm and the sacrum (pelvis). The five vertebra in the lumbar region are the largest and strongest in the spinal column.
Distribution	Distribution in pharmacology is a branch of pharmacokinetics describing reversible transfer of drug from one location to another within the body.
Biochemistry	Biochemistry studies how complex chemical reactions give rise to life. It is a hybrid branch of chemistry which specialises in the chemical processes in living organisms.
Methodology	Techniques of measurement used to collect and manipulate empirical data refer to a

methodology.

Culture Culture, generally refers to patterns of human activity and the symbolic structures that give such activity significance.

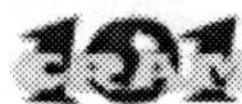

Tissue	A collection of interconnected cells that perform a similar function within an organism is called tissue.
Phosphate	A phosphate is a polyatomic ion or radical consisting of one phosphorus atom and four oxygen. In the ionic form, it carries a -3 formal charge, and is denoted PO_4^{3-}.
Reservoir	Reservoir is the source of infection. It is the environment in which microorganisms are able to live and grow.
Constant	A behavior or characteristic that does not vary from one observation to another is referred to as a constant.
Calcium	Calcium is the chemical element in the periodic table that has the symbol Ca and atomic number 20. Calcium is a soft grey alkaline earth metal that is used as a reducing agent in the extraction of thorium, zirconium and uranium. Calcium is also the fifth most abundant element in the Earth's crust.
Ion	Ion refers to an atom or molecule that has gained or lost one or more electrons, thus acquiring an electrical charge.
Muscle	Muscle is a contractile form of tissue. It is one of the four major tissue types, the other three being epithelium, connective tissue and nervous tissue. Muscle contraction is used to move parts of the body, as well as to move substances within the body.
Muscle contraction	A muscle contraction occurs when a muscle cell (called a muscle fiber) shortens. There are three general types: skeletal, heart, and smooth.
Skeletal muscle	Skeletal muscle is a type of striated muscle, attached to the skeleton. They are used to facilitate movement, by applying force to bones and joints; via contraction. They generally contract voluntarily (via nerve stimulation), although they can contract involuntarily.
Connective tissue	Connective tissue is any type of biological tissue with an extensive extracellular matrix and often serves to support, bind together, and protect organs.
Osteoblast	An osteoblast is a mononucleate cell that produces a protein that produces osteoid.
Osteon	An osteon is a predominant structure found in some lamellar or compact bone. In the center of the osteon is a central canal, called the Haversian canal. The central canal is surrounded by concentric layers of matrix called lamellae.
Capillaries	Capillaries refer to the smallest of the blood vessels and the sites of exchange between the blood and tissue cells.
Canaliculi	Canaliculi are small, microscopic canals between the various lacunae of ocified bone. The radiating processes of the osteocytes project into these canals. In cartilage, the lacunae and hence, the chondrocytes, are isolated from each other. Materials picked up by osteocytes adjacent to blood vessels, are distributed throughout the bone matrix via the canaliculi.
Metabolite	The term metabolite is usually restricted to small molecules. They are the intermediates and products of metabolism. A primary metabolite is directly involved in the normal growth, development, and reproduction. A secondary metabolite is not directly involved in those processes, but usually has important ecological function.
Capillary	A capillary is the smallest of a body's blood vessels, measuring 5-10 micro meters. They connect arteries and veins, and most closely interact with tissues. Their walls are composed of a single layer of cells, the endothelium. This layer is so thin that molecules such as oxygen, water and lipids can pass through them by diffusion and enter the tissues.
Blood	Blood is a circulating tissue composed of fluid plasma and cells. The main function of blood is to supply nutrients (oxygen, glucose) and constitutional elements to tissues and to remove waste products.

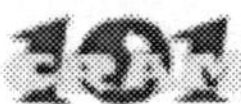

Cytoplasm — Cytoplasm refers to the contents of a cell excluding the nucleus and cell membrane. Cytoplasm is a homogeneous, generally clear jelly-like material that fills cells.

Protein — A protein is a complex, high-molecular-weight organic compound that consists of amino acids joined by peptide bonds. They are essential to the structure and function of all living cells and viruses. Many are enzymes or subunits of enzymes.

Blood vessel — A blood vessel is a part of the circulatory system and function to transport blood throughout the body. The most important types, arteries and veins, are so termed because they carry blood away from or towards the heart, respectively.

Periosteum — The periosteum is an envelope of fibrous connective tissue that is wrapped around the bone in all places except at joints.

Fixative — In biology, a fixative is a solution used to preserve or harden fresh tissue or cell specimens for microscopic examination. Usually they stabilise and firm tissues by denaturing or cross-linking constituent proteins. Formaldehyde solution is an example of a fixative.

Solution — Solution refers to homogenous mixture formed when a solute is dissolved in a solvent.

Acid — An acid is a water-soluble, sour-tasting chemical compound that when dissolved in water, gives a solution with a pH of less than 7.

Proteoglycan — Molecule consisting of one or more glycosaminoglycan chains attached to a core protein is referred to as proteoglycan.

Collagen — Collagen is the main protein of connective tissue in animals and the most abundant protein in mammals, making up about 1/4 of the total. It is one of the long, fibrous structural proteins whose functions are quite different from those of globular proteins such as enzymes.

Epithelium — Epithelium is a tissue composed of a layer of cells. Epithelium can be found lining internal (e.g. endothelium, which lines the inside of blood vessels) or external (e.g. skin) free surfaces of the body. Functions include secretion, absorption and protection.

Lacuna — Small pit or hollow cavity, as in bone or cartilage, where a cell or cells are located is referred to as the lacuna.

Extension — Movement increasing the angle between parts at a joint is referred to as extension.

Extracellular — Outside the cell is called extracellular.

Osteoid — Osteoid is a protein mixture which is secreted by osteoblasts. When it mineralizes, it becomes bone. Osteoid is primarily composed of type 1 collagen.

Salt — Salt is a term used for ionic compounds composed of positively charged cations and negatively charged anions, so that the product is neutral and without a net charge.

Lamina — A thin layer, such as the lamina of a vertebra or the lamina propria of a mucous membrane is referred to as lamina.

Tetracycline — Tetracycline is an antibiotic produced by the streptomyces bacterium, indicated for use against many bacterial infections. It is commonly used to treat acne.

Antibiotic — Antibiotic refers to substance such as penicillin or streptomycin that is toxic to microorganisms. Usually a product of a particular microorvanism or plant.

Affinity — Chemical affinity results from electronic properties by which dissimilar substances are capable of forming chemical compounds. Specifically, the term refers to the tendency of an atom or compound to combine by chemical reaction with atoms or compounds of unlike composition.

Injection — A method of rapid drug delivery that puts the substance directly in the bloodstream, in a

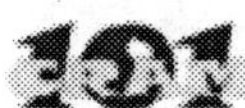

muscle, or under the skin is called injection.

Microscopy — Microscopy is any technique for producing visible images of structures or details too small to otherwise be seen by the human eye, using a microscope or other magnification tool.

Fluorescence — Fluorescence is a luminescence that is mostly found as an optical phenomenon in cold bodies, in which the molecular absorption of a photon triggers the emission of a lower-energy photon with a longer wavelength. The energy difference between the absorbed and emitted photons ends up as molecular vibrations or heat.

Biopsy — Removal of small tissue sample from the body for microscopic examination is called biopsy.

Intramembranous ossification — Intramembranous ossification is one of two types of bone formation and is process responsible for the development of flat bones, especially those found in the skull. Unlike endochondral ossification, cartilage is not involved or present in this process.

Ossification — Ossification is the process of bone formation, in which connective tissues, such as cartilage are turned to bone or bone-like tissue.

Digestion — Digestion refers to the mechanical and chemical breakdown of food into molecules small enough for the body to absorb; the second main stage of food processing, following ingestion.

Lysosome — Organelle that contains enzymes that degrade worn cell parts is called a lysosome.

Cartilage — Cartilage is a type of dense connective tissue. Cartilage is composed of cells called chondrocytes which are dispersed in a firm gel-like ground substance, called the matrix. Cartilage is avascular (contains no blood vessels) and nutrients are diffused through the matrix.

Depression — In everyday language depression refers to any downturn in mood, which may be relatively transitory and perhaps due to something trivial. This is differentiated from Clinical depression which is marked by symptoms that last two weeks or more and are so severe that they interfere with daily living.

Bone marrow — Bone marrow is the tissue comprising the center of large bones. It is the place where new blood cells are produced. Bone marrow contains two types of stem cells: hemopoietic (which can produce blood cells) and stromal (which can produce fat, cartilage and bone).

Fusion — Fusion refers to the combination of two atoms into a single atom as a result of a collision, usually accompanied by the release of energy.

Projection — Attributing one's own undesirable thoughts, impulses, traits, or behaviors to others is referred to as projection.

Organelle — Organelle refers to any structure within a cell that carries out one of its metabolic roles, such as mitochondria, centrioles, endoplasmic reticulum, and the nucleus.

Actin — A protein in a muscle fiber that, together with myosin, is responsible for contraction and relaxation is actin.

Actin filament — An actin filament is a helical protein filament formed by the polymerization of globular actin molecules. They provide mechanical support for the cell, determine the cell shape, enable cell movements; and participate in certain cell junctions.

Cytokine — A type of protein secreted by a T lymphocyte that attacks viruses, virally infected cells, and cancer cells is referred to as cytokine.

Hormone — A hormone is a chemical messenger from one cell to another. All multicellular organisms produce hormones. The best known hormones are those produced by endocrine glands of vertebrate animals, but hormones are produced by nearly every organ system and tissue type in a human or animal body. Hormone molecules are secreted directly into the bloodstream, they

move by circulation or diffusion to their target cells, which may be nearby cells in the same tissue or cells of a distant organ of the body.

Calcitonin Calcitonin is a a 32 amino acid polypeptide hormone that is produced in humans primarily by the C cells of the thyroid, and in many other animals in the ultimobranchial body.

Receptor A receptor is a protein on the cell membrane or within the cytoplasm or cell nucleus that binds to a specific molecule (a ligand), such as a neurotransmitter, hormone, or other substance, and initiates the cellular response to the ligand. Receptor, in immunology, the region of an antibody which shows recognition of an antigen.

Thyroid The thyroid is one of the larger endocrine glands in the body. It is located in the neck and produces hormones, principally thyroxine and triiodothyronine, that regulate the rate of metabolism and affect the growth and rate of function of many other systems in the body.

Parathyroid hormone Parathyroid hormone is secreted by the parathyroid glands as a polypeptide containing 84 amino acids. It acts to increase the concentration of calcium in the blood, whereas calcitonin (a hormone produced by the thyroid gland) acts to decrease calcium concentration.

Bicarbonate A Bicarbonate or, more properly, a hydrogen carbonate is a polyatomic ion. It is the intermediate form in the deprotonation of carbonic acid: removing the first proton from carbonic acid forms bicarbonate; removing the second proton leads to the carbonate ion.

Phosphorus Phosphorus is the chemical element in the periodic table that has the symbol P and atomic number 15.

Potassium Potassium is a chemical element in the periodic table. It has the symbol K (L. kalium) and atomic number 19. Potassium is a soft silvery-white metallic alkali metal that occurs naturally bound to other elements in seawater and many minerals.

Magnesium Magnesium is the chemical element in the periodic table that has the symbol Mg and atomic number 12 and an atomic mass of 24.31.

Sodium Sodium is the chemical element in the periodic table that has the symbol Na (Natrium in Latin) and atomic number 11. Sodium is a soft, waxy, silvery reactive metal belonging to the alkali metals that is abundant in natural compounds (especially halite). It is highly reactive.

Minerals Minerals refer to inorganic chemical compounds found in nature; salts.

Crystal Crystal is a solid in which the constituent atoms, molecules, or ions are packed in a regularly ordered, repeating pattern extending in all three spatial dimensions.

Collagen fibril Collagen fibril refers to extracellular structure formed by self-assembly of secreted fibrillar collagen subunits. An abundant constituent of the extracellular matrix in many animal tissues.

Hydrolase Hydrolase is a general term for any enzyme that catalyzes a hydrolysis reaction, the chemical breakdown of polymers into smaller molecules through the addition of water molecules.

Fiber Fibers used by man come from a wide variety of sources: Natural fiber include those made out of plants, animal and mineral sources. Natural fibers can be classified according to their origin.

Collagen fiber White fiber in the matrix of connective tissue, giving flexibility and strength is called collagen fiber.

Resistance Resistance refers to a nonspecific ability to ward off infection or disease regardless of whether the body has been previously exposed to it. A force that opposes the flow of a fluid such as air or blood. Compare with immunity.

Tendon	A tendon or sinew is a tough band of fibrous connective tissue that connects muscle to bone. They are similar to ligaments except that ligaments join one bone to another.
Osseous tissue	Osseous tissue, or bone tissue is the major structural and supportive connective tissue of the body. Osseous tissue forms the bones that make up the skeletal system.
Compact bone	Type of bone that contains osteons consisting of concentric layers of matrix and osteocytes in lacunae is called compact bone. It forms the stout walls of the diaphysis of long bones and a thin wall of the epiphysis of long bones
Cancellous	Cancellous bone is a spongy type of bone with a very high surface area, found at the ends of long bones. The spongy bone contains red bone marrow which leads to the production of red blood cells.
Microscope	A microscope is an instrument for viewing objects that are too small to be seen by the naked or unaided eye.
Epiphyses	Epiphyses refers to ends of long bones. The epiphyseal plate-sometimes referred to as the growth plate-is made of cartilage and allows growth of the bone to occur. During childhood, the cartilage cells multiply and absorb calcium, to develop into bone.
Spongy bone	Type of bone that has an irregular meshlike arrangement of thin plates of bone filled with red marrow is spongy bone.
Epiphysis	Epiphysis refers to the end of a long bone.
Haversian system	One of many structural units of vertebrate bone, consisting of concentric layers of mineralized bone matrix surrounding lacunae, which contain osteocytes, and a central canal, which contains blood vessels and nerves is referred to as haversian system.
Nerve	A nerve is an enclosed, cable-like bundle of nerve fibers or axons, which includes the glia that ensheath the axons in myelin.
Skull	Skull refers to a bony protective encasement of the brain and the organs of hearing and equilibrium; includes the facial bones. Also called the cranium.
Loose connective tissue	Loose connective tissue or Areolar connective tissue holds organs and epithelia in place, and has a variety of proteinaceous fibers, including collagen and elastin. It is also important in inflammation.
Histology	Histology is the study of tissue sectioned as a thin slice, using a microscope. It can be described as microscopic anatomy.
Central canal	The central canal is the cerebrospinal fluid-filled space that runs longitudinally through the length of the entire spinal cord. The central canal is contiguous with the ventricular system of the brain.
Haversian canals	Haversian canals are a series of tubes around narrow channels formed by lamellae. They are arranged in parallel to the long axis of the bone. The Haversian canals surround bloods vessels and nerve cells throughout the bone and communicate with osteocytes in lacunae through canaliculi.
Course	Pattern of development and change of a disorder over time is a course.
Helix	A helix is a twisted shape like a spring, screw or a spiral staircase. Helixes are important in biology, as DNA is helical and many proteins have helical substructures, known as alpha helices.
Variability	Statistically, variability refers to how much the scores in a distribution spread out, away from the mean.
Adaptation	A biological adaptation is an anatomical structure, physiological process or behavioral trait

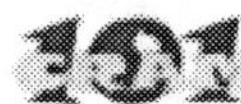

	of an organism that has evolved over a period of time by the process of natural selection such that it increases the expected long-term reproductive success of the organism.
Endochondral ossification	Endochondral ossification is one of two types of bone formation and is the process responsible for much of the bone growth in vertebrate skeletons, especially in long bones. Endochondral ossification occurs by replacement of hyaline cartilage.
Condensation	Combining several people, objects, or events into a single dream image is referred to as condensation.
Mandible	The mandible is the largest and strongest bone of the face. It forms the lower jaw and holds the lower teeth in place. In insects, the mandible is the segment forming the mouth.
Parietal	When speaking of inner organs, visceral means close to or attached to the organ, while parietal is more distant. For example, the visceral pleura is attached to the lung and the parietal pleura is attached to the chest wall.
Temporal bones	The temporal bones are situated at the sides and base of the skull. Each consists of five parts.
Parietal bone	The parietal bone is a bone in the human skull and form, by their union, the sides and roof of the cranium. Each bone is irregularly quadrilateral in form, and has two surfaces, four borders, and four angles.
Hyaline cartilage	Hyaline cartilage is the most abundant type of cartilage. Hyaline cartilage is a translucent matrix or ground substance found lining bones in joints. It is also present inside bones, serving as a center of ossification or bone growth
Cranial	In the limbs of most animals, the terms cranial and caudal are used in the regions proximal to the carpus (the wrist, in the forelimb) and the tarsus (the ankle in the hindlimb). Objects and surfaces closer to or facing towards the head are cranial; those facing away or further from the head are caudal.
Articular	The articular is a bone in the lower jaw of most tetrapods, including reptiles, birds, and amphibians, but has become a middle ear bone (the malleus) in mammals. It is the site of articulation between the lower jaw and the skull, and is connected to two other lower jaw bones, the suprangular and the angular.
Skeleton	In biology, the skeleton or skeletal system is the biological system providing physical support in living organisms.
Chondrocyte	Chondrocyte refers to a living cell of cartilage. With their extracellular secretions of collagen, chondrocytes form cartilage.
Glycogen	Glycogen refers to a complex, extensively branched polysaccharide of many glucose monomers; serves as an energy-storage molecule in liver and muscle cells.
Septa	Septa are thin walls or partitions between the internal chambers (camerae) of the shell of a cephalopod, namely nautiloids or ammonoids.
Hypothesis	A specific statement about behavior or mental processes that is testable through research is a hypothesis.
Vesicle	Membranous, cytoplasmic sac formed by an infolding of the cell membrane is called a vesicle.
Brain	The part of the central nervous system involved in regulating and controlling body activity and interpreting information from the senses transmitted through the nervous system is referred to as the brain.
Ventricle	In the heart, a ventricle is a heart chamber which collects blood from an atrium (another heart chamber) and pumps it out of the heart.

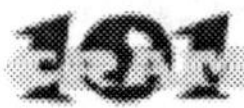

Hydrocephalus	Hydrocephalus is an abnormal accumulation of cerebrospinal fluid in the ventricles of the brain. This increase in intracranial volume results in elevated intracranial pressure and compression of the brain.
Blood clot	A blood clot is the final product of the blood coagulation step in hemostasis. It is achieved via the aggregation of platelets that form a platelet plug, and the activation of the humoral coagulation system
Hemorrhage	Loss of blood from the circulatory system is referred to as a hemorrhage.
Scar	A scar results from the biologic process of wound repair in the skin and other tissues of the body. It is a connective tissue that fills the wound.
Secondary tissue	A tissue produced by the vascular cambium or the cork cambium is referred to as secondary tissue.
Phosphatase	A phosphatase is an enzyme that hydrolyses phosphoric acid monoesters into a phosphate ion and a molecule with a free hydroxyl group.
Alkaline phosphatase	Alkaline phosphatase (ALP) (EC 3.1.3.1) is a hydrolase enzyme responsible for removing phosphate groups in the 5- and 3- positions from many types of molecules, including nucleotides, proteins, and alkaloids.
Suture	Suture refers to an immovable joint, such as that between flat bones of the skull. Also the stitches used to hold tissue together or to close a wound.
Traction	Traction refers to the set of mechanisms for straightening broken bones or relieving pressure on the skeletal system. It is largely replaced now by more modern techniques, but certain approaches are still used today for hip fractures.
Osteoporosis	Osteoporosis is a disease of bone in which bone mineral density (BMD) is reduced, bone microarchitecture is disrupted, the amount and variety of non-collagenous proteins in bone is changed, and a concomitantly fracture risk is increased.
Osteomalacia	Osteomalacia is also referred to as bow-leggedness or rickets. It is a disorder which most commonly relates directly to Vitamin D deficiency, which causes a lack of calcium being absorbed. It can also arise, however, from other etiologies such as rare mesenchymal tumors or any phosphate-wasting disease.
Gland	A gland is an organ in an animal's body that synthesizes a substance for release such as hormones, often into the bloodstream or into cavities inside the body or its outer surface.
Growth hormone	Growth hormone is a polypeptide hormone synthesised and secreted by the anterior pituitary gland which stimulates growth and cell reproduction in humans and other vertebrate animals.
Gigantism	Gigantism is a condition characterized by excessive height growth. Gigantism is rarely used except to refer to the rare condition of pituitary gigantism due to prepubertal growth hormone excess.
Acromegaly	Acromegaly is a hormonal disorder that results when the pituitary gland produces excess growth hormone (hGH). Most commonly it is a benign hGH producing tumor derived from a distinct type of cells (somatotrophs) and called pituitary adenoma.
Androgen	Androgen is the generic term for any natural or synthetic compound, usually a steroid hormone, that stimulates or controls the development and maintenance of masculine characteristics in vertebrates by binding to androgen receptors.
Estrogen	Estrogen is a steroid that functions as the primary female sex hormone. While present in both men and women, they are found in women in significantly higher quantities.
Tumor	An abnormal mass of cells that forms within otherwise normal tissue is a tumor. This growth

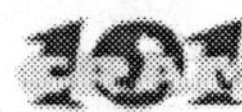

can be either malignant or benign

Cretinism
Cretinism is a condition of severely stunted physical and mental growth due to untreated congenital deficiency of thyroid hormones (hypothyroidism).

Central nervous system
The central nervous system comprized of the brain and spinal cord, represents the largest part of the nervous system. Together with the peripheral nervous system, it has a fundamental role in the control of behavior.

Nervous system
The nervous system of an animal coordinates the activity of the muscles, monitors the organs, constructs and processes input from the senses, and initiates actions.

Prohormone
A prohormone is a chemical compound that is a precursor to a hormone, usually with minimal hormonal effect by itself.

Vitamin
An organic compound other than a carbohydrate, lipid, or protein that is needed for normal metabolism but that the body cannot synthesize in adequate amounts is called a vitamin.

Steroid
A steroid is a lipid characterized by a carbon skeleton with four fused rings. Different steroids vary in the functional groups attached to these rings. Hundreds of distinct steroids have been identified in plants and animals. Their most important role in most living systems is as hormones.

Leptin
Leptin is a 16 kDa protein hormone that plays a key role in metabolism and regulation of adipose tissue. It is released by fat cells in amounts mirroring overall body fat stores. Thus, circulating leptin levels give the brain a reading of energy storage for the purposes of regulating appetite and metabolism.

Lead
Lead is a chemical element in the periodic table that has the symbol Pb and atomic number 82. A soft, heavy, toxic and malleable poor metal, lead is bluish white when freshly cut but tarnishes to dull gray when exposed to air. Lead is used in building construction, lead-acid batteries, bullets and shot, and is part of solder, pewter, and fusible alloys.

Adipose tissue
Adipose tissue is an anatomical term for loose connective tissue composed of adipocytes. Its main role is to store energy in the form of fat, although it also cushions and insulates the body. It has an important endocrine function in producing recently-discovered hormones such as leptin, resistin and TNFalpha.

Rickets
Rickets is a disorder which most commonly relates directly to Vitamin D deficiency, which causes a lack of calcium being absorbed. It can also arise, however, from other etiologies such as rare mesenchymal tumors or any phosphate-wasting disease. It is a disorder which most commonly relates directly to Vitamin D deficiency, which causes a lack of calcium being absorbed.

Young adult
An young adult is someone between the ages of 20 and 40 years old.

Synovial membrane
Membrane that forms the inner lining of the capsule of a freely movable joint is called synovial membrane. The membrane contains a fibrous outer layer, as well as an inner layer that is responsible for the production of specific components of synovial fluid, which nourishes and lubricates the joint.

Humerus
The humerus is a long bone in the arm or fore-legs (animals) that runs from the shoulder to the elbow. On a skeleton, it fits between the scapula and the radius and ulna.

Tibia
The Tibia or shin bone, in human anatomy, is the larger of the two bones in the leg below the knee. It is found medial (towards the middle) and anterior (towards the front) to the other such bone, the fibula. It is the second-longest bone in the human body.

Femur
The femur or thigh bone is the longest, most voluminous and strongest bone of the human body. It forms part of the hip and part of the knee.

Organ	Organ refers to a structure consisting of several tissues adapted as a group to perform specific functions.
Prostate	The prostate is a gland that is part of male mammalian sex organs. Its main function is to secrete and store a clear, slightly basic fluid that is part of semen. The prostate differs considerably between species anatomically, chemically and physiologically.
Kidney	The kidney is a bean-shaped excretory organ in vertebrates. Part of the urinary system, the kidneys filter wastes (especially urea) from the blood and excrete them, along with water, as urine.
Joint	A joint (articulation) is the location at which two bones make contact (articulate). They are constructed to both allow movement and provide mechanical support.
Older adult	Older adult is an adult over the age of 65.
Dense connective tissue	Dense connective tissue has collagen fibers as its main matrix element. Crowded between the collagen fibers are rows of fibroblasts, fiber-forming cells, that manufacture the fibers. Dense connective tissue forms strong, rope-like structures such as tendons and ligaments. Tendons attach skeletal muscles to bones; ligaments connect bones to bones at joints.
Ligament	A ligament is a short band of tough fibrous connective tissue composed mainly of long, stringy collagen fibres. They connect bones to other bones to form a joint. (They do not connect muscles to bones.)
Blood plasma	Blood plasma is the liquid component of blood, in which the blood cells are suspended. Serum is the same as blood plasma except that clotting factors (such as fibrin) have been removed.
Plasma	Fluid portion of circulating blood is called plasma.
Oxygen	Oxygen is a chemical element in the periodic table. It has the symbol O and atomic number 8. Oxygen is the second most common element on Earth, composing around 46% of the mass of Earth's crust and 28% of the mass of Earth as a whole, and is the third most common element in the universe.
Intervertebral disk	Layer of cartilage located between adjacent vertebrae is referred to as intervertebral disk. Each disc forms a cartilaginous joint to allow slight movement of the vertebrae, and acts as a ligament to hold the vertebrae together.
Interstice	A interstice is a small structural space between tissues or parts of an organ.
Glycosaminog-ycan	Glycosaminoglycan is a long unbranched polysaccharide, made up of repeating disaccharides that may be sulphated (e.g. glucuronic acid, iduronic acid, galactose, galactosamine, glucosamine).
Notochord	The notochord is a flexible rod-shaped body found in embryos of all chordates. It is composed of cells derived from the mesoblast and defining the primitive axis of the embryo. In lower vertebrates, it persists throughout life as the main axial support of the body, while in higher vertebrates it is replaced by the vertebral column.
Fibrocartilage	Fibrocartilage, as its name implies, is a type of cartilage arranged in a fibrous matrix that is similar to fibrous connective tissues. It is found in areas that require tensile strength, such as intervertebral disks.
Synovial joint	Synovial joint refers to freely moving joint in which two bones are separated by a cavity.
Apoptosis	In biology, apoptosis is one of the main types of programmed cell death (PCD). As such, it is a process of deliberate life relinquishment by an unwanted cell in a multicellular organism.
In vivo	In vivo is used to indicate the presence of a whole/living organism, in distinction to a partial or dead organism, or a computer model. Animal testing and clinical trials are forms

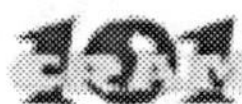

of in vivo research.

Neuron	The neuron is a major class of cells in the nervous system. In vertebrates, they are found in the brain, the spinal cord and in the nerves and ganglia of the peripheral nervous system, and their primary role is to process and transmit neural information.
Nerve tissue	Nerve tissue refers the specialized tissue making up the central and peripheral nervous systems; consists of neurons and glial cells.
Tissue	A collection of interconnected cells that perform a similar function within an organism is called tissue.
Nerve	A nerve is an enclosed, cable-like bundle of nerve fibers or axons, which includes the glia that ensheath the axons in myelin.
Peripheral nervous system	The peripheral nervous system consists of the nerves and neurons that reside or extend outside the central nervous system--to serve the limbs and organs. The peripheral nervous system is divided into the somatic nervous system and the autonomic nervous system.
Spinal cord	The spinal cord is a part of the vertebrate nervous system that is enclosed in and protected by the vertebral column (it passes through the spinal canal). It consists of nerve cells. The spinal cord carries sensory signals and motor innervation to most of the skeletal muscles in the body.
Nerve cell	A cell specialized to originate or transmit nerve impulses is referred to as nerve cell.
Fiber	Fibers used by man come from a wide variety of sources: Natural fiber include those made out of plants, animal and mineral sources. Natural fibers can be classified according to their origin.
Brain	The part of the central nervous system involved in regulating and controlling body activity and interpreting information from the senses transmitted through the nervous system is referred to as the brain.
Central nervous system	The central nervous system comprized of the brain and spinal cord, represents the largest part of the nervous system. Together with the peripheral nervous system, it has a fundamental role in the control of behavior.
Nervous system	The nervous system of an animal coordinates the activity of the muscles, monitors the organs, constructs and processes input from the senses, and initiates actions.
Taste bud	A taste bud is a small structure on the upper surface of the tongue, soft palate, and epiglottis that provides information about the taste of food being eaten. The majority on the tongue sit on raized protrusions of the tongue surface called papillae.
Eye	An eye is an organ that detects light. Different kinds of light-sensitive organs are found in a variety of creatures. The simplest eyes do nothing but detect whether the surroundings are light or dark, while more complex eyes can distinguish shapes and colors.
Afferent neurons	In the nervous system, afferent neurons--otherwise known as sensory or receptor neurons--carry nerve impulses from receptors or sense organs toward the central nervous system. This term can also be used to describe relative connections between nervous structures.
Cerebellum	The cerebellum is a region of the brain that plays an important role in the integration of sensory perception and motor output. The cerebellum integrates these two functions, using the constant feedback on body position to fine-tune motor movements.
Cortex	In anatomy and zoology the cortex is the outermost or superficial layer of an organ or the outer portion of the stem or root of a plant.
Axon	An axon is a long slender projection of a nerve cell, or neuron, which conducts electrical impulses away from the neuron's cell body or soma. They are in effect the primary transmission lines of the nervous system, and as bundles they help make up nerves.

Cerebral cortex	The cerebral cortex is a brain structure in vertebrates. It is the outermost layer of the cerebrum and has a grey color. In the "higher" animals, the surface becomes folded. The cerebral cortex, made up of four lobes, is involved in many complex brain functions including memory, attention, perceptual awareness, "thinking", language and consciousness.
Myelin	Myelin is an electrically insulating fatty layer that surrounds the axons of many neurons, especially those in the peripheral nervous system. It is an outgrowth of glial cells: Schwann cells supply the myelin for peripheral neurons while oligodendrocytes supply it to those of the central nervous system.
Oligodendrocyte	Oligodendrocyte refers to type of glial cell in the vertebrate central nervous system that forms a myelin sheath around axons.
Nucleolus	A small structure within the nucleus of a cell that contains RNA and protein is referred to as nucleolus. It is where ribonucleoprotein is formed.
Synapse	A junction, or relay point, between two neurons, or between a neuron and an effector cell. Electrical and chemical signals are relayed from one cell to another at a synapse.
Autonomic nervous system	The autonomic nervous system is the part of the nervous system that is not consciously controlled. It is commonly divided into two usually antagonistic subsystems: the sympathetic and parasympathetic nervous system.
Muscle	Muscle is a contractile form of tissue. It is one of the four major tissue types, the other three being epithelium, connective tissue and nervous tissue. Muscle contraction is used to move parts of the body, as well as to move substances within the body.
Gland	A gland is an organ in an animal's body that synthesizes a substance for release such as hormones, often into the bloodstream or into cavities inside the body or its outer surface.
Stimulus	Stimulus in a nervous system, a factor that triggers sensory transduction.
Plasma	Fluid portion of circulating blood is called plasma.
Plasma membrane	The unit membrane that encloses a cell and controls the traffic of molecules in and out of the cell is the plasma membrane.
Neural tube	The neural tube is the embryonal structure that gives rise to the brain and spinal cord. The neural tube is derived from a thickened area of ectoderm, the neural plate. The process of formation of the neural tube is called neurulation.
Subcutaneous	Subcutaneous injections are given by injecting a fluid into the subcutis. It is relatively painless and an effective way to administer particular types of medication.
Sympathetic	The sympathetic nervous system activates what is often termed the "fight or flight response". It is an automatic regulation system, that is, one that operates without the intervention of conscious thought.
Melanocyte	Melanocyte cells are located in the bottom layer of the skin's epidermis. With a process called melanogenesis, they produce melanin, a pigment in the skin, eyes, and hair.
Pia mater	The pia mater is the delicate innermost layer of the meninges - the membranes surrounding the brain and spinal cord.
Medulla	Medulla in general means the inner part, and derives from the Latin word for 'marrow'. In medicine it is contrasted to the cortex.
Adrenal	In mammals, the adrenal glands are the triangle-shaped endocrine glands that sit atop the kidneys. They are chiefly responsible for regulating the stress response through the synthesis of corticosteroids and catecholamines, including cortisol and adrenaline.
Cranial	In the limbs of most animals, the terms cranial and caudal are used in the regions proximal

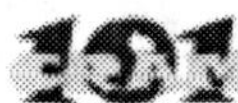

	to the carpus (the wrist, in the forelimb) and the tarsus (the ankle in the hindlimb). Objects and surfaces closer to or facing towards the head are cranial; those facing away or further from the head are caudal.
Skin	Skin is an organ of the integumentary system composed of a layer of tissues that protect underlying muscles and organs.
Chromaffin cells	Chromaffin cells are neuroendocrine cells found in the medulla of the adrenal gland and in other ganglia of the sympathetic nervous system. They are derived from the embryonic neural crest. These cells are so-named because they can be visualized by staining with chromium salts.
Adrenal medulla	Composed mainly of hormone-producing chromaffin cells, the adrenal medulla is the principal site of the conversion of the amino acid tyrosine into the catecholamines epinephrine and norepinephrine.
Chromaffin cell	Chromaffin cell refers to a neuroendocrine cell that stores adrenaline in secretory vesicles and secretes it in times of stress when stimulated by the nervous system.
Sensory neuron	Sensory neuron refers to nerve cell that transmits nerve impulses to the central nervous system after a sensory receptor has been stimulated.
Action potential	The sequence of electrical changes occurring when a nerve cell membrane is exposed to a stimulus that exceeds its threshold is called action potential.
Variable	A characteristic or aspect in which people, objects, events, or conditions vary is called variable.
Angular	The angular is a large bone in the lower jaw of amphibians, birds and reptiles, which is connected to all other lower jaw bones: the dentary (which is the entire lower jaw in mammals), the splenial, the suprangular, and the articular.
Axon terminal	A swelling at the end of an axon that is designed to release a chemical substance onto another neuron, muscle cell, or gland cell is called the axon terminal.
Neurotransmitter	A neurotransmitter is a chemical that is used to relay, amplify and modulate electrical signals between a neuron and another cell.
Olfactory	Pertaining to the sense of smell is referred to as olfactory.
Retina	The retina is a thin layer of cells at the back of the eyeball of vertebrates and some cephalopods; it is the part of the eye which converts light into nervous signals.
Mucosa	The mucosa is a lining of ectodermic origin, covered in epithelium, and involved in absorption and secretion. They line various body cavities that are exposed to the external environment and internal organs.
Olfactory mucosa	The olfactory mucosa is an organ made up of the olfactory epithelium and the mucosa, or mucus secreting glands, behind the epithelium. The mucus protects the olfactory epithelium and allows odors to dissolve so that they can be detected by olfactory receptor neurons.
Spinal nerve	The spinal nerve is usually a mized nerve, formed from the dorsal and ventral roots that come out of the spinal cord.
Dorsal root	The dorsal root is the afferent sensory root of a spinal nerve. At the distal end of the dorsal root is the dorsal root ganglion, which contains the neuron cell bodies of the nerve fibres conveyed by the root.
Dorsal	In anatomy, the dorsal is the side in which the backbone is located. This is usually the top of an animal, although in humans it refers to the back.
Muscle fiber	Cell with myofibrils containing actin and myosin filaments arranged within sarcomeres is a

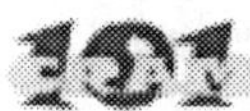

	muscle fiber.
Organ	Organ refers to a structure consisting of several tissues adapted as a group to perform specific functions.
Endocrine gland	An endocrine gland is one of a set of internal organs involved in the secretion of hormones into the blood. These glands are known as ductless, which means they do not have tubes inside them.
White matter	White matter is composed of nerve cell processes, or axons, which connect various grey matter areas of the brain to each other and carry nerve impulses between neurons.
Cytoplasm	Cytoplasm refers to the contents of a cell excluding the nucleus and cell membrane. Cytoplasm is a homogeneous, generally clear jelly-like material that fills cells.
Protein	A protein is a complex, high-molecular-weight organic compound that consists of amino acids joined by peptide bonds. They are essential to the structure and function of all living cells and viruses. Many are enzymes or subunits of enzymes.
Microscope	A microscope is an instrument for viewing objects that are too small to be seen by the naked or unaided eye.
Light microscope	An optical instrument with lenses that refract visible light to magnify images and project them into a viewer's eye or onto photographic film is referred to as light microscope.
Mitochondria	Cytoplasmic organelles responsible for ATP generation for cellular activities are referred to as mitochondria.
Fixative	In biology, a fixative is a solution used to preserve or harden fresh tissue or cell specimens for microscopic examination. Usually they stabilise and firm tissues by denaturing or cross-linking constituent proteins. Formaldehyde solution is an example of a fixative.
Silver	Silver is a chemical element with the symbol Ag. A soft white lustrous transition metal, it has the highest electrical and thermal conductivity of any metal and occurs in minerals and in free form.
Microtubule	A hollow rod of the protein tubulin in the cytoplasm is referred to as the microtubule.
Lysosome	Organelle that contains enzymes that degrade worn cell parts is called a lysosome.
Residue	A residue refers to a portion of a larger molecule, a specific monomer of a polysaccharide, protein or nucleic acid.
Purkinje cell	A purkinje cell is a class of GABAergic neurons located in the cerebellar cortex. These cells are some of the largest neurons in the brain, with an intricately elaborate dendritic arbor, characterized by a large number of dendritic spines.
Constant	A behavior or characteristic that does not vary from one observation to another is referred to as a constant.
Base	The common definition of a base is a chemical compound that absorbs hydronium ions when dissolved in water (a proton acceptor). An alkali is a special example of a base, where in an aqueous environment, hydroxide ions are donated.
Adaptation	A biological adaptation is an anatomical structure, physiological process or behavioral trait of an organism that has evolved over a period of time by the process of natural selection such that it increases the expected long-term reproductive success of the organism.
Dendritic spine	A dendritic spine is a small membranous extrusion that protrudes from a dendrite and forms one half of a synapse. Changes in dendritic spine density underlie many brain functions, including motivation, learning, and memory. In particular, long-term memory is mediated in part by the growth of new dendritic spines to reinforce a particular neural pathway.

Ion channel	A ion channel is a pore-forming protein that helps establish the small voltage gradient that exists across the membrane of all living cells, by allowing the flow of ions down their electrochemical gradient. They are present in the membranes that surround all biological cells.
Channel	Channel, in communications (sometimes called communications channel), refers to the medium used to convey information from a sender (or transmitter) to a receiver.
Ion	Ion refers to an atom or molecule that has gained or lost one or more electrons, thus acquiring an electrical charge.
Dependence	Dependence refers to a mental or physical craving for a drug and withdrawal symptoms when use of the drug is stopped.
Organelle	Organelle refers to any structure within a cell that carries out one of its metabolic roles, such as mitochondria, centrioles, endoplasmic reticulum, and the nucleus.
Macromolecule	A macromolecule is a molecule with a large molecular mass, but generally the use of the term is restricted to polymers and molecules which structurally include polymers.
Actin	A protein in a muscle fiber that, together with myosin, is responsible for contraction and relaxation is actin.
Actin filament	An actin filament is a helical protein filament formed by the polymerization of globular actin molecules. They provide mechanical support for the cell, determine the cell shape, enable cell movements; and participate in certain cell junctions.
Vesicle	Membranous, cytoplasmic sac formed by an infolding of the cell membrane is called a vesicle.
Endocytosis	Endocytosis is a process where cells absorb material (molecules or other cells) from outside by engulfing it with their cell membranes.
Toxin	Toxin refers to a microbial product or component that can injure another cell or organism at low concentrations. Often the term refers to a poisonous protein, but toxins may be lipids and other substances.
Kinesin	Kinesin is a class of motor protein dimer found in biological cells. A kinesin attaches to microtubules, and moves along the tubule in order to transport cellular cargo, such as vesicles.
ATPase	ATPase is a class of enzymes that catalyze the decomposition of adenosine triphosphate into adenosine diphosphate and a free phosphate ion. This dephosphorylation reaction releases energy, which the enzyme harnesses to drive other chemical reactions that would not otherwise occur. This process is widely used in all known forms of life.
Motor protein	Protein that uses energy derived from nucleoside triphosphate hydrolysis to propel itself along a protein filament or another polymeric molecule is called motor protein.
Membrane potential	Membrane potential is the electrical potential difference (voltage) across a cell's plasma membrane.
Extracellular fluid	Body fluids outside the individual cells are called extracellular fluid.
Extracellular	Outside the cell is called extracellular.
Presynaptic membrane	The area of the plasma membrane of a presynaptic axon that is within the synapse and has sites (active zones) especially adapted for the release of neurotransmitters is the presynaptic membrane.
Depolarization	Depolarization is a decrease in the absolute value of a cell's membrane potential. Thus, changes in membrane voltage in which the membrane potential becomes less positive or less

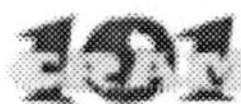

	negative are both depolarizations.
Cleft	Cleft is a congenital deformity caused by a failure in facial development during pregnancy.
Synaptic cleft	A narrow gap separating the synaptic knob of a transmitting neuron from a receiving neuron or an effector cell is a synaptic cleft.
Mitochondrion	Organelle housing enzymes that catalyze reactions of aerobic respiration is mitochondrion.
Histology	Histology is the study of tissue sectioned as a thin slice, using a microscope. It can be described as microscopic anatomy.
Potassium	Potassium is a chemical element in the periodic table. It has the symbol K (L. kalium) and atomic number 19. Potassium is a soft silvery-white metallic alkali metal that occurs naturally bound to other elements in seawater and many minerals.
Hydrophobic	Hydrophobic refers to being electrically neutral and nonpolar, and thus prefering other neutral and nonpolar solvents or molecular environments. Hydrophobic is often used interchangeably with "oily" or "lipophilic."
Anesthetic	Anesthetic refers to a substance that causes the loss of the ability to feel pain or other sensory input, e.g., ether or halothane.
Sodium	Sodium is the chemical element in the periodic table that has the symbol Na (Natrium in Latin) and atomic number 11. Sodium is a soft, waxy, silvery reactive metal belonging to the alkali metals that is abundant in natural compounds (especially halite). It is highly reactive.
Local anesthetic	Local anesthetic drugs act mainly by inhibiting sodium influx through sodium-specific ion channels in the neuronal cell membrane, in particular the so-called voltage-gated sodium channels. When the influx of sodium is interrupted, an action potential cannot arise and signal conduction is thus inhibited.
Receptor	A receptor is a protein on the cell membrane or within the cytoplasm or cell nucleus that binds to a specific molecule (a ligand), such as a neurotransmitter, hormone, or other substance, and initiates the cellular response to the ligand. Receptor, in immunology, the region of an antibody which shows recognition of an antigen.
Inhibition	The ability to prevent from making some cognitive or behavioral response is called inhibition.
Steroid	A steroid is a lipid characterized by a carbon skeleton with four fused rings. Different steroids vary in the functional groups attached to these rings. Hundreds of distinct steroids have been identified in plants and animals. Their most important role in most living systems is as hormones.
Synaptic vesicle	Small neurotransmitter-filled secretory vesicle formed at the axon terminals of nerve cells and whose contents are released into the synaptic cleft by exocytosis when an action potential reaches the axon terminal is called synaptic vesicle.
Exocytosis	Exocytosis is the process by which a cell is able to get rid of large molecules or materials including wastes through its membrane. The process involves a [vacuole], containing the material, fusing with the membrane.
Enzyme	An enzyme is a protein that catalyzes, or speeds up, a chemical reaction. They are essential to sustain life because most chemical reactions in biological cells would occur too slowly, or would lead to different products, without them.
Amino acid	An amino acid is any molecule that contains both amino and carboxylic acid functional groups. They are the basic structural building units of proteins. They form short polymer chains called peptides or polypeptides which in turn form structures called proteins.

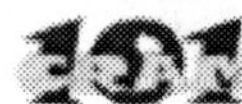

Peptide	Peptide is the family of molecules formed from the linking, in a defined order, of various amino acids. The link between one amino acid residue and the next is an amide bond, and is sometimes referred to as a peptide bond.
Amine	An organic compound with one or more amino groups is called amine. They contain nitrogen as the key atom. Structurally amines resemble ammonia, wherein one or more hydrogen atoms are replaced by organic substituents such as alkyl and aryl groups.
Acid	An acid is a water-soluble, sour-tasting chemical compound that when dissolved in water, gives a solution with a pH of less than 7.
Norepinephrine	Norepinephrine is a catecholamine and a phenethylamine with chemical formula $C_8H_{11}NO_3$. It is released from the adrenal glands as a hormone into the blood, but it is also a neurotransmitter in the nervous system where it is released from noradrenergic neurons during synaptic transmission.
Hormone	A hormone is a chemical messenger from one cell to another. All multicellular organisms produce hormones. The best known hormones are those produced by endocrine glands of vertebrate animals, but hormones are produced by nearly every organ system and tissue type in a human or animal body. Hormone molecules are secreted directly into the bloodstream, they move by circulation or diffusion to their target cells, which may be nearby cells in the same tissue or cells of a distant organ of the body.
Digestive tract	The digestive tract is the system of organs within multicellular animals which takes in food, digests it to extract energy and nutrients, and expels the remaining waste.
Acetylcholine receptor	An acetylcholine receptor is an integral membrane protein that responds to the binding of the neurotransmitter acetylcholine. They are ion channels, and, like other members of the "cys-loop" ligand-gated ion channel superfamily, are composed of five protein subunits arranged like staves around a barrel.
Acetylcholine	The chemical compound acetylcholine was the first neurotransmitter to be identified. It is a chemical transmitter in both the peripheral nervous system (PNS) and central nervous system (CNS) in many organisms including humans.
Astrocyte	An astrocyte is a characteristic star-shaped cell in the brain. They are the biggest cells found in brain tissue and outnumber the neurons ten to one. A commonly accepted function is to structure physically the brain. A second function is to provide neurons with nutrients such as glucose. They regulate the flow of nutrients provided by capillaries by forming the blood-brain barrier.
Endothelial cell	A endothelial cell also controls the passage of materials — and the transit of white blood cells — into and out of the bloodstream. In some organs, there are highly differentiated endothelial cells to perform specialized 'filtering' functions.
Blood	Blood is a circulating tissue composed of fluid plasma and cells. The main function of blood is to supply nutrients (oxygen, glucose) and constitutional elements to tissues and to remove waste products.
Physiology	The study of the function of cells, tissues, and organs is referred to as physiology.
Vasoactive intestinal peptide	Vasoactive intestinal peptide is a peptide hormone containing 28 amino acid residues.Its role in the intestine is to greatly stimulate secretion of water and electrolytes, as well as dilating intestinal smooth muscle, dilating peripheral blood vessels, and inhibiting gastrin-stimulated gastric acid secretion.
Angiotensin	Angiotensin is a polypeptide in the blood that causes vasoconstriction, increased blood pressure, and aldosterone release from the adrenal cortex. Angiotensin is produced in the liver from precursor angiotensinogen, a serum globulin. It plays an important role in the

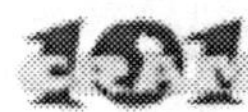

renin-angiotensin system.

Somatostatin Somatostatin is hormone secreted not only by cells of the hypothalamus but also by so called delta cells of stomach, intestine and pancreas. It binds to somatostatin receptors. All actions of the hormone are inhibitory.

Enkephalins Opiate-like brain chemicals that regulate reactions to pain and stress are enkephalins.

Opioid An opioid is any agent that binds to opioid receptors, found principally in the central nervous system and gastrointestinal tract. There are four broad classes of opioids: endogenous opioid peptides, produced in the body; opium alkaloids, such as morphine and codeine; semi-synthetic opioids such as heroin and oxycodone.

Angiotensinogen Angiotensinogen is a precursor molecule, and it is produced constitutively and released into the circulation mainly by the liver although other sites have been thought to contribute to local effects of the molecule. Biochemically it is a member of the protein family of serpins.

Ventricle In the heart, a ventricle is a heart chamber which collects blood from an atrium (another heart chamber) and pumps it out of the heart.

Central canal The central canal is the cerebrospinal fluid-filled space that runs longitudinally through the length of the entire spinal cord. The central canal is contiguous with the ventricular system of the brain.

Cerebrospinal fluid Cerebrospinal fluid is a clear bodily fluid that occupies the subarachnoid space in the brain (the space between the skull and the cerebral cortex). It is basically a saline solution and acts as a "cushion" or buffer for the cortex.

Bone marrow Bone marrow is the tissue comprising the center of large bones. It is the place where new blood cells are produced. Bone marrow contains two types of stem cells: hemopoietic (which can produce blood cells) and stromal (which can produce fat, cartilage and bone).

Cytokine A type of protein secreted by a T lymphocyte that attacks viruses, virally infected cells, and cancer cells is referred to as cytokine.

Antigen An antigen is a substance that stimulates an immune response, especially the production of antibodies. They are usually proteins or polysaccharides, but can be any type of molecule, including small molecules (haptens) coupled to a protein (carrier).

Lesion A lesion is a non-specific term referring to abnormal tissue in the body. It can be caused by any disease process including trauma (physical, chemical, electrical), infection, neoplasm, metabolic and autoimmune.

Blood vessel A blood vessel is a part of the circulatory system and function to transport blood throughout the body. The most important types, arteries and veins, are so termed because they carry blood away from or towards the heart, respectively.

Nervous tissue Tissue made up of neurons and supportive cells is referred to as nervous tissue. It forms a rapid communication network for the body.

Human immunodeficiency virus The human immunodeficiency virus is a retrovirus that primarily infects vital components of the human immune system. It is transmitted through penetrative and oral sex; blood transfusion; the sharing of contaminated needles in health care settings and through drug injection; and, between mother and infant, during pregnancy, childbirth and breastfeeding.

Infection The invasion and multiplication of microorganisms in body tissues is called an infection.

Dementia Dementia is progressive decline in cognitive function due to damage or disease in the brain beyond what might be expected from normal aging.

Virus Obligate intracellular parasite of living cells consisting of an outer capsid and an inner

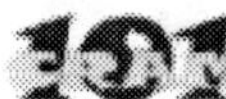

	core of nucleic acid is referred to as virus. The term virus usually refers to those particles that infect eukaryotes whilst the term bacteriophage or phage is used to describe those infecting prokaryotes.
HIV	The virus that causes AIDS is HIV (human immunodeficiency virus).
AIDS dementia complex	AIDS dementia complex (ADC) is one of the most common neurological complications of late HIV infection. It causes the loss of mental function, affecting the ability to function in a social or occupational setting.
Immunodeficiency	Immunodeficiency is a state in which the immune system's ability to fight infectious disease is compromized or entirely absent. Most cases of immunodeficiency are either congenital or acquired.
Necrosis	Necrosis is the name given to unprogrammed death of cells/living tissue. There are many causes of necrosis including injury, infection, cancer, infarction, and inflammation. Necrosis is caused by special enzymes that are released by lysosomes.
Tumor	An abnormal mass of cells that forms within otherwise normal tissue is a tumor. This growth can be either malignant or benign
Tumor necrosis factor	In medicine, tumor necrosis factor alpha (TNFá, cachexin or cachectin) is an important cytokine involved in systemic inflammation and the acute phase response.
Cerebrum	Cerebrum refers to the largest, most sophisticated, and most dominant part of the vertebrate forebrain, made up of right and left cerebral hemispheres.
Connective tissue	Connective tissue is any type of biological tissue with an extensive extracellular matrix and often serves to support, bind together, and protect organs.
Distribution	Distribution in pharmacology is a branch of pharmacokinetics describing reversible transfer of drug from one location to another within the body.
Anterior horn	Anterior horn can refer to two separate anatomical structures within the central nervous system, the anterior division of the lateral ventricle of the brain or the ventral (front) grey matter section of the spinal cord.
Staining	Staining is a biochemical technique of adding a class-specific (DNA, proteins, lipids, carbohydrates) dye to a substrate to qualify or quantify the presence of a specific compound. They are frequently used to highlight structures in tissues for viewing, often with the aid of different microscopes.
Meninges	The meninges are the system of membranes that envelop the central nervous system. The meninges consist of three layers, the dura mater, the arachnoid mater, and the pia mater.
Skull	Skull refers to a bony protective encasement of the brain and the organs of hearing and equilibrium; includes the facial bones. Also called the cranium.
Vertebral column	In human anatomy, the vertebral column is a column of vertebrae situated in the dorsal aspect of the abdomen. It houses the spinal cord in its spinal canal.
Dura mater	The dura mater is the tough and inflexible outermost of the three layers of the meninges surrounding the brain. The other two meninges are the pia mater and the arachnoid mater. The dura mater envelops and protects the brain and spinal cord.
Periosteum	The periosteum is an envelope of fibrous connective tissue that is wrapped around the bone in all places except at joints.
Dense connective tissue	Dense connective tissue has collagen fibers as its main matrix element. Crowded between the collagen fibers are rows of fibroblasts, fiber-forming cells, that manufacture the fibers. Dense connective tissue forms strong, rope-like structures such as tendons and ligaments.

Tendons attach skeletal muscles to bones; ligaments connect bones to bones at joints.

Loose connective tissue Loose connective tissue or Areolar connective tissue holds organs and epithelia in place, and has a variety of proteinaceous fibers, including collagen and elastin. It is also important in inflammation.

Vertebrae Vertebrae are the individual bones that make up the vertebral column (aka spine) - a flexuous and flexible column.

Epidural The epidural space is a part of the human spine inside the spinal canal separated from the spinal cord and its surrounding cerebrospinal fluid (CSF) by a membrane called the dura mater or simply dura.

Veins Blood vessels that return blood toward the heart from the circulation are referred to as veins.

Vein Vein in animals, is a vessel that returns blood to the heart. In plants, a vascular bundle in a leaf, composed of xylem and phloem.

Adipose tissue Adipose tissue is an anatomical term for loose connective tissue composed of adipocytes. Its main role is to store energy in the form of fat, although it also cushions and insulates the body. It has an important endocrine function in producing recently-discovered hormones such as leptin, resistin and TNFalpha.

Epithelium Epithelium is a tissue composed of a layer of cells. Epithelium can be found lining internal (e.g. endothelium, which lines the inside of blood vessels) or external (e.g. skin) free surfaces of the body. Functions include secretion, absorption and protection.

Squamous epithelium The squamous epithelium is epithelium consisting of one or more cell layers, the most superficial of which is composed of flat, scalelike or platelike cells.

Subarachnoid space Subarachnoid space is the interval between the arachnoid and pia mater. It is occupied by a spongy tissue consisting of trabeculæ of delicate connective tissue, and intercommunicating channels in which the subarachnoid fluid is contained.

Protrusion Protrusion is the anterior movement of an object. This term is often applied to the jaw.

Capillaries Capillaries refer to the smallest of the blood vessels and the sites of exchange between the blood and tissue cells.

Capillary A capillary is the smallest of a body's blood vessels, measuring 5-10 micro meters. They connect arteries and veins, and most closely interact with tissues. Their walls are composed of a single layer of cells, the endothelium. This layer is so thin that molecules such as oxygen, water and lipids can pass through them by diffusion and enter the tissues.

Antibiotic Antibiotic refers to substance such as penicillin or streptomycin that is toxic to microorganisms. Usually a product of a particular microorvanism or plant.

Occluding junction Type of cell junction that seals cells together in an epithelium, forming a barrier through which even small molecules cannot pass, is referred to as occluding junction.

Choroid The choroid is the vascular layer of the eye lying between the retina and the sclera. The choroid provides oxygen and nourishment to the outer layers of the retina.

Plexus A plexus is also a network of blood vessels, with the choroid plexuses of the brain being the most commonly mentioned example. A choroid plexus is very thin and vascular roof plates of the most anterior and most posterior cavities of the brain which expand into the interiors of the cavities.

Choroid plexus The choroid plexus is the area on the ventricles of the brain where cerebrospinal fluid (CSF) is produced. Choroid plexus is present in the superior part of the inferior horn of the

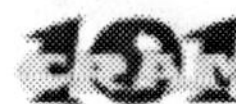

	lateral ventricles.
Metabolism	Metabolism is the biochemical modification of chemical compounds in living organisms and cells. This includes the biosynthesis of complex organic molecules (anabolism) and their breakdown (catabolism).
Shock	Circulatory shock, a state of cardiac output that is insufficient to meet the body's physiological needs, with consequences ranging from fainting to death is referred to as shock. Insulin shock, a state of severe hypoglycemia caused by administration of insulin.
Lymphocyte	A lymphocyte is a type of white blood cell involved in the human body's immune system. There are two broad categories, namely T cells and B cells.
Absorption	Absorption is a physical or chemical phenomenon or a process in which atoms, molecules, or ions enter some bulk phase - gas, liquid or solid material. In nutrition, amino acids are broken down through digestion, which begins in the stomach.
Intracranial pressure	Intracranial pressure is the pressure of the brain, Cerebrospinal fluid (CSF), and the brain's blood supply within the intracranial space.
Hydrocephalus	Hydrocephalus is an abnormal accumulation of cerebrospinal fluid in the ventricles of the brain. This increase in intracranial volume results in elevated intracranial pressure and compression of the brain.
Anatomy	Anatomy is the branch of biology that deals with the structure and organization of living things. It can be divided into animal anatomy (zootomy) and plant anatomy (phytonomy).
Peripheral nerve	A nerve that links the brain and spinal cord to the rest of the body peripheral nervous system- in vertebrates, the part of the nervous system that connects the central nervous system to the rest of the body is a peripheral nerve.
Lamina	A thin layer, such as the lamina of a vertebra or the lamina propria of a mucous membrane is referred to as lamina.
Collagen	Collagen is the main protein of connective tissue in animals and the most abundant protein in mammals, making up about 1/4 of the total. It is one of the long, fibrous structural proteins whose functions are quite different from those of globular proteins such as enzymes.
Epineurium	The epineurium is the outermost layer of connective tissue surrounding a peripheral nerve. It includes the blood vessels supplying the nerve.
Aggression	The intentional verbal or non verbal infliction of injury or harm on another person is called aggression.
Motor nerve	A motor nerve enables the brain to stimulate muscle contraction. A motor nerve is an efferent nerve that exclusively contains the axons of motorneurons, which innervate skeletal muscle.
Sensory nerves	Sensory nerves bring impulses toward the central nervous system.
Ganglion	In vertebrate anatomy, a ganglion is a tissue mass that contains the dendrites and cell bodies (or "somata") of nerve cells, in most case ones belonging to the peripheral nervous system.
Cranial nerves	Cranial nerves are nerves that emerge from the brainstem instead of the spinal cord. In human anatomy, there are exactly 12 pairs of them, traditionally abbreviated by the corresponding Roman numerals.
Cranial nerve	A cranial nerve is a nerve that emerges from the brainstem instead of the spinal cord. Nerves I and II are named as such, but are technically not nerves, as they are continuations of the central nervous system.
Ganglion cell	A ganglion cell is a type of neuron located in the retina of the eye that receives visual

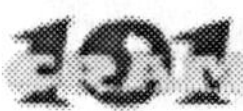

information from photoreceptors via various intermediate cells such as bipolar cells, amacrine cells, and horizontal cells. The axons are myelinated.

Autonomic ganglia Autonomic ganglia are clusters of neuronal cell bodies and their dendrites and are essentially a junction between autonomic nerves originating from the central nervous system and autonomic nerves innervating their target organs in the periphery.

Multipolar neuron A multipolar neuron is a type of neuron that possesses a single (usually long) axon and many dendrites, allowing for the integration of a great deal of information from other neurons

Modulation Modulation is the process of varying a carrier signal, typically a sinusoidal signal, in order to use that signal to convey information.

Smooth muscle Smooth muscle is a type of non-striated muscle, found within the "walls" of hollow organs; such as blood vessels, the bladder, the uterus, and the gastrointestinal tract. Smooth muscle is used to move matter within the body, via contraction; it generally operates "involuntarily", without nerve stimulation.

Homeostasis Homeostasis is the property of an open system, especially living organisms, to regulate its internal environment to maintain a stable, constant condition, by means of multiple dynamic equilibrium adjustments, controlled by interrelated regulation mechanisms.

Adjustment Adjustment is an attempt to cope with a given situation.

Reflex arc A reflex arc is the neural pathway that mediates a reflex. It generally does not involve the brain.

Internal environment Conditions and elements that make up the inside of the body are called an internal environment.

Skeletal muscle Skeletal muscle is a type of striated muscle, attached to the skeleton. They are used to facilitate movement, by applying force to bones and joints; via contraction. They generally contract voluntarily (via nerve stimulation), although they can contract involuntarily.

Micrograph A micrograph is a photograph or similar image taken through a microscope or similar device to show a magnified image of an item.

Collagen fiber White fiber in the matrix of connective tissue, giving flexibility and strength is called collagen fiber.

Concept A mental category used to class together objects, relations, events, abstractions, or qualities that have common properties is called concept.

Visceral Visceral refers to the internal organs of an animal.

Pathology Pathology is the study of the processes underlying disease and other forms of illness, harmful abnormality, or dysfunction.

Target cell Specific cell on which a hormone exerts its effect is a target cell.

Population Population refers to all members of a well-defined group of organisms, events, or things.

Biosynthesis Biosynthesis is a phenomenon where chemical compounds are produced from simpler reagents. Biosynthesis, unlike chemical synthesis, takes place within living organisms and is generally catalysed by enzymes.

Neuromuscular junction A neuromuscular junction is the junction of the axon terminal of a motoneuron with the motor end plate, the highly-excitable region of muscle fiber plasma membrane responsible for initiation of action potentials across the muscle's surface.

Multiple sclerosis Multiple sclerosis affects neurons, the cells of the brain and spinal cord that carry information, create thought and perception, and allow the brain to control the body.

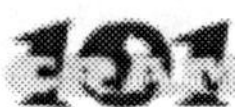

Surrounding and protecting these neurons is a layer of fat, called myelin, which helps neurons carry electrical signals. MS causes gradual destruction of myelin (demyelination) in patches throughout the brain and/or spinal cord, causing various symptoms depending upon which signals are interrupted.

Animal model

An animal model usually refers to a non-human animal with a disease that is similar to a human condition.

Anxiety

Anxiety is a complex combination of the feeling of fear, apprehension and worry often accompanied by physical sensations such as palpitations, chest pain and/or shortness of breath.

Activation

As reflected by facial expressions, the degree of arousal a person is experiencing is referred to as activation.

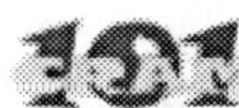

Protein	A protein is a complex, high-molecular-weight organic compound that consists of amino acids joined by peptide bonds. They are essential to the structure and function of all living cells and viruses. Many are enzymes or subunits of enzymes.
Organ	Organ refers to a structure consisting of several tissues adapted as a group to perform specific functions.
Muscle	Muscle is a contractile form of tissue. It is one of the four major tissue types, the other three being epithelium, connective tissue and nervous tissue. Muscle contraction is used to move parts of the body, as well as to move substances within the body.
Tissue	A collection of interconnected cells that perform a similar function within an organism is called tissue.
Skeletal muscle	Skeletal muscle is a type of striated muscle, attached to the skeleton. They are used to facilitate movement, by applying force to bones and joints; via contraction. They generally contract voluntarily (via nerve stimulation), although they can contract involuntarily.
Actin	A protein in a muscle fiber that, together with myosin, is responsible for contraction and relaxation is actin.
Actin filament	An actin filament is a helical protein filament formed by the polymerization of globular actin molecules. They provide mechanical support for the cell, determine the cell shape, enable cell movements; and participate in certain cell junctions.
Cardiac muscle	Cardiac muscle is a type of striated muscle found within the heart. Its function is to "pump" blood through the circulatory system. Unlike skeletal muscle, which contracts in response to nerve stimulation, and like smooth muscle, cardiac muscle is myogenic, meaning that it stimulates its own contraction without a requisite electrical impulse.
Intercalated disk	Intercalated disk refers to region that holds adjacent cardiac muscle cells together and that appear as dense bands at right angles to the muscle striations.
Fiber	Fibers used by man come from a wide variety of sources: Natural fiber include those made out of plants, animal and mineral sources. Natural fibers can be classified according to their origin.
Smooth muscle	Smooth muscle is a type of non-striated muscle, found within the "walls" of hollow organs; such as blood vessels, the bladder, the uterus, and the gastrointestinal tract. Smooth muscle is used to move matter within the body, via contraction; it generally operates "involuntarily", without nerve stimulation.
Connective tissue	Connective tissue is any type of biological tissue with an extensive extracellular matrix and often serves to support, bind together, and protect organs.
Extracellular	Outside the cell is called extracellular.
Organelle	Organelle refers to any structure within a cell that carries out one of its metabolic roles, such as mitochondria, centrioles, endoplasmic reticulum, and the nucleus.
Myofibril	Myofibril is a cylindrical organelle, found within muscle cells. They are bundles of filaments that run from one end of the cell to the other and are attached to the cell surface membrane at each end.
Cytoplasm	Cytoplasm refers to the contents of a cell excluding the nucleus and cell membrane. Cytoplasm is a homogeneous, generally clear jelly-like material that fills cells.
Plasma	Fluid portion of circulating blood is called plasma.
Muscle fiber	Cell with myofibrils containing actin and myosin filaments arranged within sarcomeres is a muscle fiber.

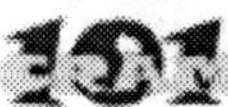

Fusion	Fusion refers to the combination of two atoms into a single atom as a result of a collision, usually accompanied by the release of energy.
Hypertrophy	Hypertrophy is the increase of the size of an organ. It should be distinguished from hyperplasia which occurs due to cell division; hypertrophy occurs due to an increase in cell size rather than division. It is most commonly seen in muscle that has been actively stimulated, the most well-known method being exercise.
Hyperplasia	Hyperplasia is a general term for an increase in the number of the cells of an organ or tissue causing it to increase in size.
Uterus	The uterus is the major female reproductive organ of most mammals. One end, the cervix, opens into the vagina; the other is connected on both sides to the fallopian tubes. The main function is to accept a fertilized ovum which becomes implanted into the endometrium, and derives nourishment from blood vessels which develop exclusively for this purpose.
Septa	Septa are thin walls or partitions between the internal chambers (camerae) of the shell of a cephalopod, namely nautiloids or ammonoids.
Dense connective tissue	Dense connective tissue has collagen fibers as its main matrix element. Crowded between the collagen fibers are rows of fibroblasts, fiber-forming cells, that manufacture the fibers. Dense connective tissue forms strong, rope-like structures such as tendons and ligaments. Tendons attach skeletal muscles to bones; ligaments connect bones to bones at joints.
Lamina	A thin layer, such as the lamina of a vertebra or the lamina propria of a mucous membrane is referred to as lamina.
Blood vessel	A blood vessel is a part of the circulatory system and function to transport blood throughout the body. The most important types, arteries and veins, are so termed because they carry blood away from or towards the heart, respectively.
Capillary	A capillary is the smallest of a body's blood vessels, measuring 5-10 micro meters. They connect arteries and veins, and most closely interact with tissues. Their walls are composed of a single layer of cells, the endothelium. This layer is so thin that molecules such as oxygen, water and lipids can pass through them by diffusion and enter the tissues.
Blood	Blood is a circulating tissue composed of fluid plasma and cells. The main function of blood is to supply nutrients (oxygen, glucose) and constitutional elements to tissues and to remove waste products.
Capillaries	Capillaries refer to the smallest of the blood vessels and the sites of exchange between the blood and tissue cells.
Microscope	A microscope is an instrument for viewing objects that are too small to be seen by the naked or unaided eye.
Nerve	A nerve is an enclosed, cable-like bundle of nerve fibers or axons, which includes the glia that ensheath the axons in myelin.
Striated muscle	Striated muscle refers to contractile tissue characterized by multinucleated cells containing highly ordered arrangements of actin and myosin microfilaments. Also known as skeletal muscle.
Collagen	Collagen is the main protein of connective tissue in animals and the most abundant protein in mammals, making up about 1/4 of the total. It is one of the long, fibrous structural proteins whose functions are quite different from those of globular proteins such as enzymes.
Collagen fiber	White fiber in the matrix of connective tissue, giving flexibility and strength is called collagen fiber.
Transverse	A transverse (also known as axial or horizontal) plane is an X-Y plane, parallel to the

	ground, which (in humans) separates the superior from the inferior, or put another way, the head from the feet.
A band	A band is a dark band corresponding to an area where actin and myosin filaments overlap in cardiac or skeletal muscle.
I band	I band refers to the area near the edge of the sarcomere where there are only thin filaments.
Tendon	A tendon or sinew is a tough band of fibrous connective tissue that connects muscle to bone. They are similar to ligaments except that ligaments join one bone to another.
Light microscope	An optical instrument with lenses that refract visible light to magnify images and project them into a viewer's eye or onto photographic film is referred to as light microscope.
Sarcomere	A sarcomere is the basic unit of a cross striated muscle's myofibril. They are multi-protein complexes composed of three different filament systems. A sarcomere is defined as the segment between two neighboring Z-lines (or Z-discs).
Phosphate	A phosphate is a polyatomic ion or radical consisting of one phosphorus atom and four oxygen. In the ionic form, it carries a -3 formal charge, and is denoted PO_4^{3-}.
Adenosine	Adenosine is a nucleoside comprized of adenine attached to a ribose (ribofuranose) moiety via a β-N_9-glycosidic bond. Adenosine plays an important role in biochemical processes, such as energy transfer - as adenosine triphosphate (ATP) and adenosine diphosphate (ADP) - as well as in signal transduction as cyclic adenosine monophosphate, cAMP.
Adenosine triphosphate	Organic molecule that stores energy and releases energy for use in cellular processes is adenosine triphosphate.
Adenosine diphosphate	Adenosine diphosphate refers to a molecule composed of the sugar ribose, the base adenine, and two phosphate groups; a component of ATP.
Muscle contraction	A muscle contraction occurs when a muscle cell (called a muscle fiber) shortens. There are three general types: skeletal, heart, and smooth.
Phosphate group	The functional group $-0P0_3H_2$; the transfer of energy from one compound to another is often accomplished by the transfer of a phosphate group.
Phosphocreatine	Phosphocreatine is a phosphorylated creatine molecule that is an important energy store in skeletal muscle. It is used to generate ATP from ADP, forming creatine for the 2 to 7 seconds following an intense effort.
Monomer	In chemistry, a monomer is a small molecule that may become chemically bonded to other monomers to form a polymer.
Physiology	The study of the function of cells, tissues, and organs is referred to as physiology.
Polypeptide	Polypeptide refers to polymer of many amino acids linked by peptide bonds.
Tropomyosin	Protein that blocks muscle contraction until calcium ions are present is referred to as tropomyosin.
Light chain	Light chain refers to one of the smaller polypeptides of a multisubunit protein such as myosin or immunoglobulin.
Troponin	A molecule found in thin filaments of muscle that helps regulate when muscle cells contract is referred to as troponin.
Projection	Attributing one's own undesirable thoughts, impulses, traits, or behaviors to others is referred to as projection.
Hydrolyze	Hydrolyze refers to break a chemical bond, as in a peptide linkage, with the insertion of the components of water, -H and -OH, at the cleaved ends of a chain. The digestion of proteins is

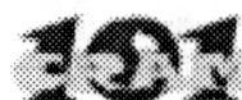

	hydrolysis.
ATPase	ATPase is a class of enzymes that catalyze the decomposition of adenosine triphosphate into adenosine diphosphate and a free phosphate ion. This dephosphorylation reaction releases energy, which the enzyme harnesses to drive other chemical reactions that would not otherwise occur. This process is widely used in all known forms of life.
Conversion	Conversion syndrome describes a condition in which physical symptoms arise for which there is no clear explanation.
Ion	Ion refers to an atom or molecule that has gained or lost one or more electrons, thus acquiring an electrical charge.
Chemical energy	Chemical energy refers to energy stored in the chemical bonds of molecules; a form of potential energy.
Depolarization	Depolarization is a decrease in the absolute value of a cell's membrane potential. Thus, changes in membrane voltage in which the membrane potential becomes less positive or less negative are both depolarizations.
Diffusion	Random movement of molecules from a region of higher concentration toward one of lower concentration is referred to as diffusion.
Lead	Lead is a chemical element in the periodic table that has the symbol Pb and atomic number 82. A soft, heavy, toxic and malleable poor metal, lead is bluish white when freshly cut but tarnishes to dull gray when exposed to air. Lead is used in building construction, lead-acid batteries, bullets and shot, and is part of solder, pewter, and fusible alloys.
Invagination	Infolding of one part of a structure into another is invagination.
Calcium	Calcium is the chemical element in the periodic table that has the symbol Ca and atomic number 20. Calcium is a soft grey alkaline earth metal that is used as a reducing agent in the extraction of thorium, zirconium and uranium. Calcium is also the fifth most abundant element in the Earth's crust.
Hypothesis	A specific statement about behavior or mental processes that is testable through research is a hypothesis.
Hydrolysis	Hydrolysis is a chemical process in which a molecule is cleaved into two parts by the addition of a molecule of water.
Cofactor	A cofactor is any substance that needs to be present in addition to an enzyme to catalyze a certain reaction.
Helix	A helix is a twisted shape like a spring, screw or a spiral staircase. Helixes are important in biology, as DNA is helical and many proteins have helical substructures, known as alpha helices.
Rigor mortis	Rigor mortis is a recognizable sign of death that is caused by a chemical change in the muscles, causing the limbs of the corpse to become stiff and difficult to move or manipulate.
Mitochondria	Cytoplasmic organelles responsible for ATP generation for cellular activities are referred to as mitochondria.
Motor nerve	A motor nerve enables the brain to stimulate muscle contraction. A motor nerve is an efferent nerve that exclusively contains the axons of motorneurons, which innervate skeletal muscle.
Myelin	Myelin is an electrically insulating fatty layer that surrounds the axons of many neurons, especially those in the peripheral nervous system. It is an outgrowth of glial cells: Schwann cells supply the myelin for peripheral neurons while oligodendrocytes supply it to those of

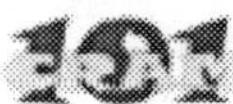

	the central nervous system.
Vesicle	Membranous, cytoplasmic sac formed by an infolding of the cell membrane is called a vesicle.
Axon	An axon is a long slender projection of a nerve cell, or neuron, which conducts electrical impulses away from the neuron's cell body or soma. They are in effect the primary transmission lines of the nervous system, and as bundles they help make up nerves.
Synaptic vesicle	Small neurotransmitter-filled secretory vesicle formed at the axon terminals of nerve cells and whose contents are released into the synaptic cleft by exocytosis when an action potential reaches the axon terminal is called synaptic vesicle.
Axon terminal	A swelling at the end of an axon that is designed to release a chemical substance onto another neuron, muscle cell, or gland cell is called the axon terminal.
Acetylcholine	The chemical compound acetylcholine was the first neurotransmitter to be identified. It is a chemical transmitter in both the peripheral nervous system (PNS) and central nervous system (CNS) in many organisms including humans.
Cleft	Cleft is a congenital deformity caused by a failure in facial development during pregnancy.
Synaptic cleft	A narrow gap separating the synaptic knob of a transmitting neuron from a receiving neuron or an effector cell is a synaptic cleft.
Glycogen	Glycogen refers to a complex, extensively branched polysaccharide of many glucose monomers; serves as an energy-storage molecule in liver and muscle cells.
Receptor	A receptor is a protein on the cell membrane or within the cytoplasm or cell nucleus that binds to a specific molecule (a ligand), such as a neurotransmitter, hormone, or other substance, and initiates the cellular response to the ligand. Receptor, in immunology, the region of an antibody which shows recognition of an antigen.
Acetylcholine receptor	An acetylcholine receptor is an integral membrane protein that responds to the binding of the neurotransmitter acetylcholine. They are ion channels, and, like other members of the "cys-loop" ligand-gated ion channel superfamily, are composed of five protein subunits arranged like staves around a barrel.
Action potential	The sequence of electrical changes occurring when a nerve cell membrane is exposed to a stimulus that exceeds its threshold is called action potential.
Motor end plate	A motor end plate is the distal end of the nerve where the nerve impulse causes emission of acetylcholine molecules into the synaptic cleft to innervate muscle fibers triggering muscle contraction.
Sodium	Sodium is the chemical element in the periodic table that has the symbol Na (Natrium in Latin) and atomic number 11. Sodium is a soft, waxy, silvery reactive metal belonging to the alkali metals that is abundant in natural compounds (especially halite). It is highly reactive.
Enzyme	An enzyme is a protein that catalyzes, or speeds up, a chemical reaction. They are essential to sustain life because most chemical reactions in biological cells would occur too slowly, or would lead to different products, without them.
Sliding filament mechanism	The sliding filament mechanism is a process used by muscles to contract.
Autoimmune	Autoimmune refers to immune reactions against normal body cells; self against self.
Myasthenia gravis	Myasthenia gravis is a neuromuscular disease leading to fluctuating weakness and fatiguability.

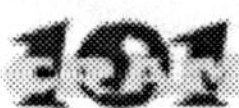

Lysosome	Organelle that contains enzymes that degrade worn cell parts is called a lysosome.
Motor unit	A motor neuron and all the muscle fibers it controls is called the motor unit.
Spinal cord	The spinal cord is a part of the vertebrate nervous system that is enclosed in and protected by the vertebral column (it passes through the spinal canal). It consists of nerve cells. The spinal cord carries sensory signals and motor innervation to most of the skeletal muscles in the body.
Muscle spindle	A muscle spindle is a specialized muscle structure innervated by both sensory and motor neuron axons. Its functions are to send proprioceptive information about the muscle to the central nervous system, and to respond to muscle stretching.
Sensory nerves	Sensory nerves bring impulses toward the central nervous system.
Variable	A characteristic or aspect in which people, objects, events, or conditions vary is called variable.
Synapse	A junction, or relay point, between two neurons, or between a neuron and an effector cell. Electrical and chemical signals are relayed from one cell to another at a synapse.
Efferent nerve	An efferent nerve carries nerve impulses away from the central nervous system. A motor nerve is an efferent nerve involved in muscular control.
Fatty acid	A fatty acid is a carboxylic acid (or organic acid), often with a long aliphatic tail (long chains), either saturated or unsaturated.
Glucose	Glucose, a simple monosaccharide sugar, is one of the most important carbohydrates and is used as a source of energy in animals and plants. Glucose is one of the main products of photosynthesis and starts respiration.
Acid	An acid is a water-soluble, sour-tasting chemical compound that when dissolved in water, gives a solution with a pH of less than 7.
Acetate	Acetate is the anion of a salt or ester of acetic acid.
Oxygen	Oxygen is a chemical element in the periodic table. It has the symbol O and atomic number 8. Oxygen is the second most common element on Earth, composing around 46% of the mass of Earth's crust and 28% of the mass of Earth as a whole, and is the third most common element in the universe.
Citric acid cycle	In aerobic organisms, the citric acid cycle is a metabolic pathway that forms part of the break down of carbohydrates, fats and proteins into carbon dioxide and water in order to generate energy. It is the second of three metabolic pathways that are involved in fuel molecule catabolism and ATP production, the other two being glycolysis and oxidative phosphorylation.
Pain	Pain is an unpleasant sensation which may be associated with actual or potential tissue damage and which may have physical and emotional components.
Oxidative phosphorylation	Oxidative phosphorylation is a biochemical process in cells. It is the final metabolic pathway of cellular respiration, after glycolysis and the citric acid cycle.
Phosphorylation	Phosphorylation refers to reaction in which a phosphate group becomes covalently coupled to another molecule.
Diagnosis	In medicine, diagnosis is the process of identifying a medical condition or disease by its signs, symptoms, and from the results of various diagnostic procedures.
Clinical significance	The degree to which research findings have useful and meaningful applications to real problems is called their clinical significance.

Paralysis	Paralysis is the complete loss of muscle function for one or more muscle groups. Paralysis may be localized, or generalized, or it may follow a certain pattern.
Atrophy	Atrophy is the partial or complete wasting away of a part of the body. Causes of atrophy include poor nourishment, poor circulation, loss of hormonal support, loss of nerve supply to the target organ, disuse or lack of exercise, or disease intrinsic to the tissue itself.
Hemoglobin	Hemoglobin is the iron-containing oxygen-transport metalloprotein in the red cells of the blood in mammals and other animals. Hemoglobin transports oxygen from the lungs to the rest of the body, such as to the muscles, where it releases the oxygen load.
Mesoderm	Mesoderm forms in the embryos of animals more complex than cnidarians. Some of the cells migrating inward to form the endoderm form an additional layer between the other two. It gives rise to muscles, bones, the dermis of the skin, and most other organs in the adult.
Myofilaments	The thick and thin filaments that form the myofibrils are referred to as myofilaments.
Desmosome	A desmosome (also known as macula adherens) is a cell structure specialized for cell-to-cell adhesion. It is a type of junctional complex.
Constant	A behavior or characteristic that does not vary from one observation to another is referred to as a constant.
Myocytes	Myocytes are modified pinacocytes which control the size of the osculum and pore openings and thus the water flow.
Aerobic	An aerobic organism is an organism that has an oxygen based metabolism. Aerobes, in a process known as cellular respiration, use oxygen to oxidize substrates (for example sugars and fats) in order to obtain energy.
Metabolism	Metabolism is the biochemical modification of chemical compounds in living organisms and cells. This includes the biosynthesis of complex organic molecules (anabolism) and their breakdown (catabolism).
Lipoprotein	A lipoprotein is a biochemical assembly that contains both proteins and lipids and may be structural or catalytic in function. They may be enzymes, proton pumps, ion pumps, or some combination of these functions.
Triglyceride	Triglyceride is a glyceride in which the glycerol is esterified with three fatty acids. They are the main constituent of vegetable oil and animal fats and play an important role in metabolism as energy sources. They contain a bit more than twice as much energy as carbohydrates and proteins.
Lipid	Lipid is one class of aliphatic hydrocarbon-containing organic compounds essential for the structure and function of living cells. They are characterized by being water-insoluble but soluble in nonpolar organic solvents.
Triglycerides	Triglycerides refer to fats and oils composed of fatty acids and glycerol; are the body's most concentrated source of energy fuel; also known as neutral fats.
Stress	Stress refers to a condition that is a response to factors that change the human systems normal state.
Fascia	Fascia is specialized connective tissue layer which surrounds muscles, bones, and joints, providing support and protection and giving structure to the body. It consists of three layers: the superficial fascia, the deep fascia and the subserous fascia. Fascia is one of the 3 types of dense connective tissue (the other two being ligaments and tendons).
Calmodulin	Calmodulin refers to ubiquitous calcium-binding protein whose binding to other proteins is governed by changes in intracellular Ca2+ concentration. Its binding modifies the activity of many target enzymes and membrane transport proteins.

Affect	Affect is the scientific term used to describe a subject's externally displayed mood. This can be assesed by the nurse by observing facial expression, tone of voice, and body language.
Hormone	A hormone is a chemical messenger from one cell to another. All multicellular organisms produce hormones. The best known hormones are those produced by endocrine glands of vertebrate animals, but hormones are produced by nearly every organ system and tissue type in a human or animal body. Hormone molecules are secreted directly into the bloodstream, they move by circulation or diffusion to their target cells, which may be nearby cells in the same tissue or cells of a distant organ of the body.
Adenosine monophosphate	Adenosine monophosphate, also known as 5'-adenylic acid and abbreviated AMP, is a nucleotide that is found in RNA. It is an ester of phosphoric acid with the nucleoside adenosine.
Estrogen	Estrogen is a steroid that functions as the primary female sex hormone. While present in both men and women, they are found in women in significantly higher quantities.
Progesterone	Progesterone is a C-21 steroid hormone involved in the female menstrual cycle, pregnancy (supports gestation) and embryogenesis of humans and other species.
Vascular smooth muscle	Vascular smooth muscle refers to the particular type of smooth muscle found within, and composing the majority of the wall of blood vessels.
Sympathetic	The sympathetic nervous system activates what is often termed the "fight or flight response". It is an automatic regulation system, that is, one that operates without the intervention of conscious thought.
Intestine	The intestine is the portion of the alimentary canal extending from the stomach to the anus and, in humans and mammals, consists of two segments, the small intestine and the large intestine. The intestine is the part of the body responsible for extracting nutrition from food.
Ureter	A ureter is a duct that carries urine from the kidneys to the urinary bladder. They are muscular tubes that can propel urine along by the motions of peristalsis.
Iris	The colored part of the vertebrate eye, formed by the anterior portion of the choroid is called the iris.
Eye	An eye is an organ that detects light. Different kinds of light-sensitive organs are found in a variety of creatures. The simplest eyes do nothing but detect whether the surroundings are light or dark, while more complex eyes can distinguish shapes and colors.
Cholinergic	A synapse is cholinergic if it uses acetylcholine as its neurotransmitter. The parasympathetic nervous system is entirely cholinergic.
Adrenergic	Pertaining to epinephrine or norepinephrine, as in adrenergic neurons that secrete one of these chemicals or adrenergic effects on a target organ is called adrenegic.
Macula	The macula is an oval yellow spot near the center of the retina of the human eye. Near its center is the fovea, a small pit that contains the largest concentration of cone cells in the eye and is responsible for central vision.
Micrograph	A micrograph is a photograph or similar image taken through a microscope or similar device to show a magnified image of an item.
Proteoglycan	Molecule consisting of one or more glycosaminoglycan chains attached to a core protein is referred to as proteoglycan.
Elastin	Elastin, is a protein in connective tissue that is elastic and allows many tissues in the body to resume their shape after stretching or contracting. Elastin helps skin to return to its original position when it is poked or pinched.

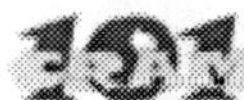

Regeneration	Regeneration is the ability to restore lost or damaged tissues, organs or limbs. It is a common feature in invertebrates, but far more limited in most vertebrates.
Scar	A scar results from the biologic process of wound repair in the skin and other tissues of the body. It is a connective tissue that fills the wound.
Population	Population refers to all members of a well-defined group of organisms, events, or things.
Trauma	Trauma refers to a severe physical injury or wound to the body caused by an external force, or a psychological shock having a lasting effect on mental life.
Silver	Silver is a chemical element with the symbol Ag. A soft white lustrous transition metal, it has the highest electrical and thermal conductivity of any metal and occurs in minerals and in free form.
Arteriole	An arteriole is a blood vessel that extends and branches out from an artery and leads to capillaries. They have thick muscular walls and are the primary site of vascular resistance.
Gland	A gland is an organ in an animal's body that synthesizes a substance for release such as hormones, often into the bloodstream or into cavities inside the body or its outer surface.
Endocrine gland	An endocrine gland is one of a set of internal organs involved in the secretion of hormones into the blood. These glands are known as ductless, which means they do not have tubes inside them.

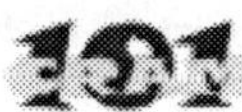

Artery	Vessel that takes blood away from the heart to the tissues and organs of the body is called an artery.
Tissue	A collection of interconnected cells that perform a similar function within an organism is called tissue.
Oxygen	Oxygen is a chemical element in the periodic table. It has the symbol O and atomic number 8. Oxygen is the second most common element on Earth, composing around 46% of the mass of Earth's crust and 28% of the mass of Earth as a whole, and is the third most common element in the universe.
Blood	Blood is a circulating tissue composed of fluid plasma and cells. The main function of blood is to supply nutrients (oxygen, glucose) and constitutional elements to tissues and to remove waste products.
Blood vessel	A blood vessel is a part of the circulatory system and function to transport blood throughout the body. The most important types, arteries and veins, are so termed because they carry blood away from or towards the heart, respectively.
Capillaries	Capillaries refer to the smallest of the blood vessels and the sites of exchange between the blood and tissue cells.
Capillary	A capillary is the smallest of a body's blood vessels, measuring 5-10 micro meters. They connect arteries and veins, and most closely interact with tissues. Their walls are composed of a single layer of cells, the endothelium. This layer is so thin that molecules such as oxygen, water and lipids can pass through them by diffusion and enter the tissues.
Channel	Channel, in communications (sometimes called communications channel), refers to the medium used to convey information from a sender (or transmitter) to a receiver.
Veins	Blood vessels that return blood toward the heart from the circulation are referred to as veins.
Vein	Vein in animals, is a vessel that returns blood to the heart. In plants, a vascular bundle in a leaf, composed of xylem and phloem.
Lymphatic system	Lymph originates as blood plasma lost from the circulatory system, which leaks out into the surrounding tissues. The lymphatic system collects this fluid by diffusion into lymph capillaries, and returns it to the circulatory system.
Endothelium	The endothelium is the layer of thin, flat cells that lines the interior surface of blood vessels, forming an interface between circulating blood in the lumen and the rest of the vessel wall.
Epithelium	Epithelium is a tissue composed of a layer of cells. Epithelium can be found lining internal (e.g. endothelium, which lines the inside of blood vessels) or external (e.g. skin) free surfaces of the body. Functions include secretion, absorption and protection.
Squamous epithelium	The squamous epithelium is epithelium consisting of one or more cell layers, the most superficial of which is composed of flat, scalelike or platelike cells.
Microscope	A microscope is an instrument for viewing objects that are too small to be seen by the naked or unaided eye.
Arteriole	An arteriole is a blood vessel that extends and branches out from an artery and leads to capillaries. They have thick muscular walls and are the primary site of vascular resistance.
Venule	A vessel that conveys blood between a capillary bed and a vein is a venule.
Circulatory system	The circulatory system or cardiovascular system is the organ system which circulates blood around the body of most animals.

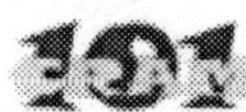

Connective tissue	Connective tissue is any type of biological tissue with an extensive extracellular matrix and often serves to support, bind together, and protect organs.
Blood pressure	Blood pressure is the pressure exerted by the blood on the walls of the blood vessels.
Adventitia	Adventitia is the outermost connective tissue covering of any organ, vessel, or other structure. For example, the connective tissue that surrounds an artery is called the adventitia because it is considered extraneous to the artery.
Fiber	Fibers used by man come from a wide variety of sources: Natural fiber include those made out of plants, animal and mineral sources. Natural fibers can be classified according to their origin.
Blood plasma	Blood plasma is the liquid component of blood, in which the blood cells are suspended. Serum is the same as blood plasma except that clotting factors (such as fibrin) have been removed.
Plasma	Fluid portion of circulating blood is called plasma.
Interstitial fluid	Interstitial fluid is one of the two components of extracellular fluid, the other being plasma. On average, a person has about 11 liters of interstitial fluid providing the cells of the body with nutrients and a means of waste removal.
Macromolecule	A macromolecule is a molecule with a large molecular mass, but generally the use of the term is restricted to polymers and molecules which structurally include polymers.
Angiotensin	Angiotensin is a polypeptide in the blood that causes vasoconstriction, increased blood pressure, and aldosterone release from the adrenal cortex. Angiotensin is produced in the liver from precursor angiotensinogen, a serum globulin. It plays an important role in the renin-angiotensin system.
Conversion	Conversion syndrome describes a condition in which physical symptoms arise for which there is no clear explanation.
Endothelial cell	A endothelial cell also controls the passage of materials — and the transit of white blood cells — into and out of the bloodstream. In some organs, there are highly differentiated endothelial cells to perform specialized 'filtering' functions.
Angiotensin II	Angiotensin II is formed by the action of renin on angiotensinogen. Renin, produced in the kidneys in response to decreased blood pressure, cleaves the peptide bond between the leucine and the valine residues on angiotensinogen.
Epinephrine	Epinephrine is a hormone and a neurotransmitter. Epinephrine plays a central role in the short-term stress reaction—the physiological response to threatening or exciting conditions (fight-or-flight response). It is secreted by the adrenal medulla.
Serotonin	Serotonin is a monoamine neurotransmitter synthesized in serotonergic neurons in the central nervous system and enterochromaffin cells in the gastrointestinal tract. It is believed to play an important part of the biochemistry of depression, migraine, bipolar disorder and anxiety.
Thrombin	Thrombin refers to an enzyme that converts fibrinogen to fibrin threads during blood clotting.
Prostaglandin	A prostaglandin is any member of a group of lipid compounds that are derived from fatty acids and have important functions in the animal body.
Triglyceride	Triglyceride is a glyceride in which the glycerol is esterified with three fatty acids. They are the main constituent of vegetable oil and animal fats and play an important role in metabolism as energy sources. They contain a bit more than twice as much energy as carbohydrates and proteins.

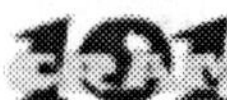

Lipoprotein	A lipoprotein is a biochemical assembly that contains both proteins and lipids and may be structural or catalytic in function. They may be enzymes, proton pumps, ion pumps, or some combination of these functions.
Cholesterol	Cholesterol is a steroid, a lipid, and an alcohol, found in the cell membranes of all body tissues, and transported in the blood plasma of all animals. It is an important component of the membranes of cells, providing stability; it makes the membrane's fluidity stable over a bigger temperature interval.
Substrate	A substrate is a molecule which is acted upon by an enzyme. Each enzyme recognizes only the specific substrate of the reaction it catalyzes. A surface in or on which an organism lives.
Steroid	A steroid is a lipid characterized by a carbon skeleton with four fused rings. Different steroids vary in the functional groups attached to these rings. Hundreds of distinct steroids have been identified in plants and animals. Their most important role in most living systems is as hormones.
Affect	Affect is the scientific term used to describe a subject's externally displayed mood. This can be assesed by the nurse by observing facial expression, tone of voice, and body language.
Enzyme	An enzyme is a protein that catalyzes, or speeds up, a chemical reaction. They are essential to sustain life because most chemical reactions in biological cells would occur too slowly, or would lead to different products, without them.
Agent	Agent refers to an epidemiological term referring to the organism or object that transmits a disease from the environment to the host.
Triglycerides	Triglycerides refer to fats and oils composed of fatty acids and glycerol; are the body's most concentrated source of energy fuel; also known as neutral fats.
Coagulation	The coagulation of blood is a complex process during which blood forms solid clots. It is an important part of haemostasis (the ceszation of blood loss from a damaged vessel) whereby a damaged blood vessel wall is covered by a fibrin clot to stop hemorrhage and aid repair of the damaged vessel.
Platelet	Cell fragment that is necessary to blood clotting is a platelet. They are the blood cell fragments that are involved in the cellular mechanisms that lead to the formation of blood clots.
Lesion	A lesion is a non-specific term referring to abnormal tissue in the body. It can be caused by any disease process including trauma (physical, chemical, electrical), infection, neoplasm, metabolic and autoimmune.
Thrombus	Blood clot that remains in the blood vessel where it formed is called a thrombus.
Intravascular	Within the arteries, vessels, veins, or capillaries is intravascular.
Embolus	Embolus refers to any abnormal traveling object in the bloodstream, such as agglutinated bacteria or blood cells, a blood clot, or an air bubble.
Tunica media	The tunica media is the middle layer of an artery. It is made up of smooth muscle cells and elastic tissue. It lays between the tunica intima on the inside and the tunica adventitia on the outside.
Muscle	Muscle is a contractile form of tissue. It is one of the four major tissue types, the other three being epithelium, connective tissue and nervous tissue. Muscle contraction is used to move parts of the body, as well as to move substances within the body.
Smooth muscle	Smooth muscle is a type of non-striated muscle, found within the "walls" of hollow organs; such as blood vessels, the bladder, the uterus, and the gastrointestinal tract. Smooth muscle is used to move matter within the body, via contraction; it generally operates

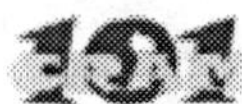

"involuntarily", without nerve stimulation.

Variable A characteristic or aspect in which people, objects, events, or conditions vary is called variable.

Lamina A thin layer, such as the lamina of a vertebra or the lamina propria of a mucous membrane is referred to as lamina.

Vascular smooth muscle Vascular smooth muscle refers to the particular type of smooth muscle found within, and composing the majority of the wall of blood vessels.

Collagen Collagen is the main protein of connective tissue in animals and the most abundant protein in mammals, making up about 1/4 of the total. It is one of the long, fibrous structural proteins whose functions are quite different from those of globular proteins such as enzymes.

Collagen fiber White fiber in the matrix of connective tissue, giving flexibility and strength is called collagen fiber.

Elastic fiber Elastic fiber is a bundles of proteins (elastin) found in connective tissue and produced by fibroblasts and smooth muscle cells in arteries.

Heterogeneous A heterogeneous compound, mixture, or other such object is one that consists of many different items, which are often not easily sorted or separated, though they are clearly distinct.

Extracellular Outside the cell is called extracellular.

Diffusion Random movement of molecules from a region of higher concentration toward one of lower concentration is referred to as diffusion.

Glycosaminog-ycan Glycosaminoglycan is a long unbranched polysaccharide, made up of repeating disaccharides that may be sulphated (e.g. glucuronic acid, iduronic acid, galactose, galactosamine, glucosamine).

Elastin Elastin, is a protein in connective tissue that is elastic and allows many tissues in the body to resume their shape after stretching or contracting. Elastin helps skin to return to its original position when it is poked or pinched.

Calcium Calcium is the chemical element in the periodic table that has the symbol Ca and atomic number 20. Calcium is a soft grey alkaline earth metal that is used as a reducing agent in the extraction of thorium, zirconium and uranium. Calcium is also the fifth most abundant element in the Earth's crust.

Ion Ion refers to an atom or molecule that has gained or lost one or more electrons, thus acquiring an electrical charge.

Lead Lead is a chemical element in the periodic table that has the symbol Pb and atomic number 82. A soft, heavy, toxic and malleable poor metal, lead is bluish white when freshly cut but tarnishes to dull gray when exposed to air. Lead is used in building construction, lead-acid batteries, bullets and shot, and is part of solder, pewter, and fusible alloys.

In vivo In vivo is used to indicate the presence of a whole/living organism, in distinction to a partial or dead organism, or a computer model. Animal testing and clinical trials are forms of in vivo research.

Intima The tunica intima (or just intima) is the innermost layer of an artery. It is made up of one layer of endothelial cells and is supported by an internal elastic lamina. The endothelial cell are in direct contact with the blood flow.

Tunica adventitia The Tunica Adventitia is the outermost layer of a blood vessel, surrounding the tunica media.

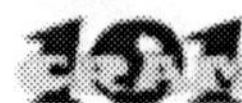

Organ	Organ refers to a structure consisting of several tissues adapted as a group to perform specific functions.
Metabolite	The term metabolite is usually restricted to small molecules. They are the intermediates and products of metabolism. A primary metabolite is directly involved in the normal growth, development, and reproduction. A secondary metabolite is not directly involved in those processes, but usually has important ecological function.
Sympathetic	The sympathetic nervous system activates what is often termed the "fight or flight response". It is an automatic regulation system, that is, one that operates without the intervention of conscious thought.
Nerve	A nerve is an enclosed, cable-like bundle of nerve fibers or axons, which includes the glia that ensheath the axons in myelin.
Neurotransmitter	A neurotransmitter is a chemical that is used to relay, amplify and modulate electrical signals between a neuron and another cell.
Vasoconstriction	Vasoconstriction refers to a decrease in the diameter of a blood vessel.
Norepinephrine	Norepinephrine is a catecholamine and a phenethylamine with chemical formula $C_8H_{11}NO_3$. It is released from the adrenal glands as a hormone into the blood, but it is also a neurotransmitter in the nervous system where it is released from noradrenergic neurons during synaptic transmission.
Efferent nerve	An efferent nerve carries nerve impulses away from the central nervous system. A motor nerve is an efferent nerve involved in muscular control.
Vasodilator	A vasodilator is a substance that causes blood vessels in the body to become wider by relaxing the smooth muscle in the vessel wall. This will reduce blood pressure (since there is more room for the blood) and might allow blood to flow around a clot.
Cholinergic	A synapse is cholinergic if it uses acetylcholine as its neurotransmitter. The parasympathetic nervous system is entirely cholinergic.
Skeletal muscle	Skeletal muscle is a type of striated muscle, attached to the skeleton. They are used to facilitate movement, by applying force to bones and joints; via contraction. They generally contract voluntarily (via nerve stimulation), although they can contract involuntarily.
Intracellular	Intracellular refers to having to do with the interior of a cell.
Acetylcholine	The chemical compound acetylcholine was the first neurotransmitter to be identified. It is a chemical transmitter in both the peripheral nervous system (PNS) and central nervous system (CNS) in many organisms including humans.
Aorta	The largest artery in the human body, the aorta originates from the left ventricle of the heart and brings oxygenated blood to all parts of the body in the systemic circulation.
Proteoglycan	Molecule consisting of one or more glycosaminoglycan chains attached to a core protein is referred to as proteoglycan.
Systole	The contraction stage of the heart cycle, when the heart chambers actively pump blood is systole.
Diastole	The stage of the heart cycle in which the heart muscle is relaxed, allowing the chambers to fill with blood is called diastole.
Involution	Shrinkage of a tissue or organ by autolysis, such as involution of the thymus after childhood and of the uterus after pregnancy is referred to as involution.
Constant	A behavior or characteristic that does not vary from one observation to another is referred to as a constant.

Histology	Histology is the study of tissue sectioned as a thin slice, using a microscope. It can be described as microscopic anatomy.
Chemoreceptor	Chemoreceptor is a cell or group of cells that transduce a chemical signal into an action potential.
Carotid body	Structure located at the branching of the carotid arteries and that contain chemoreceptors sensitive to the hydrogen ion concentration and also the level of carbon dioxide and oxygen in blood is called carotid body.
Carbon	Carbon is a chemical element in the periodic table that has the symbol C and atomic number 6. An abundant nonmetallic, tetravalent element, carbon has several allotropic forms.
Common carotid artery	In human anatomy, the common carotid artery is the blood vessel with oxygenated blood that supplies the head and neck. The left common carotid artery is one of three arteries that originate along the aortic arch. The right common carotid artery arises from the brachiocephalic artery.
Carotid artery	In human anatomy, the carotid artery refers to a number of major arteries in the head and neck.
Carbon dioxide	Carbon dioxide is an atmospheric gas comprized of one carbon and two oxygen atoms. A very widely known chemical compound, it is frequently called by its formula CO_2. In its solid state, it is commonly known as dry ice.
Adrenaline	Adrenaline is a hormone released by chromaffin cells and by some neurons in response to stress. Produces 'fight or flight' responses, including increased heart rate and blood sugar levels.
Dopamine	Dopamine is a chemical naturally produced in the body. In the brain, dopamine functions as a neurotransmitter, activating dopamine receptors. Dopamine is also a neurohormone released by the hypothalamus. Its main function as a hormone is to inhibit the release of prolactin from the anterior lobe of the pituitary.
Vesicle	Membranous, cytoplasmic sac formed by an infolding of the cell membrane is called a vesicle.
Central nervous system	The central nervous system comprized of the brain and spinal cord, represents the largest part of the nervous system. Together with the peripheral nervous system, it has a fundamental role in the control of behavior.
Afferent nerve	Axons that carry information inward to the central nervous system from the periphery of the body is called an afferent nerve.
Nervous system	The nervous system of an animal coordinates the activity of the muscles, monitors the organs, constructs and processes input from the senses, and initiates actions.
Aortic body	The aortic body is one of several small cluster of chemoreceptors, baroreceptors, and supporting cells located along the aortic arch. It measures changes in blood pressure and the composition of arterial blood flowing past it, including the partial pressures of oxygen and carbon dioxide but not pH.
Arch of the aorta	The arch of the aorta begins at the level of the upper border of the second sternocostal articulation of the right side, and runs at first upward, backward, and to the left in front of the trachea; it is then directed backward on the left side of the trachea and finally passes downward on the left side of the body of the fourth thoracic vertebra, at the lower border of which it becomes continuous with the descending aorta. It thus forms two curvatures: one with its convexity upward, the other with its convexity forward and to the left. Its upper border is usually about 2.5 cm. below the superior border to the manubrium sterni.

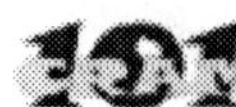

Internal carotid artery	In human anatomy, the internal carotid artery is a major artery of the head and neck. It arises from the common carotid artery when it bifurcates into an internal and external branch. It has no branches in the neck. It ascends and enters the skull through the carotid canal. Inside the cranium, it gives off the ophthalmic artery .
Sinus	A sinus is a pouch or cavity in any organ or tissue, or an abnormal cavity or passage caused by the destruction of tissue.
Brain	The part of the central nervous system involved in regulating and controlling body activity and interpreting information from the senses transmitted through the nervous system is referred to as the brain.
Endocytosis	Endocytosis is a process where cells absorb material (molecules or other cells) from outside by engulfing it with their cell membranes.
Receptor	A receptor is a protein on the cell membrane or within the cytoplasm or cell nucleus that binds to a specific molecule (a ligand), such as a neurotransmitter, hormone, or other substance, and initiates the cellular response to the ligand. Receptor, in immunology, the region of an antibody which shows recognition of an antigen.
Monocyte	A monocyte is a leukocyte, part of the human body's immune system that protect against blood-borne pathogens and move quickly to sites of infection in the tissues.
Lipid	Lipid is one class of aliphatic hydrocarbon-containing organic compounds essential for the structure and function of living cells. They are characterized by being water-insoluble but soluble in nonpolar organic solvents.
Atherosclerosis	Process by which a fatty substance or plaque builds up inside arteries to form obstructions is called atherosclerosis.
Coronary	Referring to the heart or the blood vessels of the heart is referred to as coronary.
Coronary arteries	Arteries that directly supply the heart with blood are referred to as coronary arteries.
Coronary artery	An artery that supplies blood to the wall of the heart is called a coronary artery.
Cerebrum	Cerebrum refers to the largest, most sophisticated, and most dominant part of the vertebrate forebrain, made up of right and left cerebral hemispheres.
Irrigate	To gently flush a canal with fluid is to irrigate the area.
Necrosis	Necrosis is the name given to unprogrammed death of cells/living tissue. There are many causes of necrosis including injury, infection, cancer, infarction, and inflammation. Necrosis is caused by special enzymes that are released by lysosomes.
Skin	Skin is an organ of the integumentary system composed of a layer of tissues that protect underlying muscles and organs.
Aneurysm	An aneurysm is a localized dilation or ballooning of a blood vessel by more than 50% of the diameter of the vessel. Aneurysms most commonly occur in the arteries at the base of the brain and in the aorta (the main artery coming out of the heart) - this is an aortic aneurysm.
Catecholamines	A class of compounds, including epinephrine and norepinephrine, that are synthesized from the amino acid tyrosine are called catecholamines.
Catecholamine	Catecholamine is a chemical compound derived from the amino acid tyrosine that acts as a hormone or neurotransmitter. They are examples of phenethylamines.
Conservation	Conservation refers to according to Piaget, recognition that basic properties of substances such as weight and mass remain the same when superficial features change.

Parasympathetic nervous system	The parasympathetic nervous system is one of two divisions of the autonomic nervous system. It conserves energy as it slows the heart rate, increases intestinal and gland activity, and relaxes sphincter muscles in the gastro-intestinal tract. In other words, it acts to reverse the effects of the sympathetic nervous system.
Transverse	A transverse (also known as axial or horizontal) plane is an X-Y plane, parallel to the ground, which (in humans) separates the superior from the inferior, or put another way, the head from the feet.
Mitochondria	Cytoplasmic organelles responsible for ATP generation for cellular activities are referred to as mitochondria.
Organelle	Organelle refers to any structure within a cell that carries out one of its metabolic roles, such as mitochondria, centrioles, endoplasmic reticulum, and the nucleus.
Cytoplasm	Cytoplasm refers to the contents of a cell excluding the nucleus and cell membrane. Cytoplasm is a homogeneous, generally clear jelly-like material that fills cells.
Edema	Edema is swelling of any organ or tissue due to accumulation of excess fluid. Edema has many root causes, but its common mechanism is accumulation of fluid into the tissues.
Inflammatory response	Inflammatory response refers to a complex sequence of events involving chemicals and immune cells that results in the isolation and destruction of antigens and tissues near the antigens.
Tropomyosin	Protein that blocks muscle contraction until calcium ions are present is referred to as tropomyosin.
Actin	A protein in a muscle fiber that, together with myosin, is responsible for contraction and relaxation is actin.
Somatic	The term somatic refers to the body. It also refers to the part of the nervous system that controls voluntary movement and senzation and judges relative effort and weight, called proprioception.
Visceral	Visceral refers to the internal organs of an animal.
Diaphragm	The diaphragm is a shelf of muscle extending across the bottom of the ribcage. It is critically important in respiration: in order to draw air into the lungs, the diaphragm contracts, thus enlarging the thoracic cavity and reducing intra-thoracic pressure.
Hydrophobic	Hydrophobic refers to being electrically neutral and nonpolar, and thus prefering other neutral and nonpolar solvents or molecular environments. Hydrophobic is often used interchangeably with "oily" or "lipophilic."
Bone marrow	Bone marrow is the tissue comprising the center of large bones. It is the place where new blood cells are produced. Bone marrow contains two types of stem cells: hemopoietic (which can produce blood cells) and stromal (which can produce fat, cartilage and bone).
Spleen	The spleen is a ductless, vertebrate gland that is not necessary for life but is closely associated with the circulatory system, where it functions in the destruction of old red blood cells and removal of other debris from the bloodstream, and also in holding a reservoir of blood.
Liver	The liver is an organ in vertebrates, including humans. It plays a major role in metabolism and has a number of functions in the body including drug detoxification, glycogen storage, and plasma protein synthesis. It also produces bile, which is important for digestion.
Anastomosis	An anastomosis is a connection between two structures, organs or spaces. It commonly refers to connections between blood vessels or connections between other tubular structures such as a loops of intestine.

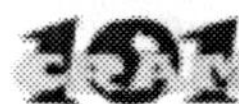

Kidney	The kidney is a bean-shaped excretory organ in vertebrates. Part of the urinary system, the kidneys filter wastes (especially urea) from the blood and excrete them, along with water, as urine.
Dense connective tissue	Dense connective tissue has collagen fibers as its main matrix element. Crowded between the collagen fibers are rows of fibroblasts, fiber-forming cells, that manufacture the fibers. Dense connective tissue forms strong, rope-like structures such as tendons and ligaments. Tendons attach skeletal muscles to bones; ligaments connect bones to bones at joints.
Metabolic rate	Energy expended by the body per unit time is called metabolic rate.
Hydrophilic	Pertaining to molecules that attract water or dissolve in it because of their polar nature is hydrophilic.
Glucose	Glucose, a simple monosaccharide sugar, is one of the most important carbohydrates and is used as a source of energy in animals and plants. Glucose is one of the main products of photosynthesis and starts respiration.
Tunica intima	The tunica intima is the innermost layer of an artery. It is made up of one layer of endothelial cells and is supported by an internal elastic lamina. The endothelial cell are in direct contact with the blood flow.
Venous blood	In the circulatory system, venous blood or peripheral blood is blood returning to the heart. With one exception (the pulmonary vein) this blood is deoxygenated and high in carbon dioxide, having released oxygen and absorbed CO_2 in the tissues.
Pericardium	The pericardium is a double-walled sac that contains the heart and the roots of the great vessels. There are two layers to this sac: the fibrous pericardium, serous pericardium.
Endocardium	In the heart, the endocardium is the innermost layer of cells, embryologically and biologically similar to the endothelium that lines blood vessels.
Myocardium	Myocardium is the muscular tissue of the heart. The myocardium is composed of specialized cardiac muscle cells with an ability not possessed by muscle tissue elsewhere in the body.
Skeleton	In biology, the skeleton or skeletal system is the biological system providing physical support in living organisms.
Glomerulus	A glomerulus is a capillary tuft surrounded by Bowman's capsule in nephrons of the vertebrate kidney. It receives its blood supply from an afferent arteriole of the renal circulation, and empties into an efferent arteriole.
Base	The common definition of a base is a chemical compound that absorbs hydronium ions when dissolved in water (a proton acceptor). An alkali is a special example of a base, where in an aqueous environment, hydroxide ions are donated.
Cardiac muscle	Cardiac muscle is a type of striated muscle found within the heart. Its function is to "pump" blood through the circulatory system. Unlike skeletal muscle, which contracts in response to nerve stimulation, and like smooth muscle, cardiac muscle is myogenic, meaning that it stimulates its own contraction without a requisite electrical impulse.
Homologous	Homologous refers to structures that have the same embryonic or evolutionary origin but not necessarily the same function, such as the scrotum and labia majora. Also refers to two chromosomes with identical structures and gene loci but not necessarily identical alleles.
Loose connective tissue	Loose connective tissue or Areolar connective tissue holds organs and epithelia in place, and has a variety of proteinaceous fibers, including collagen and elastin. It is also important in inflammation.
Purkinje cell	A purkinje cell is a class of GABAergic neurons located in the cerebellar cortex. These cells are some of the largest neurons in the brain, with an intricately elaborate dendritic arbor,

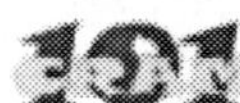

	characterized by a large number of dendritic spines.
Epicardium	Epicardium refers to the visceral portion of the pericardium on the surface of the heart.
Adipose tissue	Adipose tissue is an anatomical term for loose connective tissue composed of adipocytes. Its main role is to store energy in the form of fat, although it also cushions and insulates the body. It has an important endocrine function in producing recently-discovered hormones such as leptin, resistin and TNFalpha.
Serous	The term serous fluid is used for various bodily fluids that are typically pale yellow and transparent, and of a benign nature.
Serous membrane	Membrane that covers internal organs and lines cavities without an opening to the outside of the body is referred to as serous membrane.
Parietal	When speaking of inner organs, visceral means close to or attached to the organ, while parietal is more distant. For example, the visceral pleura is attached to the lung and the parietal pleura is attached to the chest wall.
Septum	A septum, in general, is a wall separating two cavities or two spaces containing a less dense material. The muscle wall that divides the heart chambers.
Cartilage	Cartilage is a type of dense connective tissue. Cartilage is composed of cells called chondrocytes which are dispersed in a firm gel-like ground substance, called the matrix. Cartilage is avascular (contains no blood vessels) and nutrients are diffused through the matrix.
Dense fibrous connective tissue	Dense fibrous connective tissue has collagen fibers as its main matrix element. Crowded between the collagen fibers are rows of fibroblasts, fiber-forming cells, that manufacture the fibers. Dense fibrous connective tissue forms strong, rope-like structures such as tendons and ligaments.
Fibrous connective tissue	Any connective tissue with a preponderance of fiber, such as areolar, reticular, dense regular, and dense irregular connective tissues is referred to as the fibrous connective tissue.
Ventricle	In the heart, a ventricle is a heart chamber which collects blood from an atrium (another heart chamber) and pumps it out of the heart.
Atrioventricular bundle	Atrioventricular bundle refers to group of specialized fibers that conduct impulses from the atrioventricular node to the ventricles of the heart.
Myofibril	Myofibril is a cylindrical organelle, found within muscle cells. They are bundles of filaments that run from one end of the cell to the other and are attached to the cell surface membrane at each end.
Projection	Attributing one's own undesirable thoughts, impulses, traits, or behaviors to others is referred to as projection.
Atrioventricular node	The atrioventricular node is the tissue between the atria and the ventricles of the heart, which conducts the normal electrical impulse from the atria to the ventricles.
Sinoatrial node	Sinoatrial node refers to a small mass of specialized muscle in the wall of the right atrium; generates electrical signals rhythmically and spontaneously and serves as the heart's pacemaker.
Sympathetic division	Sympathetic division refers to one of two sets of neurons in the autonomic nervous system. It generally prepares the body for energy-consuming activities, such as fleeing or fighting. It also is a subdivision of the autonomic nervous system.
Nerve cell	A cell specialized to originate or transmit nerve impulses is referred to as nerve cell.

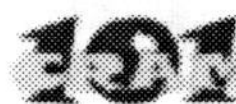

Stress	Stress refers to a condition that is a response to factors that change the human systems normal state.
Parasympathetic division	Parasympathetic division refers to one of two sets of neurons in the autonomic nervous system. It generally promotes body activities that gain and conserve energy, such as digestion and reduced heart rate.
Vagus nerve	The vagus nerve is tenth of twelve paired cranial nerves and is the only nerve that starts in the brainstem and extends all the way down past the head, right down to the abdomen. The vagus nerve is arguably the single most important nerve in the body.
Pain	Pain is an unpleasant sensation which may be associated with actual or potential tissue damage and which may have physical and emotional components.
Free nerve ending	A free nerve ending is an unspecialized, afferent nerve ending, meaning it brings information from the body's periphery to the brain. They are unencapsulated and have no complex sensory structures, unlike those found in Meissner's or Pacinian corpuscles.
Heart attack	A heart attack, is a serious, sudden heart condition usually characterized by varying degrees of chest pain or discomfort, weakness, sweating, nausea, vomiting, and arrhythmias, sometimes causing loss of consciousness. It occurs when the blood supply to a part of the heart is interrupted, causing death and scarring of the local heart tissue.
Angina	Angina pectoris is chest pain due to ischemia (a lack of blood and hence oxygen supply) to the heart muscle, generally due to obstruction or spasm of the coronary arteries (the heart's blood vessels). Coronary artery disease, the main cause of angina, is due to atherosclerosis of the cardiac arteries.
Angina pectoris	Angina pectoris is chest pain due to ischemia (a lack of blood and hence oxygen supply) to the heart muscle, generally due to obstruction or spasm of the coronary arteries (the heart's blood vessels).
Glycogen	Glycogen refers to a complex, extensively branched polysaccharide of many glucose monomers; serves as an energy-storage molecule in liver and muscle cells.
Lymph	Lymph originates as blood plasma lost from the circulatory system, which leaks out into the surrounding tissues. The lymphatic system collects this fluid by diffusion into lymph capillaries, and returns it to the circulatory system.
Jugular vein	The external and internal jugular vein bring deoxygenated blood from the head back to the heart via the superior vena cava.
Subclavian	In general, Subclavian means beneath the clavicle.
Subclavian vein	The subclavian vein is a continuation of the axillary vein and runs from the outer border of the first rib to the medial border of anterior scalene muscle. From here it joins with the internal jugular vein to form the innominate vein, also known as the brachiocephalic vein.
Thoracic duct	The thoracic duct is an important part of the lymphatic system. It is the largest lymphatic vessel in the body. It collects most of the lymph in the body, neck and head, which is collected by the right lymphatic duct) and drains into the systemic (blood) circulation.
Lymphatic circulation	Lymphatic circulation is not closed and has no central pump; the lymph moves slowly and under low pressure due mostly to the milking action of skeletal muscles. Like veins, lymph vessels have one-way valves and depend mainly on the movement of skeletal muscles to squeeze fluid through them.
Neural network	A clusters of neurons that is interconnected to process information is referred to as a neural network.
Lymphocyte	A lymphocyte is a type of white blood cell involved in the human body's immune system. There

are two broad categories, namely T cells and B cells.

Lymphoid organ

Organ other than a lymphatic vessel that is part of the lymphatic system is referred to as a lymphoid organ.

Atrial natriuretic factor

Atrial natriuretic factor is a peptide hormone involved in the homeostatic control of body water and sodium. It is released by atrial monocytes, cells in the atria of the heart, in response to signals of raized blood pressure and acts to reduce this.

Gland

A gland is an organ in an animal's body that synthesizes a substance for release such as hormones, often into the bloodstream or into cavities inside the body or its outer surface.

Salivary gland

The salivary gland produces saliva, which keeps the mouth and other parts of the digestive system moist. It also helps break down carbohydrates and lubricates the passage of food down from the oro-pharynx to the esophagus to the stomach.

Protein

A protein is a complex, high-molecular-weight organic compound that consists of amino acids joined by peptide bonds. They are essential to the structure and function of all living cells and viruses. Many are enzymes or subunits of enzymes.

Regeneration

Regeneration is the ability to restore lost or damaged tissues, organs or limbs. It is a common feature in invertebrates, but far more limited in most vertebrates.

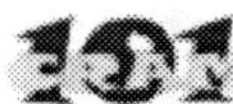

Plasma	Fluid portion of circulating blood is called plasma.
Blood	Blood is a circulating tissue composed of fluid plasma and cells. The main function of blood is to supply nutrients (oxygen, glucose) and constitutional elements to tissues and to remove waste products.
Erythrocyte	Red blood cells are the most common type of blood cell and are the vertebrate body's principal means of delivering oxygen from the lungs or gills to body tissues via the blood. Red blood cells are also known as erythrocyte.
Leukocyte	A white blood cell is a leukocyte. They help to defend the body against infectious disease and foreign materials as part of the immune system.
Platelet	Cell fragment that is necessary to blood clotting is a platelet. They are the blood cell fragments that are involved in the cellular mechanisms that lead to the formation of blood clots.
Circulatory system	The circulatory system or cardiovascular system is the organ system which circulates blood around the body of most animals.
White blood cell	The white blood cell is a a component of blood. They help to defend the body against infectious disease and foreign materials as part of the immune system.
Red blood cells	Red blood cells are the most common type of blood cell and are the vertebrate body's principal means of delivering oxygen from the lungs or gills to body tissues via the blood.
Red blood cell	The red blood cell is the most common type of blood cell and is the vertebrate body's principal means of delivering oxygen from the lungs or gills to body tissues via the blood.
Heparin	Heparin as a drug is used as an injectable anticoagulant. Heparin is a highly sulfated glycosaminoglycan widely used as an injectable anticoagulant. It is also used to form an inner anticoagulant surface on various experimental and medical devices such as test tubes and renal dialysis machines.
Anticoagulant	A biochemical that inhibits blood clotting is referred to as an anticoagulant.
Value	Value is worth in general, and it is thought to be connected to reasons for certain practices, policies, actions, beliefs or emotions. Value is "that which one acts to gain and/or keep."
Buffy coat	Buffy coat is the fraction of a centrifugated blood sample that contains most of the white blood cells. After centrifugation, one can distinguish a layer of clear fluid (the plasma), a layer of red fluid containing most of the red blood cells, and a thin layer in between, the buffy coat, with most of the white blood cells and platelets.
Eye	An eye is an organ that detects light. Different kinds of light-sensitive organs are found in a variety of creatures. The simplest eyes do nothing but detect whether the surroundings are light or dark, while more complex eyes can distinguish shapes and colors.
Capillaries	Capillaries refer to the smallest of the blood vessels and the sites of exchange between the blood and tissue cells.
Capillary	A capillary is the smallest of a body's blood vessels, measuring 5-10 micro meters. They connect arteries and veins, and most closely interact with tissues. Their walls are composed of a single layer of cells, the endothelium. This layer is so thin that molecules such as oxygen, water and lipids can pass through them by diffusion and enter the tissues.
Tissue	A collection of interconnected cells that perform a similar function within an organism is called tissue.
Venule	A vessel that conveys blood between a capillary bed and a vein is a venule.

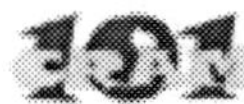

Metabolite | The term metabolite is usually restricted to small molecules. They are the intermediates and products of metabolism. A primary metabolite is directly involved in the normal growth, development, and reproduction. A secondary metabolite is not directly involved in those processes, but usually has important ecological function.

Hormone | A hormone is a chemical messenger from one cell to another. All multicellular organisms produce hormones. The best known hormones are those produced by endocrine glands of vertebrate animals, but hormones are produced by nearly every organ system and tissue type in a human or animal body. Hormone molecules are secreted directly into the bloodstream, they move by circulation or diffusion to their target cells, which may be nearby cells in the same tissue or cells of a distant organ of the body.

Carbon | Carbon is a chemical element in the periodic table that has the symbol C and atomic number 6. An abundant nonmetallic, tetravalent element, carbon has several allotropic forms.

Oxygen | Oxygen is a chemical element in the periodic table. It has the symbol O and atomic number 8. Oxygen is the second most common element on Earth, composing around 46% of the mass of Earth's crust and 28% of the mass of Earth as a whole, and is the third most common element in the universe.

Carbon dioxide | Carbon dioxide is an atmospheric gas comprized of one carbon and two oxygen atoms. A very widely known chemical compound, it is frequently called by its formula CO_2. In its solid state, it is commonly known as dry ice.

Absorption | Absorption is a physical or chemical phenomenon or a process in which atoms, molecules, or ions enter some bulk phase - gas, liquid or solid material. In nutrition, amino acids are broken down through digestion, which begins in the stomach.

Hemoglobin | Hemoglobin is the iron-containing oxygen-transport metalloprotein in the red cells of the blood in mammals and other animals. Hemoglobin transports oxygen from the lungs to the rest of the body, such as to the muscles, where it releases the oxygen load.

Solution | Solution refers to homogenous mixture formed when a solute is dissolved in a solvent.

Protein | A protein is a complex, high-molecular-weight organic compound that consists of amino acids joined by peptide bonds. They are essential to the structure and function of all living cells and viruses. Many are enzymes or subunits of enzymes.

Residue | A residue refers to a portion of a larger molecule, a specific monomer of a polysaccharide, protein or nucleic acid.

Organ | Organ refers to a structure consisting of several tissues adapted as a group to perform specific functions.

Acid | An acid is a water-soluble, sour-tasting chemical compound that when dissolved in water, gives a solution with a pH of less than 7.

Molecular weight | The molecular mass of a substance, called molecular weight and abbreviated as MW, is the mass of one molecule of that substance, relative to the unified atomic mass unit u (equal to 1/12 the mass of one atom of carbon-12).

Lipoprotein | A lipoprotein is a biochemical assembly that contains both proteins and lipids and may be structural or catalytic in function. They may be enzymes, proton pumps, ion pumps, or some combination of these functions.

Amino acid | An amino acid is any molecule that contains both amino and carboxylic acid functional groups. They are the basic structural building units of proteins. They form short polymer chains called peptides or polypeptides which in turn form structures called proteins.

Vitamin | An organic compound other than a carbohydrate, lipid, or protein that is needed for normal

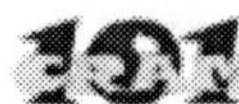

metabolism but that the body cannot synthesize in adequate amounts is called a vitamin.

Salt Salt is a term used for ionic compounds composed of positively charged cations and negatively charged anions, so that the product is neutral and without a net charge.

Organic compound An organic compound is any member of a large class of chemical compounds whose molecules contain carbon, with the exception of carbides, carbonates, carbon oxides and gases containing carbon.

Interstitial fluid Interstitial fluid is one of the two components of extracellular fluid, the other being plasma. On average, a person has about 11 liters of interstitial fluid providing the cells of the body with nutrients and a means of waste removal.

Extracellular fluid Body fluids outside the individual cells are called extracellular fluid.

Extracellular Outside the cell is called extracellular.

Prothrombin Prothrombin refers to plasma protein that is converted to thrombin during the steps of blood clotting. Prothrombin is a blood plasma protein and is synthesized in the liver.

Coagulation The coagulation of blood is a complex process during which blood forms solid clots. It is an important part of haemostasis (the ceszation of blood loss from a damaged vessel) whereby a damaged blood vessel wall is covered by a fibrin clot to stop hemorrhage and aid repair of the damaged vessel.

Albumin Albumin refers generally to any protein with water solubility, which is moderately soluble in concentrated salt solutions, and experiences heat coagulation (protein denaturation).

Inflammation Inflammation is the first response of the immune system to infection or irritation and may be referred to as the innate cascade.

Phagocytosis Phagocytosis (literally, "cell eating") is a form of endocytosis where large particles are enveloped by the cell membrane of a (usually larger) cell and internalized to form a phagosome, or "food vacuole."

Modulation Modulation is the process of varying a carrier signal, typically a sinusoidal signal, in order to use that signal to convey information.

Neutrophil Neutrophil refers to a type of phagocytic leukocyte.

Digestion Digestion refers to the mechanical and chemical breakdown of food into molecules small enough for the body to absorb; the second main stage of food processing, following ingestion.

Antibody An antibody is a protein used by the immune system to identify and neutralize foreign objects like bacteria and viruses. Each antibody recognizes a specific antigen unique to its target.

Bacteria The domain that contains procaryotic cells with primarily diacyl glycerol diesters in their membranes and with bacterial rRNA. Bacteria also is a general term for organisms that are composed of procaryotic cells and are not multicellular.

Lysosome Organelle that contains enzymes that degrade worn cell parts is called a lysosome.

Cancer Cancer is a class of diseases or disorders characterized by uncontrolled division of cells and the ability of these cells to invade other tissues, either by direct growth into adjacent tissue through invasion or by implantation into distant sites by metastasis.

Enzyme An enzyme is a protein that catalyzes, or speeds up, a chemical reaction. They are essential to sustain life because most chemical reactions in biological cells would occur too slowly, or would lead to different products, without them.

Tumor An abnormal mass of cells that forms within otherwise normal tissue is a tumor. This growth

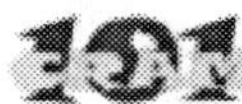

can be either malignant or benign

Virus Obligate intracellular parasite of living cells consisting of an outer capsid and an inner core of nucleic acid is referred to as virus. The term virus usually refers to those particles that infect eukaryotes whilst the term bacteriophage or phage is used to describe those infecting prokaryotes.

Osmotic pressure Osmotic pressure is the pressure produced by a solution in a space that is enclosed by a differentially permeable membrane.

Microscope A microscope is an instrument for viewing objects that are too small to be seen by the naked or unaided eye.

Staining Staining is a biochemical technique of adding a class-specific (DNA, proteins, lipids, carbohydrates) dye to a substrate to qualify or quantify the presence of a specific compound. They are frequently used to highlight structures in tissues for viewing, often with the aid of different microscopes.

Artery Vessel that takes blood away from the heart to the tissues and organs of the body is called an artery.

Gas exchange In humans and other mammals, respiratory gas exchange or ventilation is carried out by mechanisms of the lungs. The actual gas exchange occurs in the alveoli.

Ratio In number and more generally in algebra, a ratio is the linear relationship between two quantities.

Anemia Anemia is a deficiency of red blood cells and/or hemoglobin. This results in a reduced ability of blood to transfer oxygen to the tissues, and this causes hypoxia; since all human cells depend on oxygen for survival, varying degrees of anemia can have a wide range of clinical consequences.

Polycythemia Polycythemia is a condition in which there is a net increase in the total circulating red blood cell mass of the body.

Adaptation A biological adaptation is an anatomical structure, physiological process or behavioral trait of an organism that has evolved over a period of time by the process of natural selection such that it increases the expected long-term reproductive success of the organism.

Metabolism Metabolism is the biochemical modification of chemical compounds in living organisms and cells. This includes the biosynthesis of complex organic molecules (anabolism) and their breakdown (catabolism).

Glucose Glucose, a simple monosaccharide sugar, is one of the most important carbohydrates and is used as a source of energy in animals and plants. Glucose is one of the main products of photosynthesis and starts respiration.

Hexose A hexose is a monosaccharide with six carbon atoms having the chemical formula $C_6H_{12}O_6$.

In vivo In vivo is used to indicate the presence of a whole/living organism, in distinction to a partial or dead organism, or a computer model. Animal testing and clinical trials are forms of in vivo research.

Carbohydrate Carbohydrate is a chemical compound that contains oxygen, hydrogen, and carbon atoms. They consist of monosaccharide sugars of varying chain lengths and that have the general chemical formula $C_n(H_2O)_n$ or are derivatives of such.

Phospholipid Phospholipid is a class of lipids formed from four components: fatty acids, a negatively-charged phosphate group, an alcohol and a backbone. Phospholipids with a glycerol backbone are known as glycerophospholipids or phosphoglycerides.

Cholesterol	Cholesterol is a steroid, a lipid, and an alcohol, found in the cell membranes of all body tissues, and transported in the blood plasma of all animals. It is an important component of the membranes of cells, providing stability; it makes the membrane's fluidity stable over a bigger temperature interval.
Glycolipid	Glycolipid refers to lipid in plasma membranes that bears a carbohydrate chain attached to a hydrophobic tail.
Lipid	Lipid is one class of aliphatic hydrocarbon-containing organic compounds essential for the structure and function of living cells. They are characterized by being water-insoluble but soluble in nonpolar organic solvents.
Membrane protein	A membrane protein is a protein molecule that is attached to, or associated with the membrane of a cell or an organelle. Membrane proteins can be classified into two groups, based on their attachment to the membrane.
Lipid bilayer	A lipid bilayer is a membrane or zone of a membrane composed of lipid molecules (usually phospholipids). The lipid bilayer is a critical component of all biological membranes, including cell membranes, and is a prerequisite for cell-based organisms.
Skeleton	In biology, the skeleton or skeletal system is the biological system providing physical support in living organisms.
Valine	Nutritionally, valine is also an essential amino acid. It is named after the plant valerian. In sickle-cell disease, it substitutes for the hydrophilic amino acid glutamic acid in hemoglobin.
Glutamic acid	Glutamic acid is one of the 20 standard amino acids used by all organisms in their proteins. It is critical for proper cell function, but it is not an essential nutrient in humans because glutamic acid can be manufactured from other compounds.
Life span	Life span refers to the upper boundary of life, the maximum number of years an individual can live. The maximum life span of human beings is about 120 years of age.
Lead	Lead is a chemical element in the periodic table that has the symbol Pb and atomic number 82. A soft, heavy, toxic and malleable poor metal, lead is bluish white when freshly cut but tarnishes to dull gray when exposed to air. Lead is used in building construction, lead-acid batteries, bullets and shot, and is part of solder, pewter, and fusible alloys.
Blood vessel	A blood vessel is a part of the circulatory system and function to transport blood throughout the body. The most important types, arteries and veins, are so termed because they carry blood away from or towards the heart, respectively.
Anoxia	Asphyxia is a condition of severely deficient supply of oxygen to the body. In the absence of remedial action it will very rapidly lead to unconsciousness and death. Anoxia means the pathological state in which tissues do not get (enough of) oxygen. Problems during childbirth can lead to the newborn experiencing asphyxia.
Spleen	The spleen is a ductless, vertebrate gland that is not necessary for life but is closely associated with the circulatory system, where it functions in the destruction of old red blood cells and removal of other debris from the bloodstream, and also in holding a reservoir of blood.
Carbaminohem-globin	Hemoglobin involved in respiration carrying carbon dioxide is referred to as carbaminohemoglobin.
Reversibility	Reversibility according to Piaget, is recognition that processes can be undone, that things can be made as they were.
Bone marrow	Bone marrow is the tissue comprising the center of large bones. It is the place where new

	blood cells are produced. Bone marrow contains two types of stem cells: hemopoietic (which can produce blood cells) and stromal (which can produce fat, cartilage and bone).
Hemorrhage	Loss of blood from the circulatory system is referred to as a hemorrhage.
Iron	Iron is essential to all organisms, except for a few bacteria. It is mostly stably incorporated in the inside of metalloproteins, because in exposed or in free form it causes production of free radicals that are generally toxic to cells.
Cytoplasm	Cytoplasm refers to the contents of a cell excluding the nucleus and cell membrane. Cytoplasm is a homogeneous, generally clear jelly-like material that fills cells.
Mitochondria	Cytoplasmic organelles responsible for ATP generation for cellular activities are referred to as mitochondria.
Organelle	Organelle refers to any structure within a cell that carries out one of its metabolic roles, such as mitochondria, centrioles, endoplasmic reticulum, and the nucleus.
Complex oligosaccharide	Complex oligosaccharide refers to a chain of sugars attached to a glycoprotein that is generated by trimming of the original oligosaccharide attached in the endoplasmic reticulum and subsequent addition of further sugars.
Oligosaccharide	An oligosaccharide is a saccharide polymer containing a small number (typically three to six) of component sugars, also known as simple sugars. They are generally found either O- or N-linked to compatible amino acid side chains in proteins or to lipid moieties.
Apoptosis	In biology, apoptosis is one of the main types of programmed cell death (PCD). As such, it is a process of deliberate life relinquishment by an unwanted cell in a multicellular organism.
DNA	Deoxyribonucleic acid (DNA) is a nucleic acid —usually in the form of a double helix— that contains the genetic instructions specifying the biological development of all cellular forms of life, and most viruses.
Polymorphonulear leukocyte	Polymorphonuclear leukocyte refers to a leukocyte that has a variety of nuclear forms.
Blood plasma	Blood plasma is the liquid component of blood, in which the blood cells are suspended. Serum is the same as blood plasma except that clotting factors (such as fibrin) have been removed.
Granulocytes	Granulocytes are a category of white blood cells, characterised by the fact that all types have differently staining granules in their cytoplasm on light microscopy. They are also called polymorphonuclear leukocytes (PMN or PML) because of the varying shapes of the nucleus, which is usually lobed into three segments.
Granulocyte	Granulocyte is a category of white blood cells, characterized by the fact that all types have differently staining granules in their cytoplasm on light microscopy.
Polymorphonulear	Cells with nuclei having several parts or lobes are called polymorphonuclear.
Inflammatory response	Inflammatory response refers to a complex sequence of events involving chemicals and immune cells that results in the isolation and destruction of antigens and tissues near the antigens.
Substrate	A substrate is a molecule which is acted upon by an enzyme. Each enzyme recognizes only the specific substrate of the reaction it catalyzes. A surface in or on which an organism lives.
Connective tissue	Connective tissue is any type of biological tissue with an extensive extracellular matrix and often serves to support, bind together, and protect organs.
Endothelial cell	A endothelial cell also controls the passage of materials — and the transit of white blood cells — into and out of the bloodstream. In some organs, there are highly differentiated

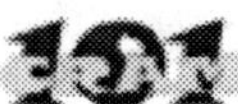

	endothelial cells to perform specialized 'filtering' functions.
Monocyte	A monocyte is a leukocyte, part of the human body's immune system that protect against blood-borne pathogens and move quickly to sites of infection in the tissues.
Microorganism	A microorganism or microbe is an organism that is so small that it is microscopic (invisible to the naked eye).
Chemotaxis	Chemotaxis is the phenomenon in which bodily cells, bacteria, and other single-celled or multicellular organisms direct their movements according to certain chemicals in their environment.
Lymphocyte	A lymphocyte is a type of white blood cell involved in the human body's immune system. There are two broad categories, namely T cells and B cells.
Phosphatase	A phosphatase is an enzyme that hydrolyses phosphoric acid monoesters into a phosphate ion and a molecule with a free hydroxyl group.
Lysozyme	Lysozyme is an enzyme (EC 3.2.1.17), commonly referred to as the "body's own antibiotic" since it kills bacteria. It is abundantly present in a number of secretions, such as tears (except bovine tears).
Myeloperoxidase	Myeloperoxidase is a peroxidase enzyme (EC 1.11.1.7) most abundantly present in neutrophil granulocytes (a subtype of white blood cells). It is a lysosomal protein stored in azurophilic granules of the neutrophil.
Population	Population refers to all members of a well-defined group of organisms, events, or things.
Light microscope	An optical instrument with lenses that refract visible light to magnify images and project them into a viewer's eye or onto photographic film is referred to as light microscope.
Glycogen	Glycogen refers to a complex, extensively branched polysaccharide of many glucose monomers; serves as an energy-storage molecule in liver and muscle cells.
Oxidation	Oxidation refers to the loss of electrons from a substance involved in a redox reaction; always accompanies reduction.
Citric acid cycle	In aerobic organisms, the citric acid cycle is a metabolic pathway that forms part of the break down of carbohydrates, fats and proteins into carbon dioxide and water in order to generate energy. It is the second of three metabolic pathways that are involved in fuel molecule catabolism and ATP production, the other two being glycolysis and oxidative phosphorylation.
Collagen	Collagen is the main protein of connective tissue in animals and the most abundant protein in mammals, making up about 1/4 of the total. It is one of the long, fibrous structural proteins whose functions are quite different from those of globular proteins such as enzymes.
Vacuole	Vacuole refers to a space or cavity within the cytoplasm of a cell.
Alkaline phosphatase	Alkaline phosphatase (ALP) (EC 3.1.3.1) is a hydrolase enzyme responsible for removing phosphate groups in the 5- and 3- positions from many types of molecules, including nucleotides, proteins, and alkaloids.
Hydrogen	Hydrogen is a chemical element in the periodic table that has the symbol H and atomic number 1. At standard temperature and pressure it is a colorless, odorless, nonmetallic, univalent, tasteless, highly flammable diatomic gas.
Anion	A negatively-charged ion, which has more electrons in its electron shell than it has protons in its nucleus, is known as an anion, for it is attracted to anodes; a positively-charged ion, which has fewer electrons than protons, is known as a cation, for it is attracted to cathodes.

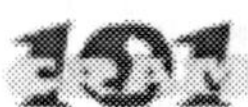

Hydrogen peroxide	Hydrogen peroxide is a clear liquid, slightly more viscous than water, that has strong oxidizing properties and is therefore a powerful bleaching agent that has found use as a disinfectant, as an oxidizer, and in rocketry (particularly in high concentrations as high-test peroxide (HTP) as a monopropellant, and in bipropellant systems.
Halide	A halide is a binary compound, of which one part is a halogen atom and the other part is an element or radical that is less electronegative than the halogen, to make a fluoride, chloride, bromide, iodide, or astatide compound. Many salts are halides.
Ion	Ion refers to an atom or molecule that has gained or lost one or more electrons, thus acquiring an electrical charge.
Cell wall	A cell wall is a more or less solid layer surrounding a cell. They are found in bacteria, archaea, fungi, plants, and algae.
Peptidoglycan	Peptidoglycan, also known as murein, is a substance that forms a homogeneous layer lying outside the plasma membrane in bacteria.
Actin	A protein in a muscle fiber that, together with myosin, is responsible for contraction and relaxation is actin.
Infection	The invasion and multiplication of microorganisms in body tissues is called an infection.
Arginine	Arginine is an α-amino acid. The L-form is one of the 20 most common natural amino acids. In mammals, arginine is classified as a semiessential or conditionally essential amino acid, depending on the developmental stage and health status of the individual.
Variable	A characteristic or aspect in which people, objects, events, or conditions vary is called variable.
Vagina	The vagina is the tubular tract leading from the uterus to the exterior of the body in female placental mammals and marsupials, or to the cloaca in female birds, monotremes, and some reptiles. Female insects and other invertebrates also have a vagina, which is the terminal part of the oviduct.
Uterus	The uterus is the major female reproductive organ of most mammals. One end, the cervix, opens into the vagina; the other is connected on both sides to the fallopian tubes. The main function is to accept a fertilized ovum which becomes implanted into the endometrium, and derives nourishment from blood vessels which develop exclusively for this purpose.
Gastrointest-nal tract	The gastrointestinal tract is the system of organs within multicellular animals which takes in food, digests it to extract energy and nutrients, and expels the remaining waste.
Antigen	An antigen is a substance that stimulates an immune response, especially the production of antibodies. They are usually proteins or polysaccharides, but can be any type of molecule, including small molecules (haptens) coupled to a protein (carrier).
Adrenal	In mammals, the adrenal glands are the triangle-shaped endocrine glands that sit atop the kidneys. They are chiefly responsible for regulating the stress response through the synthesis of corticosteroids and catecholamines, including cortisol and adrenaline.
Cortex	In anatomy and zoology the cortex is the outermost or superficial layer of an organ or the outer portion of the stem or root of a plant.
Corticosteroid	Any steroid hormone secreted by the adrenal cortex, such as aldosterone, cortisol, and sex steroids is called a corticosteroid.
Adrenal cortex	Situated along the perimeter of the adrenal gland, the adrenal cortex mediates the stress response through the production of mineralocorticoids and glucocorticoids, including aldosterone and cortisol respectively. It is also a secondary site of androgen synthesis.

Hypersensitivity	Hypersensitivity is an immune response that damages the body's own tissues. Four or five types of hypersensitivity are often described; immediate, antibody-dependent, immune complex, cell-mediated, and stimulatory.
Nucleolus	A small structure within the nucleus of a cell that contains RNA and protein is referred to as nucleolus. It is where ribonucleoprotein is formed.
Kidney	The kidney is a bean-shaped excretory organ in vertebrates. Part of the urinary system, the kidneys filter wastes (especially urea) from the blood and excrete them, along with water, as urine.
Distribution	Distribution in pharmacology is a branch of pharmacokinetics describing reversible transfer of drug from one location to another within the body.
Vesicle	Membranous, cytoplasmic sac formed by an infolding of the cell membrane is called a vesicle.
Blood clotting	A complex process by which platelets, the protein fibrin, and red blood cells block an irregular surface in or on the body, such as a damaged blood vessel, sealing the wound is referred to as blood clotting.
Invagination	Infolding of one part of a structure into another is invagination.
Channel	Channel, in communications (sometimes called communications channel), refers to the medium used to convey information from a sender (or transmitter) to a receiver.
Plasma membrane	The unit membrane that encloses a cell and controls the traffic of molecules in and out of the cell is the plasma membrane.
Microtubule	A hollow rod of the protein tubulin in the cytoplasm is referred to as the microtubule.
Glycosaminoglycan	Glycosaminoglycan is a long unbranched polysaccharide, made up of repeating disaccharides that may be sulphated (e.g. glucuronic acid, iduronic acid, galactose, galactosamine, glucosamine).
Serotonin	Serotonin is a monoamine neurotransmitter synthesized in serotonergic neurons in the central nervous system and enterochromaffin cells in the gastrointestinal tract. It is believed to play an important part of the biochemistry of depression, migraine, bipolar disorder and anxiety.
Adenosine	Adenosine is a nucleoside comprized of adenine attached to a ribose (ribofuranose) moiety via a β-N_9-glycosidic bond. Adenosine plays an important role in biochemical processes, such as energy transfer - as adenosine triphosphate (ATP) and adenosine diphosphate (ADP) - as well as in signal transduction as cyclic adenosine monophosphate, cAMP.
Calcium	Calcium is the chemical element in the periodic table that has the symbol Ca and atomic number 20. Calcium is a soft grey alkaline earth metal that is used as a reducing agent in the extraction of thorium, zirconium and uranium. Calcium is also the fifth most abundant element in the Earth's crust.
Adenosine diphosphate	Adenosine diphosphate refers to a molecule composed of the sugar ribose, the base adenine, and two phosphate groups; a component of ATP.
Endothelium	The endothelium is the layer of thin, flat cells that lines the interior surface of blood vessels, forming an interface between circulating blood in the lumen and the rest of the vessel wall.
Blood clot	A blood clot is the final product of the blood coagulation step in hemostasis. It is achieved via the aggregation of platelets that form a platelet plug, and the activation of the humoral coagulation system
Thrombus	Blood clot that remains in the blood vessel where it formed is called a thrombus.

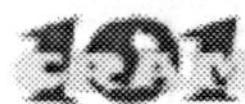

Fibrin	Fibrin is a protein involved in the clotting of blood. It is a fibrillar protein that is polymerized to form a "mesh" that forms a haemostatic plug or clot (in conjunction with platelets) over a wound site.
Fiber	Fibers used by man come from a wide variety of sources: Natural fiber include those made out of plants, animal and mineral sources. Natural fibers can be classified according to their origin.
Activation	As reflected by facial expressions, the degree of arousal a person is experiencing is referred to as activation.
Activator	Activator (proteomics), is a type of effector that increases the rate of enzyme mediated reactions.
Plasmin	Plasmin is an important degrading enzyme of many proteins of blood plasma but specifically of fibrin clots. This process is termed fibrinolysis.
Hemophilia	Hemophilia is the name of any of several hereditary genetic illnesses that impair the body's ability to control bleeding. Genetic deficiencies cause lowered plasma clotting factor activity so as to compromise blood-clotting; when a blood vessel is injured, a scab will not form and the vessel can continue to bleed excessively for a very long period of time.
Skin	Skin is an organ of the integumentary system composed of a layer of tissues that protect underlying muscles and organs.
Body cavity	A fluid-containing space between the digestive tract and the body wall is referred to as body cavity.
Joint	A joint (articulation) is the location at which two bones make contact (articulate). They are constructed to both allow movement and provide mechanical support.
Recessive gene	Recessive gene refers to a gene that will not be expressed if paired with a dominant gene but will be expressed if paired with another recessive gene.
Chromosomes	Physical structures in the cell's nucleus that house the genes. Each human cell has 23 pairs of chromosomes.
Allergy	An allergy or Type I hypersensitivity is an immune malfunction whereby a person's body is hypersensitized to react immunologically to typically nonimmunogenic substances. When a person is hypersensitized, these substances are known as allergens.

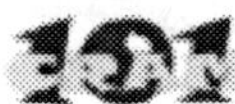

Organ	Organ refers to a structure consisting of several tissues adapted as a group to perform specific functions.
Blood	Blood is a circulating tissue composed of fluid plasma and cells. The main function of blood is to supply nutrients (oxygen, glucose) and constitutional elements to tissues and to remove waste products.
Yolk sac	The yolk sac is the first element seen in the gestational sac during pregnancy, usually at 5 weeks gestation. It is filled with fluid, the vitelline fluid, which possibly may be utilized for the nourishment of the embryo during the earlier stages of its existence.
Mesoderm	Mesoderm forms in the embryos of animals more complex than cnidarians. Some of the cells migrating inward to form the endoderm form an additional layer between the other two. It gives rise to muscles, bones, the dermis of the skin, and most other organs in the adult.
Yolk	Dense nutrient material that is present in the egg of a bird or reptile is referred to as yolk.
Embryogenesis	Embryogenesis is the process by which the embryo is formed and develops. It starts with the fertilization of the ovum, which is then called a zygote.
Bone marrow	Bone marrow is the tissue comprising the center of large bones. It is the place where new blood cells are produced. Bone marrow contains two types of stem cells: hemopoietic (which can produce blood cells) and stromal (which can produce fat, cartilage and bone).
Clavicle	In human anatomy, the clavicle or collar bone is a bone that makes up part of the shoulder girdle (pectoral girdle). It is a doubly-curved long bone that connects the arm (upper limb) to the body (trunk), located directly above the first rib.
Tissue	A collection of interconnected cells that perform a similar function within an organism is called tissue.
Spleen	The spleen is a ductless, vertebrate gland that is not necessary for life but is closely associated with the circulatory system, where it functions in the destruction of old red blood cells and removal of other debris from the bloodstream, and also in holding a reservoir of blood.
Liver	The liver is an organ in vertebrates, including humans. It plays a major role in metabolism and has a number of functions in the body including drug detoxification, glycogen storage, and plasma protein synthesis. It also produces bile, which is important for digestion.
Ossification	Ossification is the process of bone formation, in which connective tissues, such as cartilage are turned to bone or bone-like tissue.
Skeleton	In biology, the skeleton or skeletal system is the biological system providing physical support in living organisms.
Erythrocyte	Red blood cells are the most common type of blood cell and are the vertebrate body's principal means of delivering oxygen from the lungs or gills to body tissues via the blood. Red blood cells are also known as erythrocyte.
Leukocyte	A white blood cell is a leukocyte. They help to defend the body against infectious disease and foreign materials as part of the immune system.
Monocyte	A monocyte is a leukocyte, part of the human body's immune system that protect against blood-borne pathogens and move quickly to sites of infection in the tissues.
Platelet	Cell fragment that is necessary to blood clotting is a platelet. They are the blood cell fragments that are involved in the cellular mechanisms that lead to the formation of blood clots.

Constant	A behavior or characteristic that does not vary from one observation to another is referred to as a constant.
Fluorescence	Fluorescence is a luminescence that is mostly found as an optical phenomenon in cold bodies, in which the molecular absorption of a photon triggers the emission of a lower-energy photon with a longer wavelength. The energy difference between the absorbed and emitted photons ends up as molecular vibrations or heat.
Antibody	An antibody is a protein used by the immune system to identify and neutralize foreign objects like bacteria and viruses. Each antibody recognizes a specific antigen unique to its target.
Antigen	An antigen is a substance that stimulates an immune response, especially the production of antibodies. They are usually proteins or polysaccharides, but can be any type of molecule, including small molecules (haptens) coupled to a protein (carrier).
In vitro	In vitro is an experimental technique where the experiment is performed in a test tube, or generally outside a living organism or cell.
In vivo	In vivo is used to indicate the presence of a whole/living organism, in distinction to a partial or dead organism, or a computer model. Animal testing and clinical trials are forms of in vivo research.
Donor	Blood donation is a process by which a blood donor voluntarily has blood drawn for storage in a blood bank for subsequent use in a blood transfusion.
Culture	Culture, generally refers to patterns of human activity and the symbolic structures that give such activity significance.
Granulocytes	Granulocytes are a category of white blood cells, characterised by the fact that all types have differently staining granules in their cytoplasm on light microscopy. They are also called polymorphonuclear leukocytes (PMN or PML) because of the varying shapes of the nucleus, which is usually lobed into three segments.
Granulocyte	Granulocyte is a category of white blood cells, characterized by the fact that all types have differently staining granules in their cytoplasm on light microscopy.
Lymphocyte	A lymphocyte is a type of white blood cell involved in the human body's immune system. There are two broad categories, namely T cells and B cells.
Lymph node	A lymph node acts as a filter, with an internal honeycomb of connective tissue filled with lymphocytes that collect and destroy bacteria and viruses. When the body is fighting an infection, these lymphocytes multiply rapidly and produce a characteristic swelling of the lymph node.
Thymus	The thymus is a ductless gland located in the upper anterior portion of the chest cavity. It is most active during puberty, after which it shrinks in size and activity in most individuals and is replaced with fat. The thymus plays an important role in the development of the immune system.
Lymph	Lymph originates as blood plasma lost from the circulatory system, which leaks out into the surrounding tissues. The lymphatic system collects this fluid by diffusion into lymph capillaries, and returns it to the circulatory system.
Population	Population refers to all members of a well-defined group of organisms, events, or things.
Cell division	Cell division (or local doubling) is the process by which a cell, called the parent cell divides into two cells, called daughter cells. Cell division is usually a small segment of a larger cell cycle.
Red blood cells	Red blood cells are the most common type of blood cell and are the vertebrate body's principal means of delivering oxygen from the lungs or gills to body tissues via the blood.

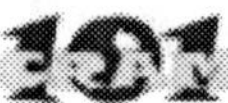

Red blood cell	The red blood cell is the most common type of blood cell and is the vertebrate body's principal means of delivering oxygen from the lungs or gills to body tissues via the blood.
Lymphoid organ	Organ other than a lymphatic vessel that is part of the lymphatic system is referred to as a lymphoid organ.
Extracellular	Outside the cell is called extracellular.
Isolation	Isolation refers to the degree to which groups do not live in the same communities.
Genes	Genes are the units of heredity in living organisms. They are encoded in the organism's genetic material (usually DNA or RNA), and control the development and behavior of the organism.
Chemotherapy	Chemotherapy is the use of chemical substances to treat disease. In its modern-day use, it refers almost exclusively to cytostatic drugs used to treat cancer.In its non-oncological use, the term may also refer to antibiotics.
Irradiation	A process in which radiation energy is applied to foods, creating compounds within the food that destroy cell membranes, break down DNA, link proteins together, limit enzyme activity, and alter a variety of other proteins and cell functions is referred to as irradiation.
Host	Host is an organism that harbors a parasite, mutual partner, or commensal partner; or a cell infected by a virus.
Suppression	Suppression is the defense mechanism where a memory is deliberately forgotten.
Bone marrow transplantation	Bone marrow transplantation (BMT) or hematopoietic stem cell transplantation (HSCT) is a medical procedure in the field of hematology and oncology that involves transplantation of hematopoietic stem cells (HSC).
Leukemia	Leukemia refers to a type of cancer of the bloodforming tissues, characterized by an excessive production of white blood cells and an abnormally high number of them in the blood; cancer of the bone marrow cells that produce leukocytes.
Anemia	Anemia is a deficiency of red blood cells and/or hemoglobin. This results in a reduced ability of blood to transfer oxygen to the tissues, and this causes hypoxia; since all human cells depend on oxygen for survival, varying degrees of anemia can have a wide range of clinical consequences.
Aplastic anemia	Aplastic anemia is a condition where the bone marrow does not produce enough, or any, new cells to replenish the blood cells.
Cancellous	Cancellous bone is a spongy type of bone with a very high surface area, found at the ends of long bones. The spongy bone contains red bone marrow which leads to the production of red blood cells.
Yellow bone marrow	Yellow bone marrow refers to a tissue found within the central cavities of long bones in adults, consisting mostly of stored fat.
Hypoxia	Hypoxia is a pathological condition in which the body as a whole or region of the body is deprived of adequate oxygen supply.
Red bone marrow	A connective tissue located within spongy bone that contains the stem cells and their differentiated forms involved in blood cell formation is red bone marrow.
Endothelium	The endothelium is the layer of thin, flat cells that lines the interior surface of blood vessels, forming an interface between circulating blood in the lumen and the rest of the vessel wall.
Cortex	In anatomy and zoology the cortex is the outermost or superficial layer of an organ or the outer portion of the stem or root of a plant.

Renal	Pertaining to the kidney is referred to as renal.
Interstitial cell	An interstitial cell are those present in the ovary, which secrete androgens.
Distribution	Distribution in pharmacology is a branch of pharmacokinetics describing reversible transfer of drug from one location to another within the body.
Anatomy	Anatomy is the branch of biology that deals with the structure and organization of living things. It can be divided into animal anatomy (zootomy) and plant anatomy (phytonomy).
Capillaries	Capillaries refer to the smallest of the blood vessels and the sites of exchange between the blood and tissue cells.
Capillary	A capillary is the smallest of a body's blood vessels, measuring 5-10 micro meters. They connect arteries and veins, and most closely interact with tissues. Their walls are composed of a single layer of cells, the endothelium. This layer is so thin that molecules such as oxygen, water and lipids can pass through them by diffusion and enter the tissues.
Fiber	Fibers used by man come from a wide variety of sources: Natural fiber include those made out of plants, animal and mineral sources. Natural fibers can be classified according to their origin.
Proteoglycan	Molecule consisting of one or more glycosaminoglycan chains attached to a core protein is referred to as proteoglycan.
Fibronectin	Fibronectin is a high molecular weight glycoprotein containing about 5% carbohydrate that bind to receptor proteins spanning the cell membrane called integrins. In addition to integrins, they also bind extracellular matrix components such as collagen, fibrin and heparin.
Collagen	Collagen is the main protein of connective tissue in animals and the most abundant protein in mammals, making up about 1/4 of the total. It is one of the long, fibrous structural proteins whose functions are quite different from those of globular proteins such as enzymes.
Laminin	Laminin is a family of heterotrimeric glycoproteins found in the basal lamina underlying epithelia. Their binding to type IV collagen contributes to the self-assembly of the basal lamina from components secreted by cells, and their recognition by growth cone integrins is important to the function of the basal lamina.
Receptor	A receptor is a protein on the cell membrane or within the cytoplasm or cell nucleus that binds to a specific molecule (a ligand), such as a neurotransmitter, hormone, or other substance, and initiates the cellular response to the ligand. Receptor, in immunology, the region of an antibody which shows recognition of an antigen.
Endothelial cell	A endothelial cell also controls the passage of materials — and the transit of white blood cells — into and out of the bloodstream. In some organs, there are highly differentiated endothelial cells to perform specialized 'filtering' functions.
Complement	Complement is a group of proteins of the complement system, found in blood serum which act in concert with antibodies to achieve the destruction of non-self particles such as foreign blood cells or bacteria.
Androgen	Androgen is the generic term for any natural or synthetic compound, usually a steroid hormone, that stimulates or controls the development and maintenance of masculine characteristics in vertebrates by binding to androgen receptors.
Protein	A protein is a complex, high-molecular-weight organic compound that consists of amino acids joined by peptide bonds. They are essential to the structure and function of all living cells and viruses. Many are enzymes or subunits of enzymes.

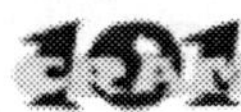

Hormone	A hormone is a chemical messenger from one cell to another. All multicellular organisms produce hormones. The best known hormones are those produced by endocrine glands of vertebrate animals, but hormones are produced by nearly every organ system and tissue type in a human or animal body. Hormone molecules are secreted directly into the bloodstream, they move by circulation or diffusion to their target cells, which may be nearby cells in the same tissue or cells of a distant organ of the body.
Toxin	Toxin refers to a microbial product or component that can injure another cell or organism at low concentrations. Often the term refers to a poisonous protein, but toxins may be lipids and other substances.
Glucocorticoid	Glucocorticoid is a class of steroid hormones characterized by the ability to bind with the cortisol receptor and trigger similar effects. They are distinguished from mineralocorticoids and sex steroids by the specific receptors, target cells, and effects.
Hemoglobin	Hemoglobin is the iron-containing oxygen-transport metalloprotein in the red cells of the blood in mammals and other animals. Hemoglobin transports oxygen from the lungs to the rest of the body, such as to the muscles, where it releases the oxygen load.
Iron	Iron is essential to all organisms, except for a few bacteria. It is mostly stably incorporated in the inside of metalloproteins, because in exposed or in free form it causes production of free radicals that are generally toxic to cells.
Motility	Motility is the ability to move spontaneously and independently. The term can apply to single cells, or to multicellular organisms.
Microscope	A microscope is an instrument for viewing objects that are too small to be seen by the naked or unaided eye.
Light microscope	An optical instrument with lenses that refract visible light to magnify images and project them into a viewer's eye or onto photographic film is referred to as light microscope.
Cytoplasm	Cytoplasm refers to the contents of a cell excluding the nucleus and cell membrane. Cytoplasm is a homogeneous, generally clear jelly-like material that fills cells.
Mitochondria	Cytoplasmic organelles responsible for ATP generation for cellular activities are referred to as mitochondria.
Organelle	Organelle refers to any structure within a cell that carries out one of its metabolic roles, such as mitochondria, centrioles, endoplasmic reticulum, and the nucleus.
Folic acid	Folic acid and folate (the anion form) are forms of a water-soluble B vitamin. These occur naturally in food and can also be taken as supplements.
Vitamin	An organic compound other than a carbohydrate, lipid, or protein that is needed for normal metabolism but that the body cannot synthesize in adequate amounts is called a vitamin.
Acid	An acid is a water-soluble, sour-tasting chemical compound that when dissolved in water, gives a solution with a pH of less than 7.
Erythropoietin	Erythropoietin is a glycoprotein hormone that is a growth factor for erythrocyte (red blood cell) precursors in the bone marrow. It increases the number of red blood cells in the blood.
Nucleolus	A small structure within the nucleus of a cell that contains RNA and protein is referred to as nucleolus. It is where ribonucleoprotein is formed.
Staining	Staining is a biochemical technique of adding a class-specific (DNA, proteins, lipids, carbohydrates) dye to a substrate to qualify or quantify the presence of a specific compound. They are frequently used to highlight structures in tissues for viewing, often with the aid of different microscopes.

Protrusion	Protrusion is the anterior movement of an object. This term is often applied to the jaw.
Neutrophil	Neutrophil refers to a type of phagocytic leukocyte.
Condensation	Combining several people, objects, or events into a single dream image is referred to as condensation.
Inflammation	Inflammation is the first response of the immune system to infection or irritation and may be referred to as the innate cascade.
Infection	The invasion and multiplication of microorganisms in body tissues is called an infection.
Buffer	A chemical substance that resists changes in pH by accepting H^+ ions from or donating H^+ ions to solutions is called a buffer.
Blood vessel	A blood vessel is a part of the circulatory system and function to transport blood throughout the body. The most important types, arteries and veins, are so termed because they carry blood away from or towards the heart, respectively.
Plasma	Fluid portion of circulating blood is called plasma.
Venule	A vessel that conveys blood between a capillary bed and a vein is a venule.
Connective tissue	Connective tissue is any type of biological tissue with an extensive extracellular matrix and often serves to support, bind together, and protect organs.
Phagocytosis	Phagocytosis (literally, "cell eating") is a form of endocytosis where large particles are enveloped by the cell membrane of a (usually larger) cell and internalized to form a phagosome, or "food vacuole."
Apoptosis	In biology, apoptosis is one of the main types of programmed cell death (PCD). As such, it is a process of deliberate life relinquishment by an unwanted cell in a multicellular organism.
Epinephrine	Epinephrine is a hormone and a neurotransmitter. Epinephrine plays a central role in the short-term stress reaction—the physiological response to threatening or exciting conditions (fight-or-flight response). It is secreted by the adrenal medulla.
Course	Pattern of development and change of a disorder over time is a course.
Peripheral lymphoid organ	Peripheral lymphoid organ refers to lymphoid organ in which T cells and B cells interact with foreign antigens. Examples are spleen, lymph nodes, and mucosal-associated lymphoid tissue.
Tonsils	The tonsils are areas of lymphoid tissue on either side of the throat. As with other organs of the lymphatic system, the tonsils act as part of the immune system to help protect against infection.
Tonsil	Tonsil refers to a patch of lymphatic tissue consisting of connective tissue that contains many lymphocytes; located in the pharynx and throat.
Aspiration	In medicine, aspiration is the entry of secretions or foreign material into the trachea and lungs.
Compact bone	Type of bone that contains osteons consisting of concentric layers of matrix and osteocytes in lacunae is called compact bone. It forms the stout walls of the diaphysis of long bones and a thin wall of the epiphysis of long bones
Sternum	Sternum or breastbone is a long, flat bone located in the center of the thorax (chest). It connects to the rib bones via cartilage, forming the rib cage with them, and thus helps to protect the lungs and heart from physical trauma.
Diagnosis	In medicine, diagnosis is the process of identifying a medical condition or disease by its signs, symptoms, and from the results of various diagnostic procedures.

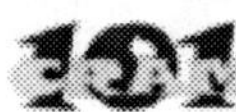

Monoclonal antibodies	Monoclonal antibodies are antibodies that are identical because they were produced by one type of immune cell, all clones of a single parent cell.
Kidney	The kidney is a bean-shaped excretory organ in vertebrates. Part of the urinary system, the kidneys filter wastes (especially urea) from the blood and excrete them, along with water, as urine.
DNA	Deoxyribonucleic acid (DNA) is a nucleic acid —usually in the form of a double helix— that contains the genetic instructions specifying the biological development of all cellular forms of life, and most viruses.
Invagination	Infolding of one part of a structure into another is invagination.
Coagulation	The coagulation of blood is a complex process during which blood forms solid clots. It is an important part of haemostasis (the ceszation of blood loss from a damaged vessel) whereby a damaged blood vessel wall is covered by a fibrin clot to stop hemorrhage and aid repair of the damaged vessel.
Plasma membrane	The unit membrane that encloses a cell and controls the traffic of molecules in and out of the cell is the plasma membrane.
Life span	Life span refers to the upper boundary of life, the maximum number of years an individual can live. The maximum life span of human beings is about 120 years of age.
Micrograph	A micrograph is a photograph or similar image taken through a microscope or similar device to show a magnified image of an item.
Pathology	Pathology is the study of the processes underlying disease and other forms of illness, harmful abnormality, or dysfunction.

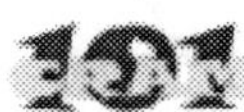

Bone marrow	Bone marrow is the tissue comprising the center of large bones. It is the place where new blood cells are produced. Bone marrow contains two types of stem cells: hemopoietic (which can produce blood cells) and stromal (which can produce fat, cartilage and bone).
Lymph node	A lymph node acts as a filter, with an internal honeycomb of connective tissue filled with lymphocytes that collect and destroy bacteria and viruses. When the body is fighting an infection, these lymphocytes multiply rapidly and produce a characteristic swelling of the lymph node.
Tissue	A collection of interconnected cells that perform a similar function within an organism is called tissue.
Thymus	The thymus is a ductless gland located in the upper anterior portion of the chest cavity. It is most active during puberty, after which it shrinks in size and activity in most individuals and is replaced with fat. The thymus plays an important role in the development of the immune system.
Spleen	The spleen is a ductless, vertebrate gland that is not necessary for life but is closely associated with the circulatory system, where it functions in the destruction of old red blood cells and removal of other debris from the bloodstream, and also in holding a reservoir of blood.
Organ	Organ refers to a structure consisting of several tissues adapted as a group to perform specific functions.
Lymph	Lymph originates as blood plasma lost from the circulatory system, which leaks out into the surrounding tissues. The lymphatic system collects this fluid by diffusion into lymph capillaries, and returns it to the circulatory system.
Blood	Blood is a circulating tissue composed of fluid plasma and cells. The main function of blood is to supply nutrients (oxygen, glucose) and constitutional elements to tissues and to remove waste products.
Connective tissue	Connective tissue is any type of biological tissue with an extensive extracellular matrix and often serves to support, bind together, and protect organs.
Lymphoid organ	Organ other than a lymphatic vessel that is part of the lymphatic system is referred to as a lymphoid organ.
Immune system	The immune system is the system of specialized cells and organs that protect an organism from outside biological influences. When the immune system is functioning properly, it protects the body against bacteria and viral infections, destroying cancer cells and foreign substances.
Distribution	Distribution in pharmacology is a branch of pharmacokinetics describing reversible transfer of drug from one location to another within the body.
Lymphocyte	A lymphocyte is a type of white blood cell involved in the human body's immune system. There are two broad categories, namely T cells and B cells.
Constant	A behavior or characteristic that does not vary from one observation to another is referred to as a constant.
Antigen	An antigen is a substance that stimulates an immune response, especially the production of antibodies. They are usually proteins or polysaccharides, but can be any type of molecule, including small molecules (haptens) coupled to a protein (carrier).
Bacteria	The domain that contains procaryotic cells with primarily diacyl glycerol diesters in their membranes and with bacterial rRNA. Bacteria also is a general term for organisms that are composed of procaryotic cells and are not multicellular.

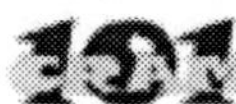

Protein	A protein is a complex, high-molecular-weight organic compound that consists of amino acids joined by peptide bonds. They are essential to the structure and function of all living cells and viruses. Many are enzymes or subunits of enzymes.
Epitope	An epitope is the part of a foreign organism or its proteins that is being recognized by the immune system and targeted by antibodies, cytotoxic T cells or both.
Tumor	An abnormal mass of cells that forms within otherwise normal tissue is a tumor. This growth can be either malignant or benign
Virus	Obligate intracellular parasite of living cells consisting of an outer capsid and an inner core of nucleic acid is referred to as virus. The term virus usually refers to those particles that infect eukaryotes whilst the term bacteriophage or phage is used to describe those infecting prokaryotes.
Antigenic determinant	The specific part of an antigen that stimulates an immune system response by binding to receptors on the surface of lymphocytes is referred to as an antigenic determinant.
Polysaccharide	A carbohydrate composed of many joined monosaccharides is called a polysaccharide.
Antibody	An antibody is a protein used by the immune system to identify and neutralize foreign objects like bacteria and viruses. Each antibody recognizes a specific antigen unique to its target.
Plasma	Fluid portion of circulating blood is called plasma.
Lipid	Lipid is one class of aliphatic hydrocarbon-containing organic compounds essential for the structure and function of living cells. They are characterized by being water-insoluble but soluble in nonpolar organic solvents.
Immune response	The body's defensive reaction to invasion by bacteria, viral agents, or other foreign substances is called immune response.
Humoral immune	Humoral immune system refers to the part of the immune system mediated by B cells; it is mediated by circulating antibodies and is active against extracellular bacterial and viral infections.
Receptor	A receptor is a protein on the cell membrane or within the cytoplasm or cell nucleus that binds to a specific molecule (a ligand), such as a neurotransmitter, hormone, or other substance, and initiates the cellular response to the ligand. Receptor, in immunology, the region of an antibody which shows recognition of an antigen.
Light chain	Light chain refers to one of the smaller polypeptides of a multisubunit protein such as myosin or immunoglobulin.
Carboxyl	A carboxyl is the univalent radical -COOH; present in and characteristic of organic acids.
Variable	A characteristic or aspect in which people, objects, events, or conditions vary is called variable.
Trimer	In biochemistry, a trimer is a macromolecular compound formed by three non-covalently bound macromolecules.
Infection	The invasion and multiplication of microorganisms in body tissues is called an infection.
Fetus	Fetus refers to a developing human from the ninth week of gestation until birth; has all the major structures of an adult.
Circulatory system	The circulatory system or cardiovascular system is the organ system which circulates blood around the body of most animals.
Placental barrier	The placental barrier between the fetus and the wall of the mother's uterus allows for the transfer of materials from mother, and eliminates waste products of fetus.

Colostrum	Thin, milky fluid rich in proteins, including antibodies, that is secreted by the mammary glands a few days prior to or after delivery before true milk is secreted is called colostrum.
Saliva	Saliva is the moist, clear, and usually somewhat frothy substance produced in the mouths of some animals, including humans.
Jugular vein	The external and internal jugular vein bring deoxygenated blood from the head back to the heart via the superior vena cava.
Polypeptide	Polypeptide refers to polymer of many amino acids linked by peptide bonds.
Tonsil	Tonsil refers to a patch of lymphatic tissue consisting of connective tissue that contains many lymphocytes; located in the pharynx and throat.
Vein	Vein in animals, is a vessel that returns blood to the heart. In plants, a vascular bundle in a leaf, composed of xylem and phloem.
Secretory IgA	Secretory IgA is the primary immunoglobulin of the secretory immune system. It correlates inversely with self-reported levels of stress and is regarded by some as a potential biomarker for stress.
Thoracic duct	The thoracic duct is an important part of the lymphatic system. It is the largest lymphatic vessel in the body. It collects most of the lymph in the body, neck and head, which is collected by the right lymphatic duct) and drains into the systemic (blood) circulation.
Affinity	Chemical affinity results from electronic properties by which dissimilar substances are capable of forming chemical compounds. Specifically, the term refers to the tendency of an atom or compound to combine by chemical reaction with atoms or compounds of unlike composition.
Anaphylaxis	Anaphylaxis refers to an immediate hypersensitivity reaction following exposure of a sensitized individual to the appropriate antigen.
Heparin	Heparin as a drug is used as an injectable anticoagulant. Heparin is a highly sulfated glycosaminoglycan widely used as an injectable anticoagulant. It is also used to form an inner anticoagulant surface on various experimental and medical devices such as test tubes and renal dialysis machines.
Blood plasma	Blood plasma is the liquid component of blood, in which the blood cells are suspended. Serum is the same as blood plasma except that clotting factors (such as fibrin) have been removed.
Plasma membrane	The unit membrane that encloses a cell and controls the traffic of molecules in and out of the cell is the plasma membrane.
Complement	Complement is a group of proteins of the complement system, found in blood serum which act in concert with antibodies to achieve the destruction of non-self particles such as foreign blood cells or bacteria.
Liver	The liver is an organ in vertebrates, including humans. It plays a major role in metabolism and has a number of functions in the body including drug detoxification, glycogen storage, and plasma protein synthesis. It also produces bile, which is important for digestion.
Complement system	Group of plasma proteins that form a nonspecific defense mechanism, often by puncturing microbes, is called the complement system. The complement system is derived from many small plasma proteins that form the complex biochemical cascade of the immune system.
Phagocytosis	Phagocytosis (literally, "cell eating") is a form of endocytosis where large particles are enveloped by the cell membrane of a (usually larger) cell and internalized to form a phagosome, or "food vacuole."

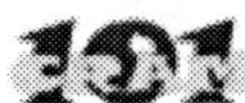

Microorganism	A microorganism or microbe is an organism that is so small that it is microscopic (invisible to the naked eye).
Enzyme	An enzyme is a protein that catalyzes, or speeds up, a chemical reaction. They are essential to sustain life because most chemical reactions in biological cells would occur too slowly, or would lead to different products, without them.
Epithelium	Epithelium is a tissue composed of a layer of cells. Epithelium can be found lining internal (e.g. endothelium, which lines the inside of blood vessels) or external (e.g. skin) free surfaces of the body. Functions include secretion, absorption and protection.
Monomer	In chemistry, a monomer is a small molecule that may become chemically bonded to other monomers to form a polymer.
Lamina	A thin layer, such as the lamina of a vertebra or the lamina propria of a mucous membrane is referred to as lamina.
Variable portion	The area on an antibody that gives it specificity in attaching to a particular antigen is a variable portion.
Activation	As reflected by facial expressions, the degree of arousal a person is experiencing is referred to as activation.
Toxin	Toxin refers to a microbial product or component that can injure another cell or organism at low concentrations. Often the term refers to a poisonous protein, but toxins may be lipids and other substances.
Neutralization	A chemical reaction involved in mixing an acid with a base which produces a salt and water is referred to as neutralization.
Agglutination	Clumping of blood cells in response to a reaction between an antibody and an antigen is called agglutination.
Inflammation	Inflammation is the first response of the immune system to infection or irritation and may be referred to as the innate cascade.
Leukocyte	A white blood cell is a leukocyte. They help to defend the body against infectious disease and foreign materials as part of the immune system.
Cytokine	A type of protein secreted by a T lymphocyte that attacks viruses, virally infected cells, and cancer cells is referred to as cytokine.
Neutrophil	Neutrophil refers to a type of phagocytic leukocyte.
Granulocyte	Granulocyte is a category of white blood cells, characterized by the fact that all types have differently staining granules in their cytoplasm on light microscopy.
Interferon	Interferon is a natural protein produced by the cells of the immune systems of most animals in response to challenges by foreign agents such as viruses, bacteria, parasites and tumor cells. They belong to the large class of glycoproteins known as cytokines.
Necrosis	Necrosis is the name given to unprogrammed death of cells/living tissue. There are many causes of necrosis including injury, infection, cancer, infarction, and inflammation. Necrosis is caused by special enzymes that are released by lysosomes.
Fever	Fever (also known as pyrexia, or a febrile response, and archaically known as ague) is a medical symptom that describes an increase in internal body temperature to levels that are above normal (37°C, 98.6°F).
Tumor necrosis factor	In medicine, tumor necrosis factor alpha (TNFá, cachexin or cachectin) is an important cytokine involved in systemic inflammation and the acute phase response.

Secondary lymphoid organs The spleen, lymph nodes, and accessory lymphoid tissue are the secondary lymphoid organs. These organs contain a scaffolding that support circulating B- and T-lymphocytes and other immune cells like macrophages and dendritic cells.

Lymphoblast Lymphoblast refers to a cell that matures into a lymphocyte after being stimulated by an antigen.

Colonize The process whereby microorganisms take up residence in a host, making the host a carrier, which does not succumb to infection is referred to colonize.

Population Population refers to all members of a well-defined group of organisms, events, or things.

Stimulus Stimulus in a nervous system, a factor that triggers sensory transduction.

Apoptosis In biology, apoptosis is one of the main types of programmed cell death (PCD). As such, it is a process of deliberate life relinquishment by an unwanted cell in a multicellular organism.

Retrovirus A retrovirus is a virus which has a genome consisting of two RNA molecules, which may or may not be identical. It relies on the enzyme reverse transcriptase to perform the reverse transcription of its genome from RNA into DNA, which can then be integrated into the host's genome with an integrase enzyme.

Syndrome Syndrome is the association of several clinically recognizable features, signs, symptoms, phenomena or characteristics which often occur together, so that the presence of one feature alerts the physician to the presence of the others

Immunodeficiency Immunodeficiency is a state in which the immune system's ability to fight infectious disease is compromized or entirely absent. Most cases of immunodeficiency are either congenital or acquired.

Histocompati-ility Histocompatibility is the property of having the same, or mostly the same, alleles of a set of genes called the major histocompatibility complex. These genes are expressed in most tissues as antigens, to which the immune system makes antibodies.

Alleles Genes coding for the same trait and found at the same locus on homologous chromosomes are called alleles.

Allele Different forms of a gene are called an allele.

Membrane protein A membrane protein is a protein molecule that is attached to, or associated with the membrane of a cell or an organelle. Membrane proteins can be classified into two groups, based on their attachment to the membrane.

Nucleic acid A nucleic acid is a complex, high-molecular-weight biochemical macromolecule composed of nucleotide chains that convey genetic information.

Acid An acid is a water-soluble, sour-tasting chemical compound that when dissolved in water, gives a solution with a pH of less than 7.

Ubiquitin Ubiquitin is a small protein that occurs in all eukaryotic cells. Its main function is to mark other proteins for destruction, known as proteolysis. Several ubiquitin molecules attach to the condemned protein, and it then moves to a proteasome, a barrel-shaped structure where the proteolysis occurs.

Peptide Peptide is the family of molecules formed from the linking, in a defined order, of various amino acids. The link between one amino acid residue and the next is an amide bond, and is sometimes referred to as a peptide bond.

Vesicle Membranous, cytoplasmic sac formed by an infolding of the cell membrane is called a vesicle.

Lead Lead is a chemical element in the periodic table that has the symbol Pb and atomic number 82. A soft, heavy, toxic and malleable poor metal, lead is bluish white when freshly cut but

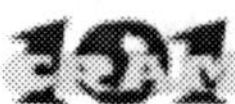

	tarnishes to dull gray when exposed to air. Lead is used in building construction, lead-acid batteries, bullets and shot, and is part of solder, pewter, and fusible alloys.
Endogenous	Originating internally, such as the endogenous cholesterol synthesized in the body in contrast to the exogenous cholesterol coming from the diet is referred to as endogenous. Compare with exogenous.
Exogenous	Exogenous refers to an action or object coming from outside a system.
Endocytosis	Endocytosis is a process where cells absorb material (molecules or other cells) from outside by engulfing it with their cell membranes.
Digestion	Digestion refers to the mechanical and chemical breakdown of food into molecules small enough for the body to absorb; the second main stage of food processing, following ingestion.
Fusion	Fusion refers to the combination of two atoms into a single atom as a result of a collision, usually accompanied by the release of energy.
Autograft	When a tissue is transplanted from one site to another on the same patient, such as a skin graft or a tissue flap, it is termed an autograft.
Isograft	A transplant in which the donor and recipient are identical twins is called an isograft.
Rejection	Rejection is a response by caregivers where they distance themselves emotionally from a chronically ill patient. Although they provide physical care they tend to scold and and correct the patient continuously.
Host	Host is an organism that harbors a parasite, mutual partner, or commensal partner; or a cell infected by a virus.
Heterograft	Xenotransplantation is the transplantation of cells, tissues or organs from one species to another such as from pigs to humans. Such cells, tissues or organs are called xenografts (xenotransplants). The terms heterograft and heterotransplant are also sometimes used, while the term homograft refers to a same-species transplant.
Homograft	Homograft is a gratf of tissue, including organs, from a member of one's own species.
Transplant rejection	Transplant rejection occurs when the immune system of the recipient of an transplant attacks the transplanted organ or tissue.
Dendritic cell	The dendritic cell is an immune cell and forms part of the mammal immune system. Once activated, they migrate to the lymphoid tissues where they interact with T cells and B cells to initiate and shape the immune response.
Heterogeneous	A heterogeneous compound, mixture, or other such object is one that consists of many different items, which are often not easily sorted or separated, though they are clearly distinct.
Langerhans cell	A Langerhans cell is an immature dendritic cell containing large granules called Birbeck granules. On infection of an area of skin, they will take up and process microbial antigens before travelling to the T-cell areas in the cortex of the draining lymph node and maturing to become fully-functional antigen-presenting cells.
Epidermis	Epidermis is the outermost layer of the skin. It forms the waterproof, protective wrap over the body's surface and is made up of stratified squamous epithelium with an underlying basement membrane. It contains no blood vessels, and is nourished by diffusion from the dermis. In plants, the outermost layer of cells covering the leaves and young parts of a plant is the epidermis.
Nervous tissue	Tissue made up of neurons and supportive cells is referred to as nervous tissue. It forms a rapid communication network for the body.

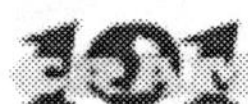

Elimination	Elimination refers to the physiologic excretion of drugs and other substances from the body.
Immunity	Resistance to the effects of specific disease-causing agents is called immunity.
Humoral immunity	Humoral immunity is the aspect of immunity that is mediated by secreted antibodies, produced in the cells of the B lymphocyte lineage (B cell). Secreted antibodies bind to antigens on the surfaces of invading microbes, which flags them for destruction.
Vaccine	A harmless variant or derivative of a pathogen used to stimulate a host organism's immune system to mount a long-term defense against the pathogen is referred to as vaccine.
Mucosa	The mucosa is a lining of ectodermic origin, covered in epithelium, and involved in absorption and secretion. They line various body cavities that are exposed to the external environment and internal organs.
Skin	Skin is an organ of the integumentary system composed of a layer of tissues that protect underlying muscles and organs.
Cell division	Cell division (or local doubling) is the process by which a cell, called the parent cell divides into two cells, called daughter cells. Cell division is usually a small segment of a larger cell cycle.
Intracellular	Intracellular refers to having to do with the interior of a cell.
Human immunodeficiency virus	The human immunodeficiency virus is a retrovirus that primarily infects vital components of the human immune system. It is transmitted through penetrative and oral sex; blood transfusion; the sharing of contaminated needles in health care settings and through drug injection; and, between mother and infant, during pregnancy, childbirth and breastfeeding.
Mutation	A change in the structure of a gene is called a mutation.
Measles	Measles refers to a highly contagious skin disease that is endemic throughout the world. It is caused by a morbilli virus in the family Paramyxoviridae, which enters the body through the respiratory tract or through the conjunctiva.
Genes	Genes are the units of heredity in living organisms. They are encoded in the organism's genetic material (usually DNA or RNA), and control the development and behavior of the organism.
Affect	Affect is the scientific term used to describe a subject's externally displayed mood. This can be assesed by the nurse by observing facial expression, tone of voice, and body language.
Autoimmune	Autoimmune refers to immune reactions against normal body cells; self against self.
Autoimmune disease	Disease that results when the immune system mistakenly attacks the body's own tissues is referred to as autoimmune disease.
Induction	A discipline technique in which a parent uses reason and explanation of the consequences for others of a child's actions is called induction.
Cytoplasm	Cytoplasm refers to the contents of a cell excluding the nucleus and cell membrane. Cytoplasm is a homogeneous, generally clear jelly-like material that fills cells.
Collagen	Collagen is the main protein of connective tissue in animals and the most abundant protein in mammals, making up about 1/4 of the total. It is one of the long, fibrous structural proteins whose functions are quite different from those of globular proteins such as enzymes.
Follicle	Follicle refers to a cluster of cells surrounding, protecting, and nourishing a developing egg cell in the ovary; also secretes estrogen. In botany, a follicle is a type of simple dry fruit produced by certain flowering plants. It is regarded as one the most primitive types of fruits, and derives from a simple pistil or carpel.

Tonsils	The tonsils are areas of lymphoid tissue on either side of the throat. As with other organs of the lymphatic system, the tonsils act as part of the immune system to help protect against infection.
Submucosa	The tissue layer just under the epithelial lining of the lumen of the digestive tract is referred to as the submucosa.
Ileum	The ileum is the final section of the small intestine. Its function is to absorb vitamin B12 and bile salts. The wall itself made up of folds, each of which has many tiny finger-like projections known as villi, on its surface.
Intestine	The intestine is the portion of the alimentary canal extending from the stomach to the anus and, in humans and mammals, consists of two segments, the small intestine and the large intestine. The intestine is the part of the body responsible for extracting nutrition from food.
M cell	Specialized cell of the intestinal mucosa and other sites, such as the urogenital tract, that delivers the antigen from the apical face of the cell to lymphocytes clustered within the pocket in its basolateral face is a the M cell.
Pinocytosis	Process by which a cell engulfs droplets of fluid from its surroundings is referred to as pinocytosis.
Digestive tract	The digestive tract is the system of organs within multicellular animals which takes in food, digests it to extract energy and nutrients, and expels the remaining waste.
Pharynx	The pharynx is the part of the digestive system and respiratory system of many animals immediately behind the mouth and in front of the esophagus.
Invagination	Infolding of one part of a structure into another is invagination.
A band	A band is a dark band corresponding to an area where actin and myosin filaments overlap in cardiac or skeletal muscle.
Tonsillitis	Tonsillitis is an inflammation of the tonsils, especially the palatine tonsils often due to S. pyogenes infection.
Purulent	Anything that creates or contains pus is purulent.
Dense connective tissue	Dense connective tissue has collagen fibers as its main matrix element. Crowded between the collagen fibers are rows of fibroblasts, fiber-forming cells, that manufacture the fibers. Dense connective tissue forms strong, rope-like structures such as tendons and ligaments. Tendons attach skeletal muscles to bones; ligaments connect bones to bones at joints.
Respiratory tract	In humans the respiratory tract is the part of the anatomy that has to do with the process of respiration or breathing.
Adenoids	Adenoids, or pharyngeal tonsils, are folds of lymphatic tissue covered by ciliated epithelium. They are found in the roof and posterior wall of the nasopharynx at the back of the throat behind the uvula.
Adenoid	An adenoid is a fold of lymphatic tissue covered by ciliated epithelium. They are found in the roof and posterior wall of the nasopharynx at the back of the throat behind the uvula. They are part of the immune system, as they trap inhaled viruses and produce antibodies, particularly in children. This function decreases with age.
Parenchyma	The parenchyma are the functional parts of an organ in the body (i.e. the nephrons of the kidney, the alveoli of the lungs). In plants parenchyma cells are thin-walled cells of the ground tissue that make up the bulk of most nonwoody structures, although sometimes their cell walls can be lignified.

Medulla | Medulla in general means the inner part, and derives from the Latin word for 'marrow'. In medicine it is contrasted to the cortex.

Cortex | In anatomy and zoology the cortex is the outermost or superficial layer of an organ or the outer portion of the stem or root of a plant.

Stellate cells | In neuroscience, stellate cells are inhibitory interneurons found within the molecular layer of the cerebellum. These cells synapse onto the dendritic arbors of Purkinje cells.

Keratin | Keratin is a family of fibrous structural proteins; tough and insoluble, they form the hard but nonmineralized structures found in reptiles, birds and mammals.

Capillaries | Capillaries refer to the smallest of the blood vessels and the sites of exchange between the blood and tissue cells.

Capillary | A capillary is the smallest of a body's blood vessels, measuring 5-10 micro meters. They connect arteries and veins, and most closely interact with tissues. Their walls are composed of a single layer of cells, the endothelium. This layer is so thin that molecules such as oxygen, water and lipids can pass through them by diffusion and enter the tissues.

Arteriole | An arteriole is a blood vessel that extends and branches out from an artery and leads to capillaries. They have thick muscular walls and are the primary site of vascular resistance.

Blood vessel | A blood vessel is a part of the circulatory system and function to transport blood throughout the body. The most important types, arteries and veins, are so termed because they carry blood away from or towards the heart, respectively.

Endothelium | The endothelium is the layer of thin, flat cells that lines the interior surface of blood vessels, forming an interface between circulating blood in the lumen and the rest of the vessel wall.

Septa | Septa are thin walls or partitions between the internal chambers (camerae) of the shell of a cephalopod, namely nautiloids or ammonoids.

Extracellular | Outside the cell is called extracellular.

Veins | Blood vessels that return blood toward the heart from the circulation are referred to as veins.

Hormone | A hormone is a chemical messenger from one cell to another. All multicellular organisms produce hormones. The best known hormones are those produced by endocrine glands of vertebrate animals, but hormones are produced by nearly every organ system and tissue type in a human or animal body. Hormone molecules are secreted directly into the bloodstream, they move by circulation or diffusion to their target cells, which may be nearby cells in the same tissue or cells of a distant organ of the body.

Staining | Staining is a biochemical technique of adding a class-specific (DNA, proteins, lipids, carbohydrates) dye to a substrate to qualify or quantify the presence of a specific compound. They are frequently used to highlight structures in tissues for viewing, often with the aid of different microscopes.

Mesentery | A mesentery is a part of the peritoneum that connects an internal organ, such as the small intestine, to the abdominal wall.

Abdomen | The abdomen is a part of the body. In humans, and in many other vertebrates, it is the region between the thorax and the pelvis. In fully developed insects, the abdomen is the third (or posterior) segment, after the head and thorax.

Course | Pattern of development and change of a disorder over time is a course.

Thorax | The thorax is a division of an animal's body that lies between the head and the abdomen. In

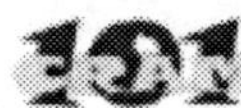

humans, the thorax is the region of the body that extends from the neck to the diaphragm, not including the upper limbs.

Depression	In everyday language depression refers to any downturn in mood, which may be relatively transitory and perhaps due to something trivial. This is differentiated from Clinical depression which is marked by symptoms that last two weeks or more and are so severe that they interfere with daily living.
Artery	Vessel that takes blood away from the heart to the tissues and organs of the body is called an artery.
Kidney	The kidney is a bean-shaped excretory organ in vertebrates. Part of the urinary system, the kidneys filter wastes (especially urea) from the blood and excrete them, along with water, as urine.
Nerve	A nerve is an enclosed, cable-like bundle of nerve fibers or axons, which includes the glia that ensheath the axons in myelin.
Elderly	Old age consists of ages nearing the average life span of human beings, and thus the end of the human life cycle. Euphemisms for older people include advanced adult, elderly, and senior or senior citizen.
Atrophy	Atrophy is the partial or complete wasting away of a part of the body. Causes of atrophy include poor nourishment, poor circulation, loss of hormonal support, loss of nerve supply to the target organ, disuse or lack of exercise, or disease intrinsic to the tissue itself.
Adipose tissue	Adipose tissue is an anatomical term for loose connective tissue composed of adipocytes. Its main role is to store energy in the form of fat, although it also cushions and insulates the body. It has an important endocrine function in producing recently-discovered hormones such as leptin, resistin and TNFalpha.
Skeleton	In biology, the skeleton or skeletal system is the biological system providing physical support in living organisms.
Fiber	Fibers used by man come from a wide variety of sources: Natural fiber include those made out of plants, animal and mineral sources. Natural fibers can be classified according to their origin.
Channel	Channel, in communications (sometimes called communications channel), refers to the medium used to convey information from a sender (or transmitter) to a receiver.
Lymph vessel	Lymph vessel refers to one of the system of vessels carrying lymph from the lymph capillaries to the veins.
Sinus	A sinus is a pouch or cavity in any organ or tissue, or an abnormal cavity or passage caused by the destruction of tissue.
Trabecula	A trabecula is a small, often microscopic, tissue element in the form of a small beam, strut or rod, generally having a mechanical function, and usually but not necessarily composed of dense collagenous tissue.
Venule	A vessel that conveys blood between a capillary bed and a vein is a venule.
Sugar	A sugar is the simplest molecule that can be identified as a carbohydrate. These include monosaccharides and disaccharides, trisaccharides and the oligosaccharides. The term "glyco-" indicates the presence of a sugar in an otherwise non-carbohydrate substance.
Endothelial cell	A endothelial cell also controls the passage of materials — and the transit of white blood cells — into and out of the bloodstream. In some organs, there are highly differentiated endothelial cells to perform specialized 'filtering' functions.

Integrin	An integrin is an integral membrane protein in the plasma membrane of cells. It plays a role in the attachment of a cell to the extracellular matrix (ECM) and in signal transduction from the ECM to the cell.
Medial	In anatomical terms of location toward or near the midline is called medial.
Muscle	Muscle is a contractile form of tissue. It is one of the four major tissue types, the other three being epithelium, connective tissue and nervous tissue. Muscle contraction is used to move parts of the body, as well as to move substances within the body.
Smooth muscle	Smooth muscle is a type of non-striated muscle, found within the "walls" of hollow organs; such as blood vessels, the bladder, the uterus, and the gastrointestinal tract. Smooth muscle is used to move matter within the body, via contraction; it generally operates "involuntarily", without nerve stimulation.
Splenic artery	The splenic artery is the blood vessel that supplies oxygenated blood to the spleen. It branches from the celiac artery, follows a course superior to the pancreas and gives off branches to the stomach, among which is the left gastroepiploic artery, and pancreas before reaching the spleen.
Granulocytes	Granulocytes are a category of white blood cells, characterised by the fact that all types have differently staining granules in their cytoplasm on light microscopy. They are also called polymorphonuclear leukocytes (PMN or PML) because of the varying shapes of the nucleus, which is usually lobed into three segments.
Erythrocyte	Red blood cells are the most common type of blood cell and are the vertebrate body's principal means of delivering oxygen from the lungs or gills to body tissues via the blood. Red blood cells are also known as erythrocyte.
Platelet	Cell fragment that is necessary to blood clotting is a platelet. They are the blood cell fragments that are involved in the cellular mechanisms that lead to the formation of blood clots.
Histology	Histology is the study of tissue sectioned as a thin slice, using a microscope. It can be described as microscopic anatomy.
Red blood cells	Red blood cells are the most common type of blood cell and are the vertebrate body's principal means of delivering oxygen from the lungs or gills to body tissues via the blood.
Red blood cell	The red blood cell is the most common type of blood cell and is the vertebrate body's principal means of delivering oxygen from the lungs or gills to body tissues via the blood.
Splenic vein	The splenic vein is the blood vessel that drains blood from spleen. It joins with the superior mesenteric vein, to form the portal vein and follows a course superior to the pancreas, along side of the similarly named artery, the splenic artery.
Life span	Life span refers to the upper boundary of life, the maximum number of years an individual can live. The maximum life span of human beings is about 120 years of age.
Leukemia	Leukemia refers to a type of cancer of the bloodforming tissues, characterized by an excessive production of white blood cells and an abnormally high number of them in the blood; cancer of the bone marrow cells that produce leukocytes.
Transmission electron microscope	Transmission electron microscope refers to a microscope that uses an electron beam to study the internal structure of thinly sectioned specimens.
Microscope	A microscope is an instrument for viewing objects that are too small to be seen by the naked or unaided eye.
Micrograph	A micrograph is a photograph or similar image taken through a microscope or similar device to

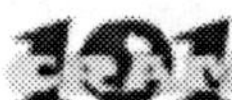

show a magnified image of an item.

Hemoglobin — Hemoglobin is the iron-containing oxygen-transport metalloprotein in the red cells of the blood in mammals and other animals. Hemoglobin transports oxygen from the lungs to the rest of the body, such as to the muscles, where it releases the oxygen load.

Amino acid — An amino acid is any molecule that contains both amino and carboxylic acid functional groups. They are the basic structural building units of proteins. They form short polymer chains called peptides or polypeptides which in turn form structures called proteins.

Iron — Iron is essential to all organisms, except for a few bacteria. It is mostly stably incorporated in the inside of metalloproteins, because in exposed or in free form it causes production of free radicals that are generally toxic to cells.

Heme — A or heme is a metal-containing cofactor that consists of an iron atom contained in the center of a large heterocyclic organic ring called a porphyrin. Although porphyrins do not necessarily contain iron, a substantial fraction of porphyrin-containing metalloproteins do in fact have heme as their prosthetic subunit. It is made a matter of common knowledge, because of its vitality as a part of hemoglobin, vital in the human body's red blood cells.

Bilirubin — A bile pigment produced from hemoglobin breakdown is bilirubin.

Bile — Bile is a bitter, greenish-yellow alkaline fluid secreted by the liver of most vertebrates. In many species, it is stored in the gallbladder between meals and upon eating is discharged into the duodenum where it aids the process of digestion.

Anemia — Anemia is a deficiency of red blood cells and/or hemoglobin. This results in a reduced ability of blood to transfer oxygen to the tissues, and this causes hypoxia; since all human cells depend on oxygen for survival, varying degrees of anemia can have a wide range of clinical consequences.

Immunology — Immunology refers to the branch of science that deals with the immune system and attempts to understand the many phenomena that are responsible for both acquired and innate immunity. It also includes the use of antibodyantigen reactions in other laboratory work .

Clonal selection — The production of a lineage of genetically identical cells that recognize and attack the specific antigen that stimulated their proliferation. Clonal selection is the mechanism that underlies the immune system's specificity and memory of antigens.

Carbohydrate — Carbohydrate is a chemical compound that contains oxygen, hydrogen, and carbon atoms. They consist of monosaccharide sugars of varying chain lengths and that have the general chemical formula $C_n(H_2O)_n$ or are derivatives of such.

Nucleic acid — A nucleic acid is a complex, high-molecular-weight biochemical macromolecule composed of nucleotide chains that convey genetic information.

Intestine — The intestine is the portion of the alimentary canal extending from the stomach to the anus and, in humans and mammals, consists of two segments, the small intestine and the large intestine. The intestine is the part of the body responsible for extracting nutrition from food.

Protein — A protein is a complex, high-molecular-weight organic compound that consists of amino acids joined by peptide bonds. They are essential to the structure and function of all living cells and viruses. Many are enzymes or subunits of enzymes.

Acid — An acid is a water-soluble, sour-tasting chemical compound that when dissolved in water, gives a solution with a pH of less than 7.

Small intestine — The small intestine is the part of the gastrointestinal tract between the stomach and the large intestine (colon). In humans over 5 years old it is about 7m long. It is divided into three structural parts: duodenum, jejunum and ileum.

Digestive tract — The digestive tract is the system of organs within multicellular animals which takes in food, digests it to extract energy and nutrients, and expels the remaining waste.

Minerals — Minerals refer to inorganic chemical compounds found in nature; salts.

Vitamin — An organic compound other than a carbohydrate, lipid, or protein that is needed for normal metabolism but that the body cannot synthesize in adequate amounts is called a vitamin.

Amino acid — An amino acid is any molecule that contains both amino and carboxylic acid functional groups. They are the basic structural building units of proteins. They form short polymer chains called peptides or polypeptides which in turn form structures called proteins.

Fatty acid — A fatty acid is a carboxylic acid (or organic acid), often with a long aliphatic tail (long chains), either saturated or unsaturated.

Digestion — Digestion refers to the mechanical and chemical breakdown of food into molecules small enough for the body to absorb; the second main stage of food processing, following ingestion.

Stomach — The stomach is an organ in the alimentary canal used to digest food. It's primary function is not the absorption of nutrients from digested food; rather, the main job of the stomach is to break down large food molecules into smaller ones, so that they can be absorbed into the blood more easily.

Monosaccharide — A monosaccharide is simplest form of a carbohydrate. They consist of one sugar and are usually colorless, water-soluble, crystalline solids. Some monosaccharides have a sweet taste. They are the building blocks of disaccharides like sucrose and polysaccharides.

Absorption — Absorption is a physical or chemical phenomenon or a process in which atoms, molecules, or ions enter some bulk phase - gas, liquid or solid material. In nutrition, amino acids are broken down through digestion, which begins in the stomach.

Large intestine — In anatomy of the digestive system, the colon, also called the large intestine or large bowel, is the part of the intestine from the cecum ('caecum' in British English) to the rectum. Its primary purpose is to extract water from feces.

Gastrointestinal tract — The gastrointestinal tract is the system of organs within multicellular animals which takes in food, digests it to extract energy and nutrients, and expels the remaining waste.

Submucosa	The tissue layer just under the epithelial lining of the lumen of the digestive tract is referred to as the submucosa.
Serosa	A serosa is a smooth membrane consisting of a thin layer of cells that excrete a fluid, known as serous fluid. Two-layered serous membranes line the cavities that contain the heart (part of the pericardium), lungs (the pleura) and intestines (the peritoneum), enclosing their contents.
Mucosa	The mucosa is a lining of ectodermic origin, covered in epithelium, and involved in absorption and secretion. They line various body cavities that are exposed to the external environment and internal organs.
Loose connective tissue	Loose connective tissue or Areolar connective tissue holds organs and epithelia in place, and has a variety of proteinaceous fibers, including collagen and elastin. It is also important in inflammation.
Lymph vessel	Lymph vessel refers to one of the system of vessels carrying lymph from the lymph capillaries to the veins.
Tissue	A collection of interconnected cells that perform a similar function within an organism is called tissue.
Lamina	A thin layer, such as the lamina of a vertebra or the lamina propria of a mucous membrane is referred to as lamina.
Muscle	Muscle is a contractile form of tissue. It is one of the four major tissue types, the other three being epithelium, connective tissue and nervous tissue. Muscle contraction is used to move parts of the body, as well as to move substances within the body.
Lymph	Lymph originates as blood plasma lost from the circulatory system, which leaks out into the surrounding tissues. The lymphatic system collects this fluid by diffusion into lymph capillaries, and returns it to the circulatory system.
Gland	A gland is an organ in an animal's body that synthesizes a substance for release such as hormones, often into the bloodstream or into cavities inside the body or its outer surface.
Blood	Blood is a circulating tissue composed of fluid plasma and cells. The main function of blood is to supply nutrients (oxygen, glucose) and constitutional elements to tissues and to remove waste products.
Connective tissue	Connective tissue is any type of biological tissue with an extensive extracellular matrix and often serves to support, bind together, and protect organs.
Smooth muscle	Smooth muscle is a type of non-striated muscle, found within the "walls" of hollow organs; such as blood vessels, the bladder, the uterus, and the gastrointestinal tract. Smooth muscle is used to move matter within the body, via contraction; it generally operates "involuntarily", without nerve stimulation.
Plexus	A plexus is also a network of blood vessels, with the choroid plexuses of the brain being the most commonly mentioned example. A choroid plexus is very thin and vascular roof plates of the most anterior and most posterior cavities of the brain which expand into the interiors of the cavities.
Nerve	A nerve is an enclosed, cable-like bundle of nerve fibers or axons, which includes the glia that ensheath the axons in myelin.
Dense connective tissue	Dense connective tissue has collagen fibers as its main matrix element. Crowded between the collagen fibers are rows of fibroblasts, fiber-forming cells, that manufacture the fibers. Dense connective tissue forms strong, rope-like structures such as tendons and ligaments. Tendons attach skeletal muscles to bones; ligaments connect bones to bones at joints.

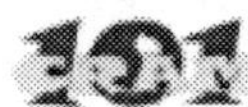

Serous	The term serous fluid is used for various bodily fluids that are typically pale yellow and transparent, and of a benign nature.
Epithelium	Epithelium is a tissue composed of a layer of cells. Epithelium can be found lining internal (e.g. endothelium, which lines the inside of blood vessels) or external (e.g. skin) free surfaces of the body. Functions include secretion, absorption and protection.
Peritoneum	In higher vertebrates, the peritoneum is the serous membrane that forms the lining of the abdominal cavity - it covers most of the intra-abdominal organs. The peritoneum both supports the abdominal organs and serves as a conduit for their blood and lymph vessels and nerves.
Mesentery	A mesentery is a part of the peritoneum that connects an internal organ, such as the small intestine, to the abdominal wall.
Serous membrane	Membrane that covers internal organs and lines cavities without an opening to the outside of the body is referred to as serous membrane.
Adipose tissue	Adipose tissue is an anatomical term for loose connective tissue composed of adipocytes. Its main role is to store energy in the form of fat, although it also cushions and insulates the body. It has an important endocrine function in producing recently-discovered hormones such as leptin, resistin and TNFalpha.
Adventitia	Adventitia is the outermost connective tissue covering of any organ, vessel, or other structure. For example, the connective tissue that surrounds an artery is called the adventitia because it is considered extraneous to the artery.
Organ	Organ refers to a structure consisting of several tissues adapted as a group to perform specific functions.
Digestive system	The organ system that ingests food, breaks it down into smaller chemical units, and absorbs the nutrient molecules is referred to as the digestive system.
Hormone	A hormone is a chemical messenger from one cell to another. All multicellular organisms produce hormones. The best known hormones are those produced by endocrine glands of vertebrate animals, but hormones are produced by nearly every organ system and tissue type in a human or animal body. Hormone molecules are secreted directly into the bloodstream, they move by circulation or diffusion to their target cells, which may be nearby cells in the same tissue or cells of a distant organ of the body.
Affect	Affect is the scientific term used to describe a subject's externally displayed mood. This can be assesed by the nurse by observing facial expression, tone of voice, and body language.
Mucus	Mucus is a slippery secretion of the lining of various membranes in the body (mucous membranes). Mucus aids in the protection of the lungs by trapping foreign particles that enter the nose during normal breathing. Additionally, it prevents tissues from drying out.
Oral cavity	The mouth, also known as the buccal cavity or the oral cavity, is the opening through which an animal or human takes in food and water. It is usually located in the head, but not always; the mouth of a planarium is in the middle of its belly.
Anal canal	The anal canal is the terminal part of the large intestine. It is situated between the rectum and anus, below the level of the pelvic diaphram.
Esophagus	The esophagus, or gullet is the muscular tube in vertebrates through which ingested food passes from the mouth area to the stomach. Food is passed through the esophagus by using the process of peristalsis.
Antibody	An antibody is a protein used by the immune system to identify and neutralize foreign objects like bacteria and viruses. Each antibody recognizes a specific antigen unique to its target.

Protease	Protease refers to an enzyme that breaks peptide bonds between amino acids of proteins.
Enzyme	An enzyme is a protein that catalyzes, or speeds up, a chemical reaction. They are essential to sustain life because most chemical reactions in biological cells would occur too slowly, or would lead to different products, without them.
Autonomic nervous system	The autonomic nervous system is the part of the nervous system that is not consciously controlled. It is commonly divided into two usually antagonistic subsystems: the sympathetic and parasympathetic nervous system.
Visceral	Visceral refers to the internal organs of an animal.
Fiber	Fibers used by man come from a wide variety of sources: Natural fiber include those made out of plants, animal and mineral sources. Natural fibers can be classified according to their origin.
Nervous system	The nervous system of an animal coordinates the activity of the muscles, monitors the organs, constructs and processes input from the senses, and initiates actions.
Variable	A characteristic or aspect in which people, objects, events, or conditions vary is called variable.
Motility	Motility is the ability to move spontaneously and independently. The term can apply to single cells, or to multicellular organisms.
Histology	Histology is the study of tissue sectioned as a thin slice, using a microscope. It can be described as microscopic anatomy.
Infection	The invasion and multiplication of microorganisms in body tissues is called an infection.
Friction	Friction is the force that opposes the relative motion or tendency of such motion of two surfaces in contact. The resulting injury to skin resembles an abrasion and can also damage superficial blood vessels directly under the skin.
Neuron	The neuron is a major class of cells in the nervous system. In vertebrates, they are found in the brain, the spinal cord and in the nerves and ganglia of the peripheral nervous system, and their primary role is to process and transmit neural information.
Medicine	Medicine is the branch of health science and the sector of public life concerned with maintaining or restoring human health through the study, diagnosis and treatment of disease and injury.
Stress	Stress refers to a condition that is a response to factors that change the human systems normal state.
Psychosomatic	A psychosomatic illness is one with physical manifestations and perhaps a supposed psychological cause. It is often diagnosed when any known or identifiable physical cause was excluded by medical examination.
Squamous epithelium	The squamous epithelium is epithelium consisting of one or more cell layers, the most superficial of which is composed of flat, scalelike or platelike cells.
Hard palate	The hard palate is a thin horizontal bony plate of the skull, located in the roof of the mouth. It spans the arch formed by the upper teeth. It forms a partition between the nasal passages and the mouth.
Keratin	Keratin is a family of fibrous structural proteins; tough and insoluble, they form the hard but nonmineralized structures found in reptiles, birds and mammals.
Gingiva	The gingiva consist of the tissue surrounding the roots of the teeth and covering the jawbone. Gingiva is considered as extensions of the skin, which, through evolution, have become mucous membranes. The gingiva are naturally transparent.

Soft palate
The soft palate, is the soft tissue comprising the back of the roof of the mouth. It is movable, consisting of muscle fibers sheathed in mucous membrane, and is responsible for closing off the nasal passages during the act of swallowing.

Dermis
The dermis is the layer of skin beneath the epidermis that consists of connective tissue and cushions the body from stress and strain.

Skin
Skin is an organ of the integumentary system composed of a layer of tissues that protect underlying muscles and organs.

Salivary gland
The salivary gland produces saliva, which keeps the mouth and other parts of the digestive system moist. It also helps break down carbohydrates and lubricates the passage of food down from the oro-pharynx to the esophagus to the stomach.

Skeletal muscle
Skeletal muscle is a type of striated muscle, attached to the skeleton. They are used to facilitate movement, by applying force to bones and joints; via contraction. They generally contract voluntarily (via nerve stimulation), although they can contract involuntarily.

Striated muscle
Striated muscle refers to contractile tissue characterized by multinucleated cells containing highly ordered arrangements of actin and myosin microfilaments. Also known as skeletal muscle.

Muscle fiber
Cell with myofibrils containing actin and myosin filaments arranged within sarcomeres is a muscle fiber.

Ventral
The surface or side of the body normally oriented upwards, away from the pull of gravity, is the dorsal side; the opposite side, typically the one closest to the ground when walking on all legs, swimming or flying, is the ventral side.

Dorsal
In anatomy, the dorsal is the side in which the backbone is located. This is usually the top of an animal, although in humans it refers to the back.

Dorsal surface
The dorsal surface is arched from above downward, and is subdivided into two unequal parts by the spine; the portion above the spine is called the supraspinatous fossa, and that below it the infraspinous fossa.

Invagination
Infolding of one part of a structure into another is invagination.

Elevation
Elevation refers to upward movement of a part of the body.

Tonsils
The tonsils are areas of lymphoid tissue on either side of the throat. As with other organs of the lymphatic system, the tonsils act as part of the immune system to help protect against infection.

Tonsil
Tonsil refers to a patch of lymphatic tissue consisting of connective tissue that contains many lymphocytes; located in the pharynx and throat.

Papilla
A papilla can be a small projection, such as a nipplelike projection on the skin, at the base of a hair or the root of a feather; the base of a new tooth.

Hydrophobic
Hydrophobic refers to being electrically neutral and nonpolar, and thus prefering other neutral and nonpolar solvents or molecular environments. Hydrophobic is often used interchangeably with "oily" or "lipophilic."

Taste bud
A taste bud is a small structure on the upper surface of the tongue, soft palate, and epiglottis that provides information about the taste of food being eaten. The majority on the tongue sit on raized protrusions of the tongue surface called papillae.

Lipase
A lipase is a water-soluble enzyme that catalyzes the hydrolysis of ester bonds in water–insoluble, lipid substrates. Most lipases act at a specific position on the glycerol backbone of a lipid substrate (A1, A2 or A3).

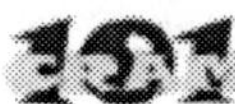

Triglyceride	Triglyceride is a glyceride in which the glycerol is esterified with three fatty acids. They are the main constituent of vegetable oil and animal fats and play an important role in metabolism as energy sources. They contain a bit more than twice as much energy as carbohydrates and proteins.
Triglycerides	Triglycerides refer to fats and oils composed of fatty acids and glycerol; are the body's most concentrated source of energy fuel; also known as neutral fats.
Ion channel	A ion channel is a pore-forming protein that helps establish the small voltage gradient that exists across the membrane of all living cells, by allowing the flow of ions down their electrochemical gradient. They are present in the membranes that surround all biological cells.
Receptor	A receptor is a protein on the cell membrane or within the cytoplasm or cell nucleus that binds to a specific molecule (a ligand), such as a neurotransmitter, hormone, or other substance, and initiates the cellular response to the ligand. Receptor, in immunology, the region of an antibody which shows recognition of an antigen.
Channel	Channel, in communications (sometimes called communications channel), refers to the medium used to convey information from a sender (or transmitter) to a receiver.
Saliva	Saliva is the moist, clear, and usually somewhat frothy substance produced in the mouths of some animals, including humans.
Ion	Ion refers to an atom or molecule that has gained or lost one or more electrons, thus acquiring an electrical charge.
Gustatory	Processes or structures associated with the sense of taste are referred to as gustatory.
Neurotransmitter	A neurotransmitter is a chemical that is used to relay, amplify and modulate electrical signals between a neuron and another cell.
Depolarization	Depolarization is a decrease in the absolute value of a cell's membrane potential. Thus, changes in membrane voltage in which the membrane potential becomes less positive or less negative are both depolarizations.
Afferent nerve	Axons that carry information inward to the central nervous system from the periphery of the body is called an afferent nerve.
Stimulus	Stimulus in a nervous system, a factor that triggers sensory transduction.
Pharynx	The pharynx is the part of the digestive system and respiratory system of many animals immediately behind the mouth and in front of the esophagus.
Larynx	The larynx is an organ in the neck of mammals involved in protection of the trachea and sound production. The larynx houses the vocal cords, and is situated at the point where the upper tract splits into the trachea and the esophagus.
Nasal cavity	The nasal cavity is a large air-filled space above and behind the nose in the middle of the face. The nasal cavity is important in warming and cleaning the air as it is inhaled. The nasal cavity also contains organs involved in olfaction.
Goblet cell	A goblet cell is a glandular simple columnar epithelial cell that is specifically designed to secrete mucus.
Blood vessel	A blood vessel is a part of the circulatory system and function to transport blood throughout the body. The most important types, arteries and veins, are so termed because they carry blood away from or towards the heart, respectively.
Coronary	Referring to the heart or the blood vessels of the heart is referred to as coronary.
Dentin	Dentin is the substance between the enamel (substance in the crown) or cementum (substance in

	the root) of a tooth and the pulp chamber. Dentin is secreted by the odontoblasts of the dental pulp.
Fibrous connective tissue	Any connective tissue with a preponderance of fiber, such as areolar, reticular, dense regular, and dense irregular connective tissues is referred to as the fibrous connective tissue.
Phospholipid	Phospholipid is a class of lipids formed from four components: fatty acids, a negatively-charged phosphate group, an alcohol and a backbone. Phospholipids with a glycerol backbone are known as glycerophospholipids or phosphoglycerides.
Collagen	Collagen is the main protein of connective tissue in animals and the most abundant protein in mammals, making up about 1/4 of the total. It is one of the long, fibrous structural proteins whose functions are quite different from those of globular proteins such as enzymes.
Ligament	A ligament is a short band of tough fibrous connective tissue composed mainly of long, stringy collagen fibres. They connect bones to other bones to form a joint. (They do not connect muscles to bones.)
Calcium	Calcium is the chemical element in the periodic table that has the symbol Ca and atomic number 20. Calcium is a soft grey alkaline earth metal that is used as a reducing agent in the extraction of thorium, zirconium and uranium. Calcium is also the fifth most abundant element in the Earth's crust.
Crystal	Crystal is a solid in which the constituent atoms, molecules, or ions are packed in a regularly ordered, repeating pattern extending in all three spatial dimensions.
Salt	Salt is a term used for ionic compounds composed of positively charged cations and negatively charged anions, so that the product is neutral and without a net charge.
Collagen fibril	Collagen fibril refers to extracellular structure formed by self-assembly of secreted fibrillar collagen subunits. An abundant constituent of the extracellular matrix in many animal tissues.
Collagen fiber	White fiber in the matrix of connective tissue, giving flexibility and strength is called collagen fiber.
Extension	Movement increasing the angle between parts at a joint is referred to as extension.
Vesicle	Membranous, cytoplasmic sac formed by an infolding of the cell membrane is called a vesicle.
Phosphate	A phosphate is a polyatomic ion or radical consisting of one phosphorus atom and four oxygen. In the ionic form, it carries a -3 formal charge, and is denoted PO_4^{3-}.
Trauma	Trauma refers to a severe physical injury or wound to the body caused by an external force, or a psychological shock having a lasting effect on mental life.
Pain	Pain is an unpleasant sensation which may be associated with actual or potential tissue damage and which may have physical and emotional components.
Theory	Theory refers to an explanatory statement, or set of statements, that concisely summarizes the state of knowledge on a phenomenon and provides direction for further study.
Caries	Caries is a progressive destruction of any kind of bone structure, including the skull, the ribs and other bones.
Sagittal	A sagittal plane is an X-Z plane, perpendicular to the ground and to the coronal plane, which separates left from right. The midsagittal plane is the specific sagittal plane that is exactly in the middle of the body.
Incisor	The incisor is the first kind of tooth in heterodont mammals. They are adapted for shearing sharply.

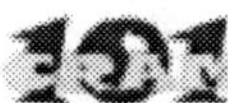

Susceptibility	The degree of resistance of a host to a pathogen is susceptibility.
Dental caries	Dental caries, also known colloquially as tooth decay, is a disease of the teeth resulting in damage to tooth structure.
Heterogeneous	A heterogeneous compound, mixture, or other such object is one that consists of many different items, which are often not easily sorted or separated, though they are clearly distinct.
Rods	Rods, are photoreceptor cells in the retina of the eye that can function in less intense light than can the other type of photoreceptor, cone cells.
Glycosaminog-ycan	Glycosaminoglycan is a long unbranched polysaccharide, made up of repeating disaccharides that may be sulphated (e.g. glucuronic acid, iduronic acid, galactose, galactosamine, glucosamine).
Myelin	Myelin is an electrically insulating fatty layer that surrounds the axons of many neurons, especially those in the peripheral nervous system. It is an outgrowth of glial cells: Schwann cells supply the myelin for peripheral neurons while oligodendrocytes supply it to those of the central nervous system.
Haversian system	One of many structural units of vertebrate bone, consisting of concentric layers of mineralized bone matrix surrounding lacunae, which contain osteocytes, and a central canal, which contains blood vessels and nerves is referred to as haversian system.
Canaliculi	Canaliculi are small, microscopic canals between the various lacunae of ocified bone. The radiating processes of the osteocytes project into these canals. In cartilage, the lacunae and hence, the chondrocytes, are isolated from each other. Materials picked up by osteocytes adjacent to blood vessels, are distributed throughout the bone matrix via the canaliculi.
Labile	Easily moved or changed, quickly shifting from one emotion to another, or easily aroused is referred to as labile.
Mastication	Mastication or chewing is the process by which food is torn and/or crushed by teeth. It is the first step of digestion and it increases the surface area of foods to allow more efficient break down by enzymes.
Atrophy	Atrophy is the partial or complete wasting away of a part of the body. Causes of atrophy include poor nourishment, poor circulation, loss of hormonal support, loss of nerve supply to the target organ, disuse or lack of exercise, or disease intrinsic to the tissue itself.
Scurvy	Scurvy refers to the deficiency disease that results after a few weeks to months of consuming a diet that lacks vitamin C; pinpoint sites of bleeding on the skin are an early sign.
Intervention	Intervention refers to a planned attempt to break through addicts' or abusers' denial and get them into treatment. Interventions most often occur when legal, workplace, health, relationship, or financial problems have become intolerable.
Periosteum	The periosteum is an envelope of fibrous connective tissue that is wrapped around the bone in all places except at joints.
Attachment	Attachment refers to the psychological tendency to seek closeness to another person, to feel secure when that person is present, and to feel anxious when that person is absent.
Sulcus	A sulcus is a depression or fissure in the surface of an organ, most especially the brain. In the brain it surrounds the gyri, creating the characteristic appearance of the brain.
Periodontal disease	A disease located around the teeth or in the periodontiumthe tissue investing and supporting the teeth, including the cementum, periodontal ligament, alveolar bone, and gingiva is referred to as the periodontal disease.

Sphincter | Muscle that surrounds a tube and closes or opens the tube by contracting and relaxing is referred to as sphincter.

Hernia | Hernia refers to abnormal protrusion of an organ or a body part through the containing wall of its cavity. Commonly referred to as a rupture, a hernia often involves protrusion of the intestine through a break in the peritoneum.

Gastroesophageal reflux | Gastroesophageal Reflux Disease (GERD; or GORD when spelling oesophageal, the BE form) is defined as chronic symptoms or mucosal damage produced by the abnormal reflux of gastric contents into the esophagus.

Heartburn | A pain emanating from the esophagus, caused by stomach acid backing up into the esophagus and irritating the esophageal tissue is heartburn.

Pepsin | Pepsin is a digestive protease released by the chief cells in the stomach that functions to degrade food proteins into peptides. It was the first animal enzyme to be discovered.

Bile | Bile is a bitter, greenish-yellow alkaline fluid secreted by the liver of most vertebrates. In many species, it is stored in the gallbladder between meals and upon eating is discharged into the duodenum where it aids the process of digestion.

Xanthine | A xanthine is a alkaloid that is commonly used for its effects as mild stimulants and as bronchodilators, notably in treating the symptoms of asthma.

Chyme | Chyme is the liquid substance found in the stomach before passing the pyloric valve and entering the duodenum. It consists of partially digested food, water, hydrochloric acid, and various digestive enzymes.

Pylorus | The pylorus is the region of the stomach that connects to the duodenum. It is divided in two parts: the pyloric antrum, which connects to the body of the stomach, and the pyloric canal, which connects to the duodenum.

Cardia | The cardia is the anatomical term for the junction orifice of the stomach and the esophagus. At the cardia, the mucosa of the esophagus transitions into gastric mucosa.

Osteoblast | An osteoblast is a mononucleate cell that produces a protein that produces osteoid.

Arteriole | An arteriole is a blood vessel that extends and branches out from an artery and leads to capillaries. They have thick muscular walls and are the primary site of vascular resistance.

Bicarbonate | A Bicarbonate or, more properly, a hydrogen carbonate is a polyatomic ion. It is the intermediate form in the deprotonation of carbonic acid: removing the first proton from carbonic acid forms bicarbonate; removing the second proton leads to the carbonate ion.

Intracellular | Intracellular refers to having to do with the interior of a cell.

Oxygen | Oxygen is a chemical element in the periodic table. It has the symbol O and atomic number 8. Oxygen is the second most common element on Earth, composing around 46% of the mass of Earth's crust and 28% of the mass of Earth as a whole, and is the third most common element in the universe.

Micronutrients | Micronutrients are essential elements only needed by life in small quantities. Vitamins and trace minerals are sometimes included in the term.

Micronutrient | Micronutrient refers to an element that an organism needs in very small amounts and that functions as a component or cofactor of enzymes.

Endogenous | Originating internally, such as the endogenous cholesterol synthesized in the body in contrast to the exogenous cholesterol coming from the diet is referred to as endogenous. Compare with exogenous.

Hydrochloric | The chemical substance hydrochloric acid is the aqueous solution of hydrogen chloride gas. It

acid	is a strong acid, the major component of gastric acid.
Ethanol	Ethanol is a flammable, colorless chemical compound, one of the alcohols that is most often found in alcoholic beverages. In common parlance, it is often referred to simply as alcohol. Its chemical formula is C_2H_5OH, also written as C_2H_6O.
Base	The common definition of a base is a chemical compound that absorbs hydronium ions when dissolved in water (a proton acceptor). An alkali is a special example of a base, where in an aqueous environment, hydroxide ions are donated.
Lead	Lead is a chemical element in the periodic table that has the symbol Pb and atomic number 82. A soft, heavy, toxic and malleable poor metal, lead is bluish white when freshly cut but tarnishes to dull gray when exposed to air. Lead is used in building construction, lead-acid batteries, bullets and shot, and is part of solder, pewter, and fusible alloys.
Helicobacter pylori	Helicobacter pylori is a bacterium that infects the mucus lining of the human stomach. This bacterium lives in the human stomach exclusively and is the only known organism that can thrive in that highly acidic environment..
Microorganism	A microorganism or microbe is an organism that is so small that it is microscopic (invisible to the naked eye).
Inflammation	Inflammation is the first response of the immune system to infection or irritation and may be referred to as the innate cascade.
Ulcer	An ulcer is an open sore of the skin, eyes or mucous membrane, often caused by an initial abrasion and generally maintained by an inflammation and/or an infection.
Agent	Agent refers to an epidemiological term referring to the organism or object that transmits a disease from the environment to the host.
Defense mechanism	Defense mechanism refers to in psychodynamic theory, an unconscious function of the ego that protects it from anxiety-evoking material by preventing accurate recognition of this material.
Aggression	The intentional verbal or non verbal infliction of injury or harm on another person is called aggression.
Prostaglandin	A prostaglandin is any member of a group of lipid compounds that are derived from fatty acids and have important functions in the animal body.
Gastric gland	A tubular structure in the vertebrate stomach that secretes gastric juice is referred to as a gastric gland.
Parietal	When speaking of inner organs, visceral means close to or attached to the organ, while parietal is more distant. For example, the visceral pleura is attached to the lung and the parietal pleura is attached to the chest wall.
Parietal cell	The parietal cell is a located in the stomach epithelium. They produce gastric acid (hydrochloric acid) in response to histamine (via H2 receptors), acetylcholine (M3 receptors) and gastrin (gastrin receptors).
Lysozyme	Lysozyme is an enzyme (EC 3.2.1.17), commonly referred to as the "body's own antibiotic" since it kills bacteria. It is abundantly present in a number of secretions, such as tears (except bovine tears).
Distribution	Distribution in pharmacology is a branch of pharmacokinetics describing reversible transfer of drug from one location to another within the body.
Isthmus	An isthmus is a narrow strip of land that is bordered on two sides by water and connects two larger land masses. It is the inverse of a strait (which lies between two land masses and

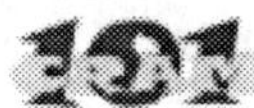

	connects two larger bodies of water).
Capillaries	Capillaries refer to the smallest of the blood vessels and the sites of exchange between the blood and tissue cells.
Capillary	A capillary is the smallest of a body's blood vessels, measuring 5-10 micro meters. They connect arteries and veins, and most closely interact with tissues. Their walls are composed of a single layer of cells, the endothelium. This layer is so thin that molecules such as oxygen, water and lipids can pass through them by diffusion and enter the tissues.
Mitochondria	Cytoplasmic organelles responsible for ATP generation for cellular activities are referred to as mitochondria.
Cytoplasm	Cytoplasm refers to the contents of a cell excluding the nucleus and cell membrane. Cytoplasm is a homogeneous, generally clear jelly-like material that fills cells.
Gastritis	Gastritis is a medical term for inflammation of the lining of the stomach. It means that white blood cells move into the wall of the stomach as a response to some type of injury.
Gastric juice	Gastric juice is a strong acidic liquid, pH 1 to 3, which is close to being colorless. It is secreted by the glands in the lining of the stomach.
Intrinsic factor	A substance produced by the gastric glands that promotes absorption of vitamin is called an intrinsic factor.
Pinocytosis	Process by which a cell engulfs droplets of fluid from its surroundings is referred to as pinocytosis.
Ileum	The ileum is the final section of the small intestine. Its function is to absorb vitamin B12 and bile salts. The wall itself made up of folds, each of which has many tiny finger-like projections known as villi, on its surface.
Autoimmune	Autoimmune refers to immune reactions against normal body cells; self against self.
Anemia	Anemia is a deficiency of red blood cells and/or hemoglobin. This results in a reduced ability of blood to transfer oxygen to the tissues, and this causes hypoxia; since all human cells depend on oxygen for survival, varying degrees of anemia can have a wide range of clinical consequences.
Autoimmune disease	Disease that results when the immune system mistakenly attacks the body's own tissues is referred to as autoimmune disease.
Polypeptide	Polypeptide refers to polymer of many amino acids linked by peptide bonds.
Cholinergic	A synapse is cholinergic if it uses acetylcholine as its neurotransmitter. The parasympathetic nervous system is entirely cholinergic.
Gastrin	In humans, gastrin is a hormone that stimulates secretion of gastric acid by the stomach. It is released by G cells in the stomach.
Pepsinogen	The inactive form of pepsin that is first secreted by specialized cells located in gastric pits of the stomach is pepsinogen.
Specificity	A medical diagnostic test for a certain disease, specificity is the proportion of true negatives of all the negative samples tested.
Micrograph	A micrograph is a photograph or similar image taken through a microscope or similar device to show a magnified image of an item.
Serotonin	Serotonin is a monoamine neurotransmitter synthesized in serotonergic neurons in the central nervous system and enterochromaffin cells in the gastrointestinal tract. It is believed to play an important part of the biochemistry of depression, migraine, bipolar disorder and

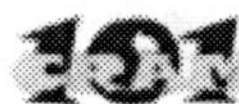

	anxiety.
Vasoconstriction	Vasoconstriction refers to a decrease in the diameter of a blood vessel.
Amine	An organic compound with one or more amino groups is called amine. They contain nitrogen as the key atom. Structurally amines resemble ammonia, wherein one or more hydrogen atoms are replaced by organic substituents such as alkyl and aryl groups.
Somatostatin	Somatostatin is hormone secreted not only by cells of the hypothalamus but also by so called delta cells of stomach, intestine and pancreas. It binds to somatostatin receptors. All actions of the hormone are inhibitory.
Diffusion	Random movement of molecules from a region of higher concentration toward one of lower concentration is referred to as diffusion.
ATPase	ATPase is a class of enzymes that catalyze the decomposition of adenosine triphosphate into adenosine diphosphate and a free phosphate ion. This dephosphorylation reaction releases energy, which the enzyme harnesses to drive other chemical reactions that would not otherwise occur. This process is widely used in all known forms of life.
Active transport	Process that requires an expenditure of energy to move a substance across a cell membrane is referred to as active transport.
Carbonic acid	A weak acid formed when carbon dioxide dissolves in water is referred to as carbonic acid.
Proton	Positive subatomic particle, located in the nucleus and having a weight of approximately one atomic mass unit is referred to as a proton.
Pyloric sphincter	Pyloric sphincter in the vertebrate digestive tract, a muscular ring that regulates the passage of food out of the stomach and into the small intestine.
Duodenum	The duodenum is a hollow jointed tube connecting the stomach to the jejunum. It is the first part of the small intestine. Two very important ducts open into the duodenum, namely the bile duct and the pancreatic duct. The duodenum is largely responsible for the breakdown of food in the small intestine.
Jejunum	The jejunum is the central of the three divisions of the small intestine. The inner surface of the jejunum, its mucous membrane, is covered in projections called villi, which increase the surface area of tissue available to absorb nutrients from the gut contents.
Substance p	Substance p is a protein substance that stimulates nerve endings at an injury site and within the spinal cord, increasing pain messages.
Gallbladder	The gallbladder is a pear-shaped organ that stores bile until the body needs it for digestion. It is connected to the liver and the duodenum by the biliary tract.
Insulin	Insulin is a polypeptide hormone that regulates carbohydrate metabolism. Apart from being the primary effector in carbohydrate homeostasis, it also has a substantial effect on small vessel muscle tone, controls storage and release of fat (triglycerides) and cellular uptake of both amino acids and some electrolytes.
Protrusion	Protrusion is the anterior movement of an object. This term is often applied to the jaw.
Actin	A protein in a muscle fiber that, together with myosin, is responsible for contraction and relaxation is actin.
Brush border	Brush border refers to dense covering of microvilli on the apical surface of epithelial cells in the intestine and kidney. The microvilli aid absorption by increasing the surface area of the cell.
Disaccharide	A disaccharide is a sugar (a carbohydrate) composed of two monosaccharides. The two monosaccharides are bonded via a condensation reaction.

Hydrolyze — Hydrolyze refers to break a chemical bond, as in a peptide linkage, with the insertion of the components of water, -H and -OH, at the cleaved ends of a chain. The digestion of proteins is hydrolysis.

Dipeptide — Two amino acids connected by a peptide bond is referred to as a dipeptide.

Lipid — Lipid is one class of aliphatic hydrocarbon-containing organic compounds essential for the structure and function of living cells. They are characterized by being water-insoluble but soluble in nonpolar organic solvents.

Pancreatic lipase — Pancreatic lipase is an enzyme secreted from the pancreas that uses hydrolysis to break apart fat molecules.

Syndrome — Syndrome is the association of several clinically recognizable features, signs, symptoms, phenomena or characteristics which often occur together, so that the presence of one feature alerts the physician to the presence of the others

Bacteria — The domain that contains procaryotic cells with primarily diacyl glycerol diesters in their membranes and with bacterial rRNA. Bacteria also is a general term for organisms that are composed of procaryotic cells and are not multicellular.

Lymphocyte — A lymphocyte is a type of white blood cell involved in the human body's immune system. There are two broad categories, namely T cells and B cells.

Plasma — Fluid portion of circulating blood is called plasma.

Peptide — Peptide is the family of molecules formed from the linking, in a defined order, of various amino acids. The link between one amino acid residue and the next is an amide bond, and is sometimes referred to as a peptide bond.

Endocrinology — Endocrinology is a branch of medicine dealing with disorders of the endocrine system and its specific secretions called hormones.

Staining — Staining is a biochemical technique of adding a class-specific (DNA, proteins, lipids, carbohydrates) dye to a substrate to qualify or quantify the presence of a specific compound. They are frequently used to highlight structures in tissues for viewing, often with the aid of different microscopes.

Actin filament — An actin filament is a helical protein filament formed by the polymerization of globular actin molecules. They provide mechanical support for the cell, determine the cell shape, enable cell movements; and participate in certain cell junctions.

Fibrin — Fibrin is a protein involved in the clotting of blood. It is a fibrillar protein that is polymerized to form a "mesh" that forms a haemostatic plug or clot (in conjunction with platelets) over a wound site.

Hydrolysis — Hydrolysis is a chemical process in which a molecule is cleaved into two parts by the addition of a molecule of water.

Carbon — Carbon is a chemical element in the periodic table that has the symbol C and atomic number 6. An abundant nonmetallic, tetravalent element, carbon has several allotropic forms.

Atom — An atom is the smallest possible particle of a chemical element that retains its chemical properties.

Villus — Villus refers to a fingerlike projection of the inner surface of the small intestine. A fingerlike projection of the chorion of the mammalian placenta. Large numbers of villus increase the surface areas of these organs.

Constant — A behavior or characteristic that does not vary from one observation to another is referred to as a constant.

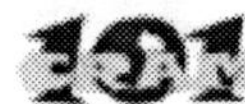

Microscope	A microscope is an instrument for viewing objects that are too small to be seen by the naked or unaided eye.
M cell	Specialized cell of the intestinal mucosa and other sites, such as the urogenital tract, that delivers the antigen from the apical face of the cell to lymphocytes clustered within the pocket in its basolateral face is a the M cell.
Antigen	An antigen is a substance that stimulates an immune response, especially the production of antibodies. They are usually proteins or polysaccharides, but can be any type of molecule, including small molecules (haptens) coupled to a protein (carrier).
Eye	An eye is an organ that detects light. Different kinds of light-sensitive organs are found in a variety of creatures. The simplest eyes do nothing but detect whether the surroundings are light or dark, while more complex eyes can distinguish shapes and colors.
Venule	A vessel that conveys blood between a capillary bed and a vein is a venule.
Veins	Blood vessels that return blood toward the heart from the circulation are referred to as veins.
Vein	Vein in animals, is a vessel that returns blood to the heart. In plants, a vascular bundle in a leaf, composed of xylem and phloem.
Macromolecule	A macromolecule is a molecule with a large molecular mass, but generally the use of the term is restricted to polymers and molecules which structurally include polymers.
Lacteal	A lacteal is a lymphatic vessel that absorbs dietary fats in the small intestine. Individual lacteals merge to form larger lymphatic vessels that transport the fats to the thoracic duct which empties into the jugular vein.
Chemoreceptor	Chemoreceptor is a cell or group of cells that transduce a chemical signal into an action potential.
Mechanoreceptor	A mechanoreceptor is a sensory receptor that responds to mechanical pressure or distortion. There are four main types: Pacinian corpuscles, Meissner's corpuscles, Merkel's discs, and the tympanic membrane.
Sensory neuron	Sensory neuron refers to nerve cell that transmits nerve impulses to the central nervous system after a sensory receptor has been stimulated.
Nerve cell	A cell specialized to originate or transmit nerve impulses is referred to as nerve cell.
Sympathetic	The sympathetic nervous system activates what is often termed the "fight or flight response". It is an automatic regulation system, that is, one that operates without the intervention of conscious thought.
Adrenergic	Pertaining to epinephrine or norepinephrine, as in adrenergic neurons that secrete one of these chemicals or adrenergic effects on a target organ is called adrenegic.
Sodium	Sodium is the chemical element in the periodic table that has the symbol Na (Natrium in Latin) and atomic number 11. Sodium is a soft, waxy, silvery reactive metal belonging to the alkali metals that is abundant in natural compounds (especially halite). It is highly reactive.
Population	Population refers to all members of a well-defined group of organisms, events, or things.
Apoptosis	In biology, apoptosis is one of the main types of programmed cell death (PCD). As such, it is a process of deliberate life relinquishment by an unwanted cell in a multicellular organism.
Chemotherapy	Chemotherapy is the use of chemical substances to treat disease. In its modern-day use, it refers almost exclusively to cytostatic drugs used to treat cancer.In its non-oncological use, the term may also refer to antibiotics.

Cancer	Cancer is a class of diseases or disorders characterized by uncontrolled division of cells and the ability of these cells to invade other tissues, either by direct growth into adjacent tissue through invasion or by implantation into distant sites by metastasis.
Regeneration	Regeneration is the ability to restore lost or damaged tissues, organs or limbs. It is a common feature in invertebrates, but far more limited in most vertebrates.
Tumor	An abnormal mass of cells that forms within otherwise normal tissue is a tumor. This growth can be either malignant or benign
Glandular epithelium	Columnar epithelium with goblet cells is called glandular epithelium. Some parts of the glandular epithelium consist of such a large number of goblet cells that there are only a few normal epithelial cells left. Columnar and cuboidal epithelial cells often become specialized as gland cells which are capable of synthesising and secreting certain substances such as enzymes, hormones, milk, mucus, sweat, wax and saliva.
Diagnosis	In medicine, diagnosis is the process of identifying a medical condition or disease by its signs, symptoms, and from the results of various diagnostic procedures.
Adaptation	A biological adaptation is an anatomical structure, physiological process or behavioral trait of an organism that has evolved over a period of time by the process of natural selection such that it increases the expected long-term reproductive success of the organism.
Physiology	The study of the function of cells, tissues, and organs is referred to as physiology.
Gastroenterology	Gastroenterology or gastrology is the medical specialty concerned with the field of digestive diseases. Traditionally, these are separated by anatomic or functional category.

Carbohydrate	Carbohydrate is a chemical compound that contains oxygen, hydrogen, and carbon atoms. They consist of monosaccharide sugars of varying chain lengths and that have the general chemical formula $C_n(H_2O)_n$ or are derivatives of such.
Digestion	Digestion refers to the mechanical and chemical breakdown of food into molecules small enough for the body to absorb; the second main stage of food processing, following ingestion.
Lysozyme	Lysozyme is an enzyme (EC 3.2.1.17), commonly referred to as the "body's own antibiotic" since it kills bacteria. It is abundantly present in a number of secretions, such as tears (except bovine tears).
Amylase	Amylase is a digestive enzyme classified as a saccharidase. It is mainly a constituent of pancreatic juice and saliva, needed for the breakdown of long-chain carbohydrates (such as starch) into smaller units.
Saliva	Saliva is the moist, clear, and usually somewhat frothy substance produced in the mouths of some animals, including humans.
Lipase	A lipase is a water-soluble enzyme that catalyzes the hydrolysis of ester bonds in water–insoluble, lipid substrates. Most lipases act at a specific position on the glycerol backbone of a lipid substrate (A1, A2 or A3).
Lipid	Lipid is one class of aliphatic hydrocarbon-containing organic compounds essential for the structure and function of living cells. They are characterized by being water-insoluble but soluble in nonpolar organic solvents.
Gland	A gland is an organ in an animal's body that synthesizes a substance for release such as hormones, often into the bloodstream or into cavities inside the body or its outer surface.
Salivary gland	The salivary gland produces saliva, which keeps the mouth and other parts of the digestive system moist. It also helps break down carbohydrates and lubricates the passage of food down from the oro-pharynx to the esophagus to the stomach.
Proline	Proline is one of the twenty proteinogenic units which are used in living organisms as the building blocks of proteins. The other nineteen units are all primary amino acids, but due to the (3-carbon) cyclic sidechain binding back to the nitrogen of the backbone, proline lacks a primary amine group ($-NH_2$).
Protein	A protein is a complex, high-molecular-weight organic compound that consists of amino acids joined by peptide bonds. They are essential to the structure and function of all living cells and viruses. Many are enzymes or subunits of enzymes.
Calcium	Calcium is the chemical element in the periodic table that has the symbol Ca and atomic number 20. Calcium is a soft grey alkaline earth metal that is used as a reducing agent in the extraction of thorium, zirconium and uranium. Calcium is also the fifth most abundant element in the Earth's crust.
Evaporative cooling	Evaporative cooling is a system in which latent heat of evaporation is used to carry heat away from an object to cool it. The latent heat contains a considerable amount of energy, and carries away more heat than if the same temperature liquid was simply removed physically.
Intestine	The intestine is the portion of the alimentary canal extending from the stomach to the anus and, in humans and mammals, consists of two segments, the small intestine and the large intestine. The intestine is the part of the body responsible for extracting nutrition from food.
Glucagon	A peptide hormone secreted by islet cells in the pancreas that raises the level of glucose in the blood is referred to as glucagon. Glucagon is a 29 amino acid polypeptide acting as an important hormone in carbohydrate metabolism.

Pancreas | The pancreas is a retroperitoneal organ that serves two functions: exocrine - it produces pancreatic juice containing digestive enzymes, and endocrine - it produces several important hormones, namely insulin.

Hormone | A hormone is a chemical messenger from one cell to another. All multicellular organisms produce hormones. The best known hormones are those produced by endocrine glands of vertebrate animals, but hormones are produced by nearly every organ system and tissue type in a human or animal body. Hormone molecules are secreted directly into the bloodstream, they move by circulation or diffusion to their target cells, which may be nearby cells in the same tissue or cells of a distant organ of the body.

Insulin | Insulin is a polypeptide hormone that regulates carbohydrate metabolism. Apart from being the primary effector in carbohydrate homeostasis, it also has a substantial effect on small vessel muscle tone, controls storage and release of fat (triglycerides) and cellular uptake of both amino acids and some electrolytes.

Enzyme | An enzyme is a protein that catalyzes, or speeds up, a chemical reaction. They are essential to sustain life because most chemical reactions in biological cells would occur too slowly, or would lead to different products, without them.

Small intestine | The small intestine is the part of the gastrointestinal tract between the stomach and the large intestine (colon). In humans over 5 years old it is about 7m long. It is divided into three structural parts: duodenum, jejunum and ileum.

Metabolism | Metabolism is the biochemical modification of chemical compounds in living organisms and cells. This includes the biosynthesis of complex organic molecules (anabolism) and their breakdown (catabolism).

Liver | The liver is an organ in vertebrates, including humans. It plays a major role in metabolism and has a number of functions in the body including drug detoxification, glycogen storage, and plasma protein synthesis. It also produces bile, which is important for digestion.

Bile | Bile is a bitter, greenish-yellow alkaline fluid secreted by the liver of most vertebrates. In many species, it is stored in the gallbladder between meals and upon eating is discharged into the duodenum where it aids the process of digestion.

Coagulation | The coagulation of blood is a complex process during which blood forms solid clots. It is an important part of haemostasis (the ceszation of blood loss from a damaged vessel) whereby a damaged blood vessel wall is covered by a fibrin clot to stop hemorrhage and aid repair of the damaged vessel.

Blood | Blood is a circulating tissue composed of fluid plasma and cells. The main function of blood is to supply nutrients (oxygen, glucose) and constitutional elements to tissues and to remove waste products.

Iron | Iron is essential to all organisms, except for a few bacteria. It is mostly stably incorporated in the inside of metalloproteins, because in exposed or in free form it causes production of free radicals that are generally toxic to cells.

Iron metabolism | The system of iron metabolism has been of special interest to hematologists because iron is essential to red blood cells, the bulk of the body's iron is contained in red blood cells' hemoglobin, and iron-deficiency is the most common cause of anemia.

Gallbladder | The gallbladder is a pear-shaped organ that stores bile until the body needs it for digestion. It is connected to the liver and the duodenum by the biliary tract.

Oral cavity | The mouth, also known as the buccal cavity or the oral cavity, is the opening through which an animal or human takes in food and water. It is usually located in the head, but not always; the mouth of a planarium is in the middle of its belly.

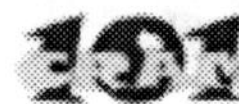

Sublingual	Area beneath the tongue is called sublingual.
Parotid	The parotid gland is the largest of the salivary glands. It is found in the subcutaneous tissue of the face, overlying the mandibular ramus and anterior and inferior to the external
Sublingual gland	The sublingual gland is a salivary gland in the mouth. They lie anterior to the submandibular gland under the tongue, beneath the mucous membrane of the floor of the mouth. They are drained by 8-20 excretory ducts.
Mucus	Mucus is a slippery secretion of the lining of various membranes in the body (mucous membranes). Mucus aids in the protection of the lungs by trapping foreign particles that enter the nose during normal breathing. Additionally, it prevents tissues from drying out.
Collagen	Collagen is the main protein of connective tissue in animals and the most abundant protein in mammals, making up about 1/4 of the total. It is one of the long, fibrous structural proteins whose functions are quite different from those of globular proteins such as enzymes.
Tissue	A collection of interconnected cells that perform a similar function within an organism is called tissue.
Fiber	Fibers used by man come from a wide variety of sources: Natural fiber include those made out of plants, animal and mineral sources. Natural fibers can be classified according to their origin.
Connective tissue	Connective tissue is any type of biological tissue with an extensive extracellular matrix and often serves to support, bind together, and protect organs.
Collagen fiber	White fiber in the matrix of connective tissue, giving flexibility and strength is called collagen fiber.
Parenchyma	The parenchyma are the functional parts of an organ in the body (i.e. the nephrons of the kidney, the alveoli of the lungs). In plants parenchyma cells are thin-walled cells of the ground tissue that make up the bulk of most nonwoody structures, although sometimes their cell walls can be lignified.
Base	The common definition of a base is a chemical compound that absorbs hydronium ions when dissolved in water (a proton acceptor). An alkali is a special example of a base, where in an aqueous environment, hydroxide ions are donated.
Serous	The term serous fluid is used for various bodily fluids that are typically pale yellow and transparent, and of a benign nature.
Myoepithelial cell	Myoepithelial cell refers to type of unstriated muscle cell found in epithelia, e.g. In the iris of the eye and in glandular tissue.
Striation	Striation refers to the tiny grooves of muscle across major muscle groups characteristic of a well-developed body.
Mitochondria	Cytoplasmic organelles responsible for ATP generation for cellular activities are referred to as mitochondria.
Microscope	A microscope is an instrument for viewing objects that are too small to be seen by the naked or unaided eye.
Plasma	Fluid portion of circulating blood is called plasma.
Ion	Ion refers to an atom or molecule that has gained or lost one or more electrons, thus acquiring an electrical charge.
Plasma membrane	The unit membrane that encloses a cell and controls the traffic of molecules in and out of the cell is the plasma membrane.

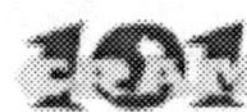

Epithelium	Epithelium is a tissue composed of a layer of cells. Epithelium can be found lining internal (e.g. endothelium, which lines the inside of blood vessels) or external (e.g. skin) free surfaces of the body. Functions include secretion, absorption and protection.
Invagination	Infolding of one part of a structure into another is invagination.
Squamous epithelium	The squamous epithelium is epithelium consisting of one or more cell layers, the most superficial of which is composed of flat, scalelike or platelike cells.
Nerve	A nerve is an enclosed, cable-like bundle of nerve fibers or axons, which includes the glia that ensheath the axons in myelin.
Plexus	A plexus is also a network of blood vessels, with the choroid plexuses of the brain being the most commonly mentioned example. A choroid plexus is very thin and vascular roof plates of the most anterior and most posterior cavities of the brain which expand into the interiors of the cavities.
Autonomic nervous system	The autonomic nervous system is the part of the nervous system that is not consciously controlled. It is commonly divided into two usually antagonistic subsystems: the sympathetic and parasympathetic nervous system.
Capillaries	Capillaries refer to the smallest of the blood vessels and the sites of exchange between the blood and tissue cells.
Capillary	A capillary is the smallest of a body's blood vessels, measuring 5-10 micro meters. They connect arteries and veins, and most closely interact with tissues. Their walls are composed of a single layer of cells, the endothelium. This layer is so thin that molecules such as oxygen, water and lipids can pass through them by diffusion and enter the tissues.
Nervous system	The nervous system of an animal coordinates the activity of the muscles, monitors the organs, constructs and processes input from the senses, and initiates actions.
Vasodilation	An increase in the diameter of superficial blood vessels triggered by nerve signals that relax the smooth muscles of the vessel walls is referred to as vasodilation.
Sympathetic	The sympathetic nervous system activates what is often termed the "fight or flight response". It is an automatic regulation system, that is, one that operates without the intervention of conscious thought.
Parotid gland	The parotid gland is the largest of the salivary glands. It is found in the subcutaneous tissue of the face, overlying the mandibular ramus and anterior and inferior to the external
Stomach	The stomach is an organ in the alimentary canal used to digest food. It's primary function is not the absorption of nutrients from digested food; rather, the main job of the stomach is to break down large food molecules into smaller ones, so that they can be absorbed into the blood more easily.
Gastric juice	Gastric juice is a strong acidic liquid, pH 1 to 3, which is close to being colorless. It is secreted by the glands in the lining of the stomach.
Organ	Organ refers to a structure consisting of several tissues adapted as a group to perform specific functions.
Digestive tract	The digestive tract is the system of organs within multicellular animals which takes in food, digests it to extract energy and nutrients, and expels the remaining waste.
Lymphocyte	A lymphocyte is a type of white blood cell involved in the human body's immune system. There are two broad categories, namely T cells and B cells.
Pathogen	A pathogen or infectious agent is a biological agent that causes disease or illness to its host.The term is most often used for agents that disrupt the normal physiology of a

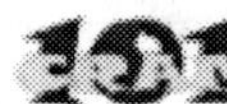

	multicellular animal or plant.
Defense mechanism	Defense mechanism refers to in psychodynamic theory, an unconscious function of the ego that protects it from anxiety-evoking material by preventing accurate recognition of this material.
Submandibular gland	The submandibular gland is one of the salivary glands, responsible for producing saliva. It lies inferior to the mylohyoid muscles and superior to the digastric muscle.
Cytoplasm	Cytoplasm refers to the contents of a cell excluding the nucleus and cell membrane. Cytoplasm is a homogeneous, generally clear jelly-like material that fills cells.
Electrolyte	An electrolyte is a substance that dissociates into free ions when dissolved (or molten), to produce an electrically conductive medium. Because they generally consist of ions in solution, they are also known as ionic solutions.
Hydrolyze	Hydrolyze refers to break a chemical bond, as in a peptide linkage, with the insertion of the components of water, -H and -OH, at the cleaved ends of a chain. The digestion of proteins is hydrolysis.
Bacteria	The domain that contains procaryotic cells with primarily diacyl glycerol diesters in their membranes and with bacterial rRNA. Bacteria also is a general term for organisms that are composed of procaryotic cells and are not multicellular.
Submucosa	The tissue layer just under the epithelial lining of the lumen of the digestive tract is referred to as the submucosa.
Islets of Langerhans	The endocrine (i.e., hormone-producing) cells of the pancreas are grouped in the Islets of Langerhans.
Atrophy	Atrophy is the partial or complete wasting away of a part of the body. Causes of atrophy include poor nourishment, poor circulation, loss of hormonal support, loss of nerve supply to the target organ, disuse or lack of exercise, or disease intrinsic to the tissue itself.
Caries	Caries is a progressive destruction of any kind of bone structure, including the skull, the ribs and other bones.
Dental caries	Dental caries, also known colloquially as tooth decay, is a disease of the teeth resulting in damage to tooth structure.
Radiation	The emission of electromagnetic waves by all objects warmer than absolute zero is referred to as radiation.
Syndrome	Syndrome is the association of several clinically recognizable features, signs, symptoms, phenomena or characteristics which often occur together, so that the presence of one feature alerts the physician to the presence of the others
Elderly	Old age consists of ages nearing the average life span of human beings, and thus the end of the human life cycle. Euphemisms for older people include advanced adult, elderly, and senior or senior citizen.
Lamina	A thin layer, such as the lamina of a vertebra or the lamina propria of a mucous membrane is referred to as lamina.
Zymogen	An inactive precursor of a digestive enzyme secreted into the lumen of the gut, where a protease cleaves it to form the active enzyme is called zymogen.
Septa	Septa are thin walls or partitions between the internal chambers (camerae) of the shell of a cephalopod, namely nautiloids or ammonoids.
Pancreatic duct	The pancreatic duct joins the pancreas to the bile duct to supply pancreatic juice which aid in digestion provided by the "exocrine pancreas".

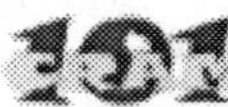

Triglyceride | Triglyceride is a glyceride in which the glycerol is esterified with three fatty acids. They are the main constituent of vegetable oil and animal fats and play an important role in metabolism as energy sources. They contain a bit more than twice as much energy as carbohydrates and proteins.

Trypsinogen | Trypsinogen is the precursor form of the pancreatic enzyme trypsin. It is found in pancreatic juice, along with amylase, lipase, and chymotrypsinogen. It is activated by enterokinase, which is found in the intestinal mucosa, to form trypsin.

Hydrolase | Hydrolase is a general term for any enzyme that catalyzes a hydrolysis reaction, the chemical breakdown of polymers into smaller molecules through the addition of water molecules.

Isosmotic | Isosmotic refers to having the same osmotic concentration or pressure as a reference solution.

Carboxyl | A carboxyl is the univalent radical -COOH; present in and characteristic of organic acids.

Nuclease | Enzyme that cleaves phosphodiester bonds in nucleic acids is referred to as nuclease.

Protease | Protease refers to an enzyme that breaks peptide bonds between amino acids of proteins.

Deoxyribonuc-ease | A deoxyribonuclease is any enzyme that catalyzes the hydrolytic cleavage of phosphodiester linkages in the DNA backbone. Deoxyribonuclease is thus one type of nuclease.

Chymotrypsinogen | Chymotrypsinogen is a precursor of the digestive enzyme chymotrypsin (zymogen). This molecule is inactive and must be cleaved by trypsin, and then by other chymotrypsin molecules before it can reach its full activity.

Enterokinase | Enterokinase is a kinase released by the intestinal glands in the small intestine that activates trypsinogen, a zymogen, to trypsin.

Trypsin | The enzyme trypsin is produced in the pancreas in the form of trypsinogen, and is then transported to the small intestine, where begins the digestion of proteins to polypeptides and amino acids.

Pancreatitis | Pancreatitis is inflammation of the pancreas. The most common causes of pancreatitis are gallstones and frequent and excessive consumption of alcohol (80% of cases), and less common causes are drugs or medication.

Acute | In medicine, an acute disease is a disease with either or both of: a rapid onset; and a short course (as opposed to a chronic course).

Alcoholism | A disorder that involves long-term, repeated, uncontrolled, compulsive, and excessive use of alcoholic beverages and that impairs the drinker's health and work and social relationships is called alcoholism.

Infection | The invasion and multiplication of microorganisms in body tissues is called an infection.

Gallstone | A gallstone is a crystalline body formed within the body by accretion or concretion of normal or abnormal bile components. They can occur anywhere within the biliary tree, including the gallbladder and the common bile duct.

Trauma | Trauma refers to a severe physical injury or wound to the body caused by an external force, or a psychological shock having a lasting effect on mental life.

Vagus nerve | The vagus nerve is tenth of twelve paired cranial nerves and is the only nerve that starts in the brainstem and extends all the way down past the head, right down to the abdomen. The vagus nerve is arguably the single most important nerve in the body.

Duodenum | The duodenum is a hollow jointed tube connecting the stomach to the jejunum. It is the first part of the small intestine. Two very important ducts open into the duodenum, namely the bile duct and the pancreatic duct. The duodenum is largely responsible for the breakdown of food

	in the small intestine.
Jejunum	The jejunum is the central of the three divisions of the small intestine. The inner surface of the jejunum, its mucous membrane, is covered in projections called villi, which increase the surface area of tissue available to absorb nutrients from the gut contents.
Mucosa	The mucosa is a lining of ectodermic origin, covered in epithelium, and involved in absorption and secretion. They line various body cavities that are exposed to the external environment and internal organs.
Cholecystokinin	Cholecystokinin is a peptide hormone of the gastrointestinal system responsible for stimulating the digestion of fat and protein. It is secreted by the duodenum and causes the release of digestive enzymes and bile from the pancreas and gall bladder. It also acts as a hunger suppresant.
Stimulus	Stimulus in a nervous system, a factor that triggers sensory transduction.
Secretin	Secretin is a peptide hormone produced in the S cells of the duodenum. It is secreted in response to low duodenal pH or the presence of fatty acids in the duodenum, and stimulates the secretion of bicarbonate from the liver, pancreas, and duodenal Brunner's glands.
Acid	An acid is a water-soluble, sour-tasting chemical compound that when dissolved in water, gives a solution with a pH of less than 7.
Electrolytes	Electrolytes refers to compounds that separate into ions in water and, in turn, are able to conduct an electrical current. These include sodium, chloride, and potassium.
Bicarbonate	A Bicarbonate or, more properly, a hydrogen carbonate is a polyatomic ion. It is the intermediate form in the deprotonation of carbonic acid: removing the first proton from carbonic acid forms bicarbonate; removing the second proton leads to the carbonate ion.
Enzyme activity	Enzyme activity is the catalytic effect exerted by an enzyme.
Micrograph	A micrograph is a photograph or similar image taken through a microscope or similar device to show a magnified image of an item.
Exocytosis	Exocytosis is the process by which a cell is able to get rid of large molecules or materials including wastes through its membrane. The process involves a [vacuole], containing the material, fusing with the membrane.
Vacuole	Vacuole refers to a space or cavity within the cytoplasm of a cell.
Amino acid	An amino acid is any molecule that contains both amino and carboxylic acid functional groups. They are the basic structural building units of proteins. They form short polymer chains called peptides or polypeptides which in turn form structures called proteins.
Fatty acid	A fatty acid is a carboxylic acid (or organic acid), often with a long aliphatic tail (long chains), either saturated or unsaturated.
Essential amino acid	An essential amino acid for an organism is an amino acid that cannot be synthesized by the organism from other available resources, and therefore must be supplied as part of its diet.
Pancreatic juice	Pancreatic juice is a juice produced by the pancreas. It contains a variety of enzymes. They include trypsinogen, chymotrypsinogen, pancreatic lipase, and amylase.
Malnutrition	Malnutrition is a general term for the medical condition in a person or animal caused by an unbalanced diet—either too little or too much food, or a diet missing one or more important nutrients.
Kwashiorkor	Kwashiorkor is a childhood disorder caused by lack of nutrients, including protein in the diet. Symptoms of kwashiorkor include a swollen abdomen, reddish discoloration of the hair and depigmented skin.

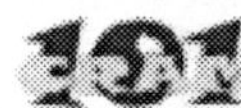

Skin	Skin is an organ of the integumentary system composed of a layer of tissues that protect underlying muscles and organs.
Diaphragm	The diaphragm is a shelf of muscle extending across the bottom of the ribcage. It is critically important in respiration: in order to draw air into the lungs, the diaphragm contracts, thus enlarging the thoracic cavity and reducing intra-thoracic pressure.
Digestive system	The organ system that ingests food, breaks it down into smaller chemical units, and absorbs the nutrient molecules is referred to as the digestive system.
Portal vein	The portal vein is the largest vein in the human body draining blood from the digestive system and its associated glands. It is formed by the union of the splenic vein and superior mesenteric vein and divides into a right and a left branch, before entering the liver.
Artery	Vessel that takes blood away from the heart to the tissues and organs of the body is called an artery.
Spleen	The spleen is a ductless, vertebrate gland that is not necessary for life but is closely associated with the circulatory system, where it functions in the destruction of old red blood cells and removal of other debris from the bloodstream, and also in holding a reservoir of blood.
Vein	Vein in animals, is a vessel that returns blood to the heart. In plants, a vascular bundle in a leaf, composed of xylem and phloem.
Hepatic artery	Hepatic artery distributes blood to the liver, pancreas and gallbladder as well as to the stomach and duodenal portion of the small intestine.
Lymph vessel	Lymph vessel refers to one of the system of vessels carrying lymph from the lymph capillaries to the veins.
Chylomicron	Particles of lipid coated with protein, produced in by the absorptive cells of the small intestine and secreted into the extracellular fluids are referred to as chylomicron.
Lymph	Lymph originates as blood plasma lost from the circulatory system, which leaks out into the surrounding tissues. The lymphatic system collects this fluid by diffusion into lymph capillaries, and returns it to the circulatory system.
Metabolite	The term metabolite is usually restricted to small molecules. They are the intermediates and products of metabolism. A primary metabolite is directly involved in the normal growth, development, and reproduction. A secondary metabolite is not directly involved in those processes, but usually has important ecological function.
Circulatory system	The circulatory system or cardiovascular system is the organ system which circulates blood around the body of most animals.
Elimination	Elimination refers to the physiologic excretion of drugs and other substances from the body.
Albumin	Albumin refers generally to any protein with water solubility, which is moderately soluble in concentrated salt solutions, and experiences heat coagulation (protein denaturation).
Carrier	Person in apparent health whose chromosomes contain a pathologic mutant gene that may be transmitted to his or her children is a carrier.
Hepatocyte	Hepatocyte cells make up 60-80% of the cytoplasmic mass of the liver. They are involved in protein synthesis, protein storage and transformation of carbohydrates, synthesis of cholesterol, bile salts and phospholipids, and detoxification, modification and excretion of exogenous and endogenous substances.
Endothelial cell	A endothelial cell also controls the passage of materials — and the transit of white blood cells — into and out of the bloodstream. In some organs, there are highly differentiated

	endothelial cells to perform specialized 'filtering' functions.
Blood vessel	A blood vessel is a part of the circulatory system and function to transport blood throughout the body. The most important types, arteries and veins, are so termed because they carry blood away from or towards the heart, respectively.
Bile duct	A bile duct is any of a number of long tube-like structures that carry bile. The top half of the common bile duct is associated with the liver, while the bottom half of the common bile duct is associated with the pancreas, through which it passes on its way to the intestine. It opens in the part of the intestine called the duodenum into a structure called the ampulla of Vater.
Arteriole	An arteriole is a blood vessel that extends and branches out from an artery and leads to capillaries. They have thick muscular walls and are the primary site of vascular resistance.
Venule	A vessel that conveys blood between a capillary bed and a vein is a venule.
Splenic vein	The splenic vein is the blood vessel that drains blood from spleen. It joins with the superior mesenteric vein, to form the portal vein and follows a course superior to the pancreas, along side of the similarly named artery, the splenic artery.
Veins	Blood vessels that return blood toward the heart from the circulation are referred to as veins.
Oxygen	Oxygen is a chemical element in the periodic table. It has the symbol O and atomic number 8. Oxygen is the second most common element on Earth, composing around 46% of the mass of Earth's crust and 28% of the mass of Earth as a whole, and is the third most common element in the universe.
Aorta	The largest artery in the human body, the aorta originates from the left ventricle of the heart and brings oxygenated blood to all parts of the body in the systemic circulation.
Abdominal aorta	The abdominal aorta travels down the posterior wall of the abdomen, the abdominal aorta runs on the left of the inferior vena cava, giving off major blood vessels to the gut organs and kidneys.
Hepatic duct	Hepatic duct refers to the duct that conveys bile from the liver to the gallbladder.
Canaliculi	Canaliculi are small, microscopic canals between the various lacunae of ocified bone. The radiating processes of the osteocytes project into these canals. In cartilage, the lacunae and hence, the chondrocytes, are isolated from each other. Materials picked up by osteocytes adjacent to blood vessels, are distributed throughout the bone matrix via the canaliculi.
Histology	Histology is the study of tissue sectioned as a thin slice, using a microscope. It can be described as microscopic anatomy.
Kupffer cell	Kupffer cell is a specialized macrophage located in the liver that forms part of the reticuloendothelial system.
Population	Population refers to all members of a well-defined group of organisms, events, or things.
Phagocytosis	Phagocytosis (literally, "cell eating") is a form of endocytosis where large particles are enveloped by the cell membrane of a (usually larger) cell and internalized to form a phagosome, or "food vacuole."
Proteoglycan	Molecule consisting of one or more glycosaminoglycan chains attached to a core protein is referred to as proteoglycan.
Cytokine	A type of protein secreted by a T lymphocyte that attacks viruses, virally infected cells, and cancer cells is referred to as cytokine.
Extracellular	Outside the cell is called extracellular.

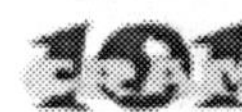

Alcoholic	An alcoholic is dependent on alcohol as characterized by craving, loss of control, physical dependence and withdrawal symptoms, and tolerance.
Fibrosis	Replacement of damaged tissue with fibrous scar tissue rather than by the original tissue type is called fibrosis.
Hepatic vein	A hepatic vein refers to blood vessels that drain de-oxygenated blood from the liver and blood cleaned by the liver into the inferior vena cava.
Inferior vena cava	The inferior vena cava is a large vein that carries de-oxygenated blood from the lower half of the body into the heart. It is formed by the left and right common iliac veins and transports blood to the right atrium of the heart.
Venous blood	In the circulatory system, venous blood or peripheral blood is blood returning to the heart. With one exception (the pulmonary vein) this blood is deoxygenated and high in carbon dioxide, having released oxygen and absorbed CO_2 in the tissues.
Irrigate	To gently flush a canal with fluid is to irrigate the area.
Endothelium	The endothelium is the layer of thin, flat cells that lines the interior surface of blood vessels, forming an interface between circulating blood in the lumen and the rest of the vessel wall.
Chromosomes	Physical structures in the cell's nucleus that house the genes. Each human cell has 23 pairs of chromosomes.
Haploid	The single set of chromosomes in a gamete (sperm or egg) is called a haploid set of chromosomes. In humans a haploid set of chromosomes contains 23 chromosomes.
Labile	Easily moved or changed, quickly shifting from one emotion to another, or easily aroused is referred to as labile.
Hydrophobic	Hydrophobic refers to being electrically neutral and nonpolar, and thus prefering other neutral and nonpolar solvents or molecular environments. Hydrophobic is often used interchangeably with "oily" or "lipophilic."
Bilirubin	A bile pigment produced from hemoglobin breakdown is bilirubin.
Glycogen	Glycogen refers to a complex, extensively branched polysaccharide of many glucose monomers; serves as an energy-storage molecule in liver and muscle cells.
Glucose	Glucose, a simple monosaccharide sugar, is one of the most important carbohydrates and is used as a source of energy in animals and plants. Glucose is one of the main products of photosynthesis and starts respiration.
Jaundice	Jaundice is yellowing of the skin, sclera (the white of the eyes) and mucous membranes caused by increased levels of bilirubin in the human body.
Hyperbilirub-nemia	With high doses of bilirubin (severe hyperbilirubinemia) there can be a complication known as kernicterus. This is the chief reason for neonatal jaundice to be treated.
Cellular component	The cellular component involves the movement of white blood cells from blood vessels into the inflamed tissue. The white blood cells, or leukocytes, take on an important role in inflammation; they extravasate (filter out) from the capillaries into tissue, and act as phagocytes, picking up bacteria and cellular debris. They may also aid by walling off an infection and preventing its spread.
Organelle	Organelle refers to any structure within a cell that carries out one of its metabolic roles, such as mitochondria, centrioles, endoplasmic reticulum, and the nucleus.
Lysosome	Organelle that contains enzymes that degrade worn cell parts is called a lysosome.

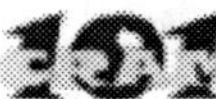

Intracellular	Intracellular refers to having to do with the interior of a cell.
Cholesterol	Cholesterol is a steroid, a lipid, and an alcohol, found in the cell membranes of all body tissues, and transported in the blood plasma of all animals. It is an important component of the membranes of cells, providing stability; it makes the membrane's fluidity stable over a bigger temperature interval.
Oxidation	Oxidation refers to the loss of electrons from a substance involved in a redox reaction; always accompanies reduction.
Uric acid	An insoluble precipitate of nitrogenous waste excreted by land snails, insects, birds, and some reptiles is called uric acid.
Bile acid	A bile acid is a steroid acid found predominantly in bile of mammals. They are produced in liver by oxidation of cholesterol, in the form of their salts are stored in gallbladder and secreted into the intestine. They act as surfactants, emulsifying lipids and assisting with their digestion and absorption.
Hydrogen	Hydrogen is a chemical element in the periodic table that has the symbol H and atomic number 1. At standard temperature and pressure it is a colorless, odorless, nonmetallic, univalent, tasteless, highly flammable diatomic gas.
Myelin	Myelin is an electrically insulating fatty layer that surrounds the axons of many neurons, especially those in the peripheral nervous system. It is an outgrowth of glial cells: Schwann cells supply the myelin for peripheral neurons while oligodendrocytes supply it to those of the central nervous system.
Purine	Purine refers to one of two families of nitrogenous bases found in nucleotides. Adenine and guanine are purines.
Hydrogen peroxide	Hydrogen peroxide is a clear liquid, slightly more viscous than water, that has strong oxidizing properties and is therefore a powerful bleaching agent that has found use as a disinfectant, as an oxidizer, and in rocketry (particularly in high concentrations as high-test peroxide (HTP) as a monopropellant, and in bipropellant systems.
Microscopy	Microscopy is any technique for producing visible images of structures or details too small to otherwise be seen by the human eye, using a microscope or other magnification tool.
Desmosome	A desmosome (also known as macula adherens) is a cell structure specialized for cell-to-cell adhesion. It is a type of junctional complex.
Lipoprotein	A lipoprotein is a biochemical assembly that contains both proteins and lipids and may be structural or catalytic in function. They may be enzymes, proton pumps, ion pumps, or some combination of these functions.
Complement	Complement is a group of proteins of the complement system, found in blood serum which act in concert with antibodies to achieve the destruction of non-self particles such as foreign blood cells or bacteria.
Complement system	Group of plasma proteins that form a nonspecific defense mechanism, often by puncturing microbes, is called the complement system. The complement system is derived from many small plasma proteins that form the complex biochemical cascade of the immune system.
Mutation	A change in the structure of a gene is called a mutation.
Excretion	Excretion is the biological process by which an organism chemically separates waste products from its body. The waste products are then usually expelled from the body by elimination.
Phospholipid	Phospholipid is a class of lipids formed from four components: fatty acids, a negatively-charged phosphate group, an alcohol and a backbone. Phospholipids with a glycerol backbone are known as glycerophospholipids or phosphoglycerides.

Lecithin	Lecithin refers to a group of phospholipids containing two fatty acids, a phosphate group, and a choline molecule. They are a group of compounds, since they can differ based on the types of fatty acids found on each lecithin molecule.
Absorption	Absorption is a physical or chemical phenomenon or a process in which atoms, molecules, or ions enter some bulk phase - gas, liquid or solid material. In nutrition, amino acids are broken down through digestion, which begins in the stomach.
Cholic acid	Cholic acid is one of the four main acids produced by the liver where it is synthesized from cholesterol. It is soluble in alcohol and acetic acid. It forms a conjugate with taurine, yielding taurocholic acid.
Glycine	Glycine (Gly, G) is a nonpolar amino acid. It is the simplest of the 20 standard (proteinogenic) amino acids: its side chain is a hydrogen atom. Because there is a second hydrogen atom at the α carbon, glycine is not optically active.
Taurocholic acid	Taurocholic acid is a deliquescent yellowish crystalline bile acid involved in the emulsification of fats. It occurs as a sodium salt in the bile of mammals. It is a conjugate of cholic acid with taurine.
Hemoglobin	Hemoglobin is the iron-containing oxygen-transport metalloprotein in the red cells of the blood in mammals and other animals. Hemoglobin transports oxygen from the lungs to the rest of the body, such as to the muscles, where it releases the oxygen load.
Red blood cells	Red blood cells are the most common type of blood cell and are the vertebrate body's principal means of delivering oxygen from the lungs or gills to body tissues via the blood.
Red blood cell	The red blood cell is the most common type of blood cell and is the vertebrate body's principal means of delivering oxygen from the lungs or gills to body tissues via the blood.
Facilitated transport	Use of a plasma membrane carrier to move a substance into or out of a cell from higher to lower concentration: no energy required is referred to as facilitated transport.
Glucuronic acid	Glucuronic acid is a carboxylic acid that has the structure of a glucose molecule that has had its sixth carbon atom (of six total) oxidized. Its formula is $C_6H_{10}O_7$.
Prothrombin	Prothrombin refers to plasma protein that is converted to thrombin during the steps of blood clotting. Prothrombin is a blood plasma protein and is synthesized in the liver.
Serum	Serum is the same as blood plasma except that clotting factors (such as fibrin) have been removed. Blood plasma contains fibrinogen.
Triglycerides	Triglycerides refer to fats and oils composed of fatty acids and glycerol; are the body's most concentrated source of energy fuel; also known as neutral fats.
Vitamin	An organic compound other than a carbohydrate, lipid, or protein that is needed for normal metabolism but that the body cannot synthesize in adequate amounts is called a vitamin.
Gluconeogenesis	Gluconeogenesis, ultimately, is the generation of glucose from noncarbohydrate sources like lactate, glycerol, and amino acids. The vast majority of gluconeogenesis takes place in the liver and, to a smaller extent, in the kidney.
Urea	Urea is an organic compound of carbon, nitrogen, oxygen and hydrogen, CON_2H_4 or $(NH_2)_2CO$. Urea is essentially a waste product: it has no physiological function. It is dissolved in blood and excreted by the kidney.
Kidney	The kidney is a bean-shaped excretory organ in vertebrates. Part of the urinary system, the kidneys filter wastes (especially urea) from the blood and excrete them, along with water, as urine.
Methylation	In biochemistry, methylation refers to the replacement of a hydrogen atom (H) with a methyl

	group (CH_3), regardless of the substrate.
Lesion	A lesion is a non-specific term referring to abnormal tissue in the body. It can be caused by any disease process including trauma (physical, chemical, electrical), infection, neoplasm, metabolic and autoimmune.
Lead	Lead is a chemical element in the periodic table that has the symbol Pb and atomic number 82. A soft, heavy, toxic and malleable poor metal, lead is bluish white when freshly cut but tarnishes to dull gray when exposed to air. Lead is used in building construction, lead-acid batteries, bullets and shot, and is part of solder, pewter, and fusible alloys.
Osmotic pressure	Osmotic pressure is the pressure produced by a solution in a space that is enclosed by a differentially permeable membrane.
Vesicle	Membranous, cytoplasmic sac formed by an infolding of the cell membrane is called a vesicle.
Barbiturate	A barbiturate is a drug that acts as a central nervous system (CNS) depressant, and by virtue of this produces a wide spectrum of effects, from mild sedation to anesthesia.
Regeneration	Regeneration is the ability to restore lost or damaged tissues, organs or limbs. It is a common feature in invertebrates, but far more limited in most vertebrates.
Tumor	An abnormal mass of cells that forms within otherwise normal tissue is a tumor. This growth can be either malignant or benign
Alcohol	Alcohol is a general term, applied to any organic compound in which a hydroxyl group (-OH) is bound to a carbon atom, which in turn is bound to other hydrogen and/or carbon atoms. The general formula for a simple acyclic alcohol is $C_nH_{2n+1}OH$.
Eye	An eye is an organ that detects light. Different kinds of light-sensitive organs are found in a variety of creatures. The simplest eyes do nothing but detect whether the surroundings are light or dark, while more complex eyes can distinguish shapes and colors.
Cirrhosis	Cirrhosis is a chronic disease of the liver in which liver tissue is replaced by connective tissue, resulting in the loss of liver function. Cirrhosis is caused by damage from toxins (including alcohol), metabolic problems, chronic viral hepatitis or other causes
Ethanol	Ethanol is a flammable, colorless chemical compound, one of the alcohols that is most often found in alcoholic beverages. In common parlance, it is often referred to simply as alcohol. Its chemical formula is C_2H_5OH, also written as C_2H_6O.
Affect	Affect is the scientific term used to describe a subject's externally displayed mood. This can be assesed by the nurse by observing facial expression, tone of voice, and body language.
Cystic duct	The cystic duct is the short duct that joins the gall bladder to the common bile duct. It usually lies next to the cystic artery.
Hepatitis	Hepatitis is a gastroenterological disease, featuring inflammation of the liver. The clinical signs and prognosis, as well as the therapy, depend on the cause.
Common hepatic duct	The common hepatic duct is the duct formed by the junction of the right hepatic duct (which drains bile from the right functional lobe of the liver) and the left hepatic duct (which drains bile from the left functional lobe of the liver). The common hepatic duct then joins the cystic duct coming from the gallbladder to form the common bile duct.
Common bile duct	The common bile duct begins at the junction of the common hepatic duct and the cystic duct and ends at the Ampulla of Vater which drains into the second part of the duodenum. It carries bile from the liver and gallbladder to the gastrointestinal tract.
Muscle	Muscle is a contractile form of tissue. It is one of the four major tissue types, the other three being epithelium, connective tissue and nervous tissue. Muscle contraction is used to

move parts of the body, as well as to move substances within the body.

Egg An egg is the zygote, resulting from fertilization of the ovum. It nourishes and protects the embryo.

Sphincter Muscle that surrounds a tube and closes or opens the tube by contracting and relaxing is referred to as sphincter.

Serosa A serosa is a smooth membrane consisting of a thin layer of cells that excrete a fluid, known as serous fluid. Two-layered serous membranes line the cavities that contain the heart (part of the pericardium), lungs (the pleura) and intestines (the peritoneum), enclosing their contents.

Smooth muscle Smooth muscle is a type of non-striated muscle, found within the "walls" of hollow organs; such as blood vessels, the bladder, the uterus, and the gastrointestinal tract. Smooth muscle is used to move matter within the body, via contraction; it generally operates "involuntarily", without nerve stimulation.

Serous membrane Membrane that covers internal organs and lines cavities without an opening to the outside of the body is referred to as serous membrane.

Sodium Sodium is the chemical element in the periodic table that has the symbol Na (Natrium in Latin) and atomic number 11. Sodium is a soft, waxy, silvery reactive metal belonging to the alkali metals that is abundant in natural compounds (especially halite). It is highly reactive.

Carcinoma Cancer that originates in the coverings of the body, such as the skin or the lining of the intestinal tract is a carcinoma.

Viral Viral phenomena are objects or patterns able to replicate themselves or convert other objects into copies of themselves when these objects are exposed to them.

Digestive gland An enzyme-producing gland in several groups of invertebrates where digestion and absorption take place is referred to as a digestive gland.

Mortality The incidence of death in a population is mortality.

Mortality rate Mortality rate is the number of deaths (from a disease or in general) per 1000 people and typically reported on an annual basis.

Physiology The study of the function of cells, tissues, and organs is referred to as physiology.

Health Health is a term that refers to a combination of the absence of illness, the ability to cope with everyday activities, physical fitness, and high quality of life.

Gastrointestinal tract The gastrointestinal tract is the system of organs within multicellular animals which takes in food, digests it to extract energy and nutrients, and expels the remaining waste.

Hypertrophy Hypertrophy is the increase of the size of an organ. It should be distinguished from hyperplasia which occurs due to cell division; hypertrophy occurs due to an increase in cell size rather than division. It is most commonly seen in muscle that has been actively stimulated, the most well-known method being exercise.

Biochemistry Biochemistry studies how complex chemical reactions give rise to life. It is a hybrid branch of chemistry which specialises in the chemical processes in living organisms.

Morphology The scientific study of organic form, including both its development and function is morphology.

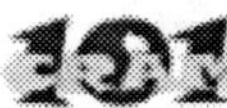

Ventilation	Ventilation refers to a mechanism that provides contact between an animal's respiratory surface and the air or water to which it is exposed. It is also called breathing.
Diaphragm	The diaphragm is a shelf of muscle extending across the bottom of the ribcage. It is critically important in respiration: in order to draw air into the lungs, the diaphragm contracts, thus enlarging the thoracic cavity and reducing intra-thoracic pressure.
Collagen	Collagen is the main protein of connective tissue in animals and the most abundant protein in mammals, making up about 1/4 of the total. It is one of the long, fibrous structural proteins whose functions are quite different from those of globular proteins such as enzymes.
Muscle	Muscle is a contractile form of tissue. It is one of the four major tissue types, the other three being epithelium, connective tissue and nervous tissue. Muscle contraction is used to move parts of the body, as well as to move substances within the body.
Lungs	Lungs are the essential organs of respiration in air-breathing vertebrates. Their principal function is to transport oxygen from the atmosphere into the bloodstream, and to excrete carbon dioxide from the bloodstream into the atmosphere.
Nasal cavity	The nasal cavity is a large air-filled space above and behind the nose in the middle of the face. The nasal cavity is important in warming and cleaning the air as it is inhaled. The nasal cavity also contains organs involved in olfaction.
Nasopharynx	Nasopharynx lies behind the nasal cavity. Postero-superiorly this extends from the level of the junction of the hard and soft palates to the base of skull, laterally to include the fossa of Rosenmuller. The inferior wall consists of the superior surface of the soft palate.
Trachea	Trachea is an airway through which respiratory gas transport takes place in organisms. In terrestrial vertebrates, such as birds and humans, the trachea lets air move from the throat to the lungs. In terrestrial invertebrates, such as onychophorans and beetles, they conduct air from outside the organism directly to all of its internal tissues.
Larynx	The larynx is an organ in the neck of mammals involved in protection of the trachea and sound production. The larynx houses the vocal cords, and is situated at the point where the upper tract splits into the trachea and the esophagus.
Conducting portion	The portion of the respiratory system in lung-breathing vertebrates that carries air to the lungs is the conducting portion. It includes the nasal cavity, paranasal sinuses, nasopharynx, larynx, trachea, and bronchi.
Gas exchange	In humans and other mammals, respiratory gas exchange or ventilation is carried out by mechanisms of the lungs. The actual gas exchange occurs in the alveoli.
Bronchioles	The bronchioles are the first airway branches that no longer contain cartilage. They are branches of the bronchi, and are smaller than one millimetre in diameter.
Bronchiole	The bronchiole is the first airway branch that no longer contains cartilage. They are branches of the bronchi, and are smaller than one millimetre in diameter.
Alveoli	Alveoli are anatomical structures that have the form of a hollow cavity. In the lung, the pulmonary alveoli are spherical outcroppings of the respiratory bronchioles and are the primary sites of gas exchange with the blood.
Alveolar duct	The alveolar duct is a tiny end tubule of the branching airways that fill the lungs. Each lung holds approximately 1.5 to 2 million of them. The tubules divide into alveolar sacs at the distal end.
Cartilage	Cartilage is a type of dense connective tissue. Cartilage is composed of cells called chondrocytes which are dispersed in a firm gel-like ground substance, called the matrix. Cartilage is avascular (contains no blood vessels) and nutrients are diffused through the

matrix.

Fiber Fibers used by man come from a wide variety of sources: Natural fiber include those made out of plants, animal and mineral sources. Natural fibers can be classified according to their origin.

Collagen fiber White fiber in the matrix of connective tissue, giving flexibility and strength is called collagen fiber.

Smooth muscle Smooth muscle is a type of non-striated muscle, found within the "walls" of hollow organs; such as blood vessels, the bladder, the uterus, and the gastrointestinal tract. Smooth muscle is used to move matter within the body, via contraction; it generally operates "involuntarily", without nerve stimulation.

Goblet cell A goblet cell is a glandular simple columnar epithelial cell that is specifically designed to secrete mucus.

Epithelium Epithelium is a tissue composed of a layer of cells. Epithelium can be found lining internal (e.g. endothelium, which lines the inside of blood vessels) or external (e.g. skin) free surfaces of the body. Functions include secretion, absorption and protection.

Microscope A microscope is an instrument for viewing objects that are too small to be seen by the naked or unaided eye.

Population Population refers to all members of a well-defined group of organisms, events, or things.

Mitochondria Cytoplasmic organelles responsible for ATP generation for cellular activities are referred to as mitochondria.

Adenosine Adenosine is a nucleoside comprized of adenine attached to a ribose (ribofuranose) moiety via a β-N_9-glycosidic bond. Adenosine plays an important role in biochemical processes, such as energy transfer - as adenosine triphosphate (ATP) and adenosine diphosphate (ADP) - as well as in signal transduction as cyclic adenosine monophosphate, cAMP.

Cilia Microscopic, hairlike processes on the exposed surfaces of certain epithelial cells are cilia.

Adenosine triphosphate Organic molecule that stores energy and releases energy for use in cellular processes is adenosine triphosphate.

Bronchus A bronchus is a caliber of airway in the respiratory tract that conducts air into the lungs. No gas exchange takes place in this part of the lungs.

Nerve A nerve is an enclosed, cable-like bundle of nerve fibers or axons, which includes the glia that ensheath the axons in myelin.

Respiratory tract In humans the respiratory tract is the part of the anatomy that has to do with the process of respiration or breathing.

Afferent nerve Axons that carry information inward to the central nervous system from the periphery of the body is called an afferent nerve.

Mucus Mucus is a slippery secretion of the lining of various membranes in the body (mucous membranes). Mucus aids in the protection of the lungs by trapping foreign particles that enter the nose during normal breathing. Additionally, it prevents tissues from drying out.

Respiratory system The respiratory system is the biological system of any organism that engages in gas exchange.In humans and other mammals, the respiratory system consists of the airways, the lungs, and the respiratory muscles that mediate the movement of air into and out of the body.

Tissue A collection of interconnected cells that perform a similar function within an organism is called tissue.

Connective tissue	Connective tissue is any type of biological tissue with an extensive extracellular matrix and often serves to support, bind together, and protect organs.
Lamina	A thin layer, such as the lamina of a vertebra or the lamina propria of a mucous membrane is referred to as lamina.
Granule cell	A granule cell receives excitatory input . They are tiny cells found within the granular layer of the cerebellum. These cells account for nearly half of the neurons in the central nervous system.
Neuroendocrine system	The network of neurons and glands that make and secrete hormones is referred to as the neuroendocrine system.
Squamous epithelium	The squamous epithelium is epithelium consisting of one or more cell layers, the most superficial of which is composed of flat, scalelike or platelike cells.
Vestibule	Vestibule refers to the cavity enclosed by the labia minora, it is the space into which the vagina and urethral opening empty.
Integument	Integument refers to the natural outer covering layers of an animal. Develops from the ectoderm.
Sweat gland	Gland responsible for the loss of a watery fluid, consisting mainly of sodium chloride (commonly known as salt) and urea in solution, that is secreted through the skin is a sweat gland.
Sebaceous	The sebaceous glands are glands found in the skin of mammals. They secrete an oily substance called sebum that is made of fat (lipids) and the debris of dead fat-producing cells.
Gland	A gland is an organ in an animal's body that synthesizes a substance for release such as hormones, often into the bloodstream or into cavities inside the body or its outer surface.
Nasal septum	The nasal septum separates the left and right airways in the nose, dividing the two nostrils. The nasal septum is comprized of the ethmoid bone, vomer bone and the quadrangular cartilage.
Septum	A septum, in general, is a wall separating two cavities or two spaces containing a less dense material. The muscle wall that divides the heart chambers.
Skull	Skull refers to a bony protective encasement of the brain and the organs of hearing and equilibrium; includes the facial bones. Also called the cranium.
Projection	Attributing one's own undesirable thoughts, impulses, traits, or behaviors to others is referred to as projection.
Conditioning	Processes by which behaviors can be learned or modified through interaction with the environment are conditioning.
Blood	Blood is a circulating tissue composed of fluid plasma and cells. The main function of blood is to supply nutrients (oxygen, glucose) and constitutional elements to tissues and to remove waste products.
Periosteum	The periosteum is an envelope of fibrous connective tissue that is wrapped around the bone in all places except at joints.
Lead	Lead is a chemical element in the periodic table that has the symbol Pb and atomic number 82. A soft, heavy, toxic and malleable poor metal, lead is bluish white when freshly cut but tarnishes to dull gray when exposed to air. Lead is used in building construction, lead-acid batteries, bullets and shot, and is part of solder, pewter, and fusible alloys.
Chemoreceptor	Chemoreceptor is a cell or group of cells that transduce a chemical signal into an action potential.

Inflammation	Inflammation is the first response of the immune system to infection or irritation and may be referred to as the innate cascade.
Engorgement	Breast engorgement occurs in the mammary glands when too much breast milk is contained within them. It is caused by insufficient breastfeeding and/or blocked milk ducts.
Olfaction	Olfaction, the sense of odor, is the detection of chemicals dissolved in air.In vertebrates smells are sensed by the olfactory epithelium located in the nasal cavity and first processed by the olfactory bulb in the olfactory system. In insects smells are sensed by sensilia located on the antenna and first processed by the antennal lobe.
Olfactory	Pertaining to the sense of smell is referred to as olfactory.
Olfactory epithelium	The olfactory epithelium is a specialized epithelial tissue inside the nasal cavity that is involved in smell. In humans, it measures about 1 inch wide by 2 inches long and lies on the roof of the nasal cavity about 3 inches above and behind the nostrils.
Mucosa	The mucosa is a lining of ectodermic origin, covered in epithelium, and involved in absorption and secretion. They line various body cavities that are exposed to the external environment and internal organs.
Base	The common definition of a base is a chemical compound that absorbs hydronium ions when dissolved in water (a proton acceptor). An alkali is a special example of a base, where in an aqueous environment, hydroxide ions are donated.
Olfactory mucosa	The olfactory mucosa is an organ made up of the olfactory epithelium and the mucosa, or mucus secreting glands, behind the epithelium. The mucus protects the olfactory epithelium and allows odors to dissolve so that they can be detected by olfactory receptor neurons.
Neuron	The neuron is a major class of cells in the nervous system. In vertebrates, they are found in the brain, the spinal cord and in the nerves and ganglia of the peripheral nervous system, and their primary role is to process and transmit neural information.
Receptor	A receptor is a protein on the cell membrane or within the cytoplasm or cell nucleus that binds to a specific molecule (a ligand), such as a neurotransmitter, hormone, or other substance, and initiates the cellular response to the ligand. Receptor, in immunology, the region of an antibody which shows recognition of an antigen.
Synapse	A junction, or relay point, between two neurons, or between a neuron and an effector cell. Electrical and chemical signals are relayed from one cell to another at a synapse.
Brain	The part of the central nervous system involved in regulating and controlling body activity and interpreting information from the senses transmitted through the nervous system is referred to as the brain.
Axon	An axon is a long slender projection of a nerve cell, or neuron, which conducts electrical impulses away from the neuron's cell body or soma. They are in effect the primary transmission lines of the nervous system, and as bundles they help make up nerves.
Olfactory lobe	Cranial lobe projecting from the anterior lower part of each cerebral hemisphere of the brain is the olfactory lobe.
Serous	The term serous fluid is used for various bodily fluids that are typically pale yellow and transparent, and of a benign nature.
Paranasal sinuses	The paranasal sinuses are eight (four pairs) air-filled spaces, or sinuses, within the bones of the skull and face. These are divided into subgroups that are named according to which bones they lie under.
Sphenoid bone	The sphenoid bone is a bone situated at the base of the skull in front of the temporals and basilar part of the occipital. It somewhat resembles a butterfly with its wings extended, and

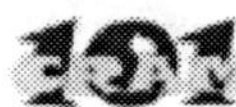

	is divided into a median portion or body, two great wings and two small wings extending outward from the sides of the body, and two pterygoid processes which project from it below.
Sinusitis	Sinusitis is inflammation, either bacterial, fungal, viral, allergic or autoimmune, of the paranasal sinuses.
Bronchitis	Bronchitis is an obstructive pulmonary disease characterized by inflammation of the bronchi of the lungs.
Syndrome	Syndrome is the association of several clinically recognizable features, signs, symptoms, phenomena or characteristics which often occur together, so that the presence of one feature alerts the physician to the presence of the others
Pharynx	The pharynx is the part of the digestive system and respiratory system of many animals immediately behind the mouth and in front of the esophagus.
Organ	Organ refers to a structure consisting of several tissues adapted as a group to perform specific functions.
Soft palate	The soft palate, is the soft tissue comprising the back of the roof of the mouth. It is movable, consisting of muscle fibers sheathed in mucous membrane, and is responsible for closing off the nasal passages during the act of swallowing.
Thyroid	The thyroid is one of the larger endocrine glands in the body. It is located in the neck and produces hormones, principally thyroxine and triiodothyronine, that regulate the rate of metabolism and affect the growth and rate of function of many other systems in the body.
Epiglottis	The epiglottis is a thin, lid-like flap of cartilage tissue covered with a mucous membrane, attached to the root of the tongue, that guards the entrance of the glottis, the opening between the vocal cords.
Elastic cartilage	Elastic cartilage is a stiff yet elastic tissue found in the pinna of the ear and several tubes, such as the walls of the auditory and eustachian canals and larynx.
Vocal cord	Vocal cord refers to one of a pair of stringlike tissues in the larynx. Air rushing past the tensed vocal cords makes them vibrate, producing sounds.
Ligament	A ligament is a short band of tough fibrous connective tissue composed mainly of long, stringy collagen fibres. They connect bones to other bones to form a joint. (They do not connect muscles to bones.)
Skeletal muscle	Skeletal muscle is a type of striated muscle, attached to the skeleton. They are used to facilitate movement, by applying force to bones and joints; via contraction. They generally contract voluntarily (via nerve stimulation), although they can contract involuntarily.
Hyaline cartilage	Hyaline cartilage is the most abundant type of cartilage. Hyaline cartilage is a translucent matrix or ground substance found lining bones in joints. It is also present inside bones, serving as a center of ossification or bone growth
Artery	Vessel that takes blood away from the heart to the tissues and organs of the body is called an artery.
Veins	Blood vessels that return blood toward the heart from the circulation are referred to as veins.
Vein	Vein in animals, is a vessel that returns blood to the heart. In plants, a vascular bundle in a leaf, composed of xylem and phloem.
Course	Pattern of development and change of a disorder over time is a course.
Fetus	Fetus refers to a developing human from the ninth week of gestation until birth; has all the major structures of an adult.

Septa	Septa are thin walls or partitions between the internal chambers (camerae) of the shell of a cephalopod, namely nautiloids or ammonoids.
Respiratory zone	The respiratory zone is the site of O_2 and CO_2 exchange with the blood. The respiratory bronchioles and the alveolar ducts are responsible for 10% of the gas exchange. The alveoli are responsible for the other 90%.
Elastic fiber	Elastic fiber is a bundles of proteins (elastin) found in connective tissue and produced by fibroblasts and smooth muscle cells in arteries.
Lymphocyte	A lymphocyte is a type of white blood cell involved in the human body's immune system. There are two broad categories, namely T cells and B cells.
Protein	A protein is a complex, high-molecular-weight organic compound that consists of amino acids joined by peptide bonds. They are essential to the structure and function of all living cells and viruses. Many are enzymes or subunits of enzymes.
Blood vessel	A blood vessel is a part of the circulatory system and function to transport blood throughout the body. The most important types, arteries and veins, are so termed because they carry blood away from or towards the heart, respectively.
Antigen	An antigen is a substance that stimulates an immune response, especially the production of antibodies. They are usually proteins or polysaccharides, but can be any type of molecule, including small molecules (haptens) coupled to a protein (carrier).
Sympathetic nervous system	The sympathetic nervous system activates what is often termed the "fight or flight response". Messages travel through in a bidirectional flow. Efferent messages can trigger changes in different parts of the body simultaneously.
Vagus nerve	The vagus nerve is tenth of twelve paired cranial nerves and is the only nerve that starts in the brainstem and extends all the way down past the head, right down to the abdomen. The vagus nerve is arguably the single most important nerve in the body.
Sympathetic	The sympathetic nervous system activates what is often termed the "fight or flight response". It is an automatic regulation system, that is, one that operates without the intervention of conscious thought.
Nervous system	The nervous system of an animal coordinates the activity of the muscles, monitors the organs, constructs and processes input from the senses, and initiates actions.
Asthma	Asthma is a complex disease characterized by bronchial hyperresponsiveness (BHR), inflammation, mucus production and intermittent airway obstruction.
Resistance	Resistance refers to a nonspecific ability to ward off infection or disease regardless of whether the body has been previously exposed to it. A force that opposes the flow of a fluid such as air or blood. Compare with immunity.
Airway resistance	Airway resistance is the opposition of the tracheobronchial tree to air flow: the mouth-to-alveoli pressure difference divided by the air flow.
Atrium	The atrium is the blood collection chamber of a heart. It has a thin-walled structure that allows blood to return to the heart. There is at least one atrium in an animal with a closed circulatory system
Inspiration	Inspiration begins with the onset of contraction of the diaphragm, which results in expansion of the intrapleural space and an increase in negative pressure according to Boyle's Law.
Expiration	In respiration, expiration is initiated by a decrease in volume and positive pressure exerted upon the intrapleural space upon diaphragm relaxation.
Capillaries	Capillaries refer to the smallest of the blood vessels and the sites of exchange between the

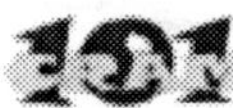

	blood and tissue cells.
Capillary	A capillary is the smallest of a body's blood vessels, measuring 5-10 micro meters. They connect arteries and veins, and most closely interact with tissues. Their walls are composed of a single layer of cells, the endothelium. This layer is so thin that molecules such as oxygen, water and lipids can pass through them by diffusion and enter the tissues.
Diffusion	Random movement of molecules from a region of higher concentration toward one of lower concentration is referred to as diffusion.
Internal environment	Conditions and elements that make up the inside of the body are called an internal environment.
Cytoplasm	Cytoplasm refers to the contents of a cell excluding the nucleus and cell membrane. Cytoplasm is a homogeneous, generally clear jelly-like material that fills cells.
Endothelial cell	A endothelial cell also controls the passage of materials — and the transit of white blood cells — into and out of the bloodstream. In some organs, there are highly differentiated endothelial cells to perform specialized 'filtering' functions.
Leukocyte	A white blood cell is a leukocyte. They help to defend the body against infectious disease and foreign materials as part of the immune system.
Arteriole	An arteriole is a blood vessel that extends and branches out from an artery and leads to capillaries. They have thick muscular walls and are the primary site of vascular resistance.
Pulmonary alveoli	In the lung, the pulmonary alveoli are spherical outcroppings of the respiratory bronchioles and are the primary sites of gas exchange with the blood.
Surfactant	A substance that decreases the surface tension of a liquid, allowing easier spreading, and the interfacial tension between two liquids is a surfactant.
Erythrocyte	Red blood cells are the most common type of blood cell and are the vertebrate body's principal means of delivering oxygen from the lungs or gills to body tissues via the blood. Red blood cells are also known as erythrocyte.
Plasma	Fluid portion of circulating blood is called plasma.
Endothelium	The endothelium is the layer of thin, flat cells that lines the interior surface of blood vessels, forming an interface between circulating blood in the lumen and the rest of the vessel wall.
Physiology	The study of the function of cells, tissues, and organs is referred to as physiology.
Fusion	Fusion refers to the combination of two atoms into a single atom as a result of a collision, usually accompanied by the release of energy.
Enzyme	An enzyme is a protein that catalyzes, or speeds up, a chemical reaction. They are essential to sustain life because most chemical reactions in biological cells would occur too slowly, or would lead to different products, without them.
Organelle	Organelle refers to any structure within a cell that carries out one of its metabolic roles, such as mitochondria, centrioles, endoplasmic reticulum, and the nucleus.
Vesicle	Membranous, cytoplasmic sac formed by an infolding of the cell membrane is called a vesicle.
Desmosome	A desmosome (also known as macula adherens) is a cell structure specialized for cell-to-cell adhesion. It is a type of junctional complex.
Occluding junction	Type of cell junction that seals cells together in an epithelium, forming a barrier through which even small molecules cannot pass, is referred to as occluding junction.
Phospholipid	Phospholipid is a class of lipids formed from four components: fatty acids, a negatively-

	charged phosphate group, an alcohol and a backbone. Phospholipids with a glycerol backbone are known as glycerophospholipids or phosphoglycerides.
Glycosaminoglycan	Glycosaminoglycan is a long unbranched polysaccharide, made up of repeating disaccharides that may be sulphated (e.g. glucuronic acid, iduronic acid, galactose, galactosamine, glucosamine).
Gestation	Gestation refers to pregnancy; the state of carrying developing young within the female reproductive tract.
Choline	Choline is a nutrient, essential for cardiovascular and brain function, and for cellular membrane composition and repair.
Lipid	Lipid is one class of aliphatic hydrocarbon-containing organic compounds essential for the structure and function of living cells. They are characterized by being water-insoluble but soluble in nonpolar organic solvents.
Exocytosis	Exocytosis is the process by which a cell is able to get rid of large molecules or materials including wastes through its membrane. The process involves a [vacuole], containing the material, fusing with the membrane.
Lipoprotein	A lipoprotein is a biochemical assembly that contains both proteins and lipids and may be structural or catalytic in function. They may be enzymes, proton pumps, ion pumps, or some combination of these functions.
Respiratory distress syndrome	Infant respiratory distress syndrome is a syndrome caused by developmental lack of surfactant and structural immaturity in the lungs of premature infants. The syndrome is more frequent in infants of diabetic mothers and in the second born of premature twins.
Congestive heart failure	Congestive heart failure is the inability of the heart to pump a sufficient amount of blood throughout the body, or requiring elevated filling pressures in order to pump effectively.
Ion	Ion refers to an atom or molecule that has gained or lost one or more electrons, thus acquiring an electrical charge.
Incidence	In epidemiological studies of a particular disorder, the rate at which new cases occur in a given place at a given time is called incidence.
Sputum	The mucous secretion from the lungs, bronchi, and trachea that is ejected through the mouth is sputum.
Iron	Iron is essential to all organisms, except for a few bacteria. It is mostly stably incorporated in the inside of metalloproteins, because in exposed or in free form it causes production of free radicals that are generally toxic to cells.
Fibrosis	Replacement of damaged tissue with fibrous scar tissue rather than by the original tissue type is called fibrosis.
Fibrin	Fibrin is a protein involved in the clotting of blood. It is a fibrillar protein that is polymerized to form a "mesh" that forms a haemostatic plug or clot (in conjunction with platelets) over a wound site.
Regeneration	Regeneration is the ability to restore lost or damaged tissues, organs or limbs. It is a common feature in invertebrates, but far more limited in most vertebrates.
Lysozyme	Lysozyme is an enzyme (EC 3.2.1.17), commonly referred to as the "body's own antibiotic" since it kills bacteria. It is abundantly present in a number of secretions, such as tears (except bovine tears).
Emphysema	Emphysema is a chronic lung disease. It is often caused by exposure to toxic chemicals or long-term exposure to tobacco smoke..

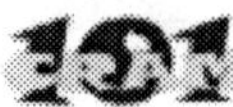

Pulmonary artery	The pulmonary artery carrys blood from the heart to the lungs. They are the only arteries (other than umbilical arteries in the fetus) that carry deoxygenated blood.
Pulmonary circuit	Pulmonary circuit refers to one of two main blood circuits in terrestrial vertebrates; conveys blood between the heart and the lungs.
Adventitia	Adventitia is the outermost connective tissue covering of any organ, vessel, or other structure. For example, the connective tissue that surrounds an artery is called the adventitia because it is considered extraneous to the artery.
Histology	Histology is the study of tissue sectioned as a thin slice, using a microscope. It can be described as microscopic anatomy.
Parenchyma	The parenchyma are the functional parts of an organ in the body (i.e. the nephrons of the kidney, the alveoli of the lungs). In plants parenchyma cells are thin-walled cells of the ground tissue that make up the bulk of most nonwoody structures, although sometimes their cell walls can be lignified.
Venule	A vessel that conveys blood between a capillary bed and a vein is a venule.
Lymph node	A lymph node acts as a filter, with an internal honeycomb of connective tissue filled with lymphocytes that collect and destroy bacteria and viruses. When the body is fighting an infection, these lymphocytes multiply rapidly and produce a characteristic swelling of the lymph node.
Lymph	Lymph originates as blood plasma lost from the circulatory system, which leaks out into the surrounding tissues. The lymphatic system collects this fluid by diffusion into lymph capillaries, and returns it to the circulatory system.
Visceral	Visceral refers to the internal organs of an animal.
Pain	Pain is an unpleasant sensation which may be associated with actual or potential tissue damage and which may have physical and emotional components.
Serous membrane	Membrane that covers internal organs and lines cavities without an opening to the outside of the body is referred to as serous membrane.
Parietal	When speaking of inner organs, visceral means close to or attached to the organ, while parietal is more distant. For example, the visceral pleura is attached to the lung and the parietal pleura is attached to the chest wall.
Visceral pleura	Visceral pleura refer to a membrane that covers the surfaces of the lungs.
Pleural cavity	The lungs are surrounded by two membranes, the pleura. The outer is attached to the chest wall and is known as the parietal pleura; the inner is attached to the lung and other visceral tissues and is known as the visceral pleura. In between the two is a thin space known as the pleural cavity or pleural space. It is filled with pleural fluid, a serous fluid produced by the pleura.
Pleural effusion	Pleural effusion is excess fluid that accumulates in the pleural cavity, the fluid-filled space that surrounds the lungs.
Inhalation	Inhalation is the movement of air from the external environment, through the airways, into the alveoli during breathing.
Intercostal muscles	Intercostal muscles are several groups of muscles that run between the ribs. They contract to pull the ribcage upwards and outwards, increasing the volume of the thorax and drawing in
Thoracic cavity	The thoracic cavity is the chamber of the human body (and other animal bodies) that is protected by the thoracic wall (thoracic cage and associated skin, muscle, and fascia).
Defense	Defense mechanism refers to in psychodynamic theory, an unconscious function of the ego that

mechanism	protects it from anxiety-evoking material by preventing accurate recognition of this material.
Microorganism	A microorganism or microbe is an organism that is so small that it is microscopic (invisible to the naked eye).
Agent	Agent refers to an epidemiological term referring to the organism or object that transmits a disease from the environment to the host.
Squamous cell carcinoma	In medicine, squamous cell carcinoma is a form of cancer of the carcinoma type that may occur in many different organs, including the skin, the esophagus, the lungs, and the cervix.
Carcinoma	Cancer that originates in the coverings of the body, such as the skin or the lining of the intestinal tract is a carcinoma.
Tumor	An abnormal mass of cells that forms within otherwise normal tissue is a tumor. This growth can be either malignant or benign
Acute	In medicine, an acute disease is a disease with either or both of: a rapid onset; and a short course (as opposed to a chronic course).
Lipopolysacc-aride	A lipopolysaccharide is a large molecule that contains both lipid and a carbohydrate. They are a major suprastructure of Gram-negative bacteria which contributes greatly to the structural integrity of the bacteria, and protects them from host immune defenses.
Health	Health is a term that refers to a combination of the absence of illness, the ability to cope with everyday activities, physical fitness, and high quality of life.
Reservoir	Reservoir is the source of infection. It is the environment in which microorganisms are able to live and grow.

Epidermis	Epidermis is the outermost layer of the skin. It forms the waterproof, protective wrap over the body's surface and is made up of stratified squamous epithelium with an underlying basement membrane. It contains no blood vessels, and is nourished by diffusion from the dermis. In plants, the outermost layer of cells covering the leaves and young parts of a plant is the epidermis.
Dermis	The dermis is the layer of skin beneath the epidermis that consists of connective tissue and cushions the body from stress and strain.
Tissue	A collection of interconnected cells that perform a similar function within an organism is called tissue.
Connective tissue	Connective tissue is any type of biological tissue with an extensive extracellular matrix and often serves to support, bind together, and protect organs.
Projection	Attributing one's own undesirable thoughts, impulses, traits, or behaviors to others is referred to as projection.
Skin	Skin is an organ of the integumentary system composed of a layer of tissues that protect underlying muscles and organs.
Sweat gland	Gland responsible for the loss of a watery fluid, consisting mainly of sodium chloride (commonly known as salt) and urea in solution, that is secreted through the skin is a sweat gland.
Sebaceous	The sebaceous glands are glands found in the skin of mammals. They secrete an oily substance called sebum that is made of fat (lipids) and the debris of dead fat-producing cells.
Gland	A gland is an organ in an animal's body that synthesizes a substance for release such as hormones, often into the bloodstream or into cavities inside the body or its outer surface.
Hypodermis	The hypodermis, also called the hypoderm, is the lowermost layer of the integumentary system in vertebrates. It is derived from the mesoderm, but unlike the dermis, it is not derived from the dermatome region of the mesoderm. In arthropods, the hypodermis is an epidermal layer of cells that secretes the chitinous cuticle. The term also refers to a layer of cells lying immediately below the epidermis of plants.
Loose connective tissue	Loose connective tissue or Areolar connective tissue holds organs and epithelia in place, and has a variety of proteinaceous fibers, including collagen and elastin. It is also important in inflammation.
Subcutaneous	Subcutaneous injections are given by injecting a fluid into the subcutis. It is relatively painless and an effective way to administer particular types of medication.
Panniculus	Panniculus is a dense layer of fatty tissue growth, usually in the abdominal cavity. It generally coincides with morbid obesity and can be mistaken for a tumor or hernia. Abdominal panniculus (the "apron" in lay term) can be removed during Abdominal Panniculectomy.
Anatomy	Anatomy is the branch of biology that deals with the structure and organization of living things. It can be divided into animal anatomy (zootomy) and plant anatomy (phytonomy).
Fascia	Fascia is specialized connective tissue layer which surrounds muscles, bones, and joints, providing support and protection and giving structure to the body. It consists of three layers: the superficial fascia, the deep fascia and the subserous fascia. Fascia is one of the 3 types of dense connective tissue (the other two being ligaments and tendons).
Superficial Fascia	The Superficial Fascia is located directly under the subcutis of the skin. Its functions include the storage of fat and water and it also provides passageways for nerves and blood vessels. In some areas of the body, it also houses a layer of skeletal muscle, allowing for movement of the skin.

Friction | Friction is the force that opposes the relative motion or tendency of such motion of two surfaces in contact. The resulting injury to skin resembles an abrasion and can also damage superficial blood vessels directly under the skin.

Receptor | A receptor is a protein on the cell membrane or within the cytoplasm or cell nucleus that binds to a specific molecule (a ligand), such as a neurotransmitter, hormone, or other substance, and initiates the cellular response to the ligand. Receptor, in immunology, the region of an antibody which shows recognition of an antigen.

Organ | Organ refers to a structure consisting of several tissues adapted as a group to perform specific functions.

Melanin | Broadly, melanin is any of the polyacetylene, polyaniline, and polypyrrole "blacks" or their mixed copolymers. The most common form of biological melanin is a polymer of either or both of two monomer molecules: indolequinone, and dihydroxyindole carboxylic acid.

Blood vessel | A blood vessel is a part of the circulatory system and function to transport blood throughout the body. The most important types, arteries and veins, are so termed because they carry blood away from or towards the heart, respectively.

Metabolism | Metabolism is the biochemical modification of chemical compounds in living organisms and cells. This includes the biosynthesis of complex organic molecules (anabolism) and their breakdown (catabolism).

Excretion | Excretion is the biological process by which an organism chemically separates waste products from its body. The waste products are then usually expelled from the body by elimination.

Blood | Blood is a circulating tissue composed of fluid plasma and cells. The main function of blood is to supply nutrients (oxygen, glucose) and constitutional elements to tissues and to remove waste products.

Thermoregulation | Thermoregulation is the ability of an organism to keep its body temperature within certain boundaries, even when temperature surrounding is very different.

Adipose tissue | Adipose tissue is an anatomical term for loose connective tissue composed of adipocytes. Its main role is to store energy in the form of fat, although it also cushions and insulates the body. It has an important endocrine function in producing recently-discovered hormones such as leptin, resistin and TNFalpha.

Radiation | The emission of electromagnetic waves by all objects warmer than absolute zero is referred to as radiation.

Vitamin | An organic compound other than a carbohydrate, lipid, or protein that is needed for normal metabolism but that the body cannot synthesize in adequate amounts is called a vitamin.

Edema | Edema is swelling of any organ or tissue due to accumulation of excess fluid. Edema has many root causes, but its common mechanism is accumulation of fluid into the tissues.

Langerhans cell | A Langerhans cell is an immature dendritic cell containing large granules called Birbeck granules. On infection of an area of skin, they will take up and process microbial antigens before travelling to the T-cell areas in the cortex of the draining lymph node and maturing to become fully-functional antigen-presenting cells.

Epithelium | Epithelium is a tissue composed of a layer of cells. Epithelium can be found lining internal (e.g. endothelium, which lines the inside of blood vessels) or external (e.g. skin) free surfaces of the body. Functions include secretion, absorption and protection.

Melanocyte | Melanocyte cells are located in the bottom layer of the skin's epidermis. With a process called melanogenesis, they produce melanin, a pigment in the skin, eyes, and hair.

Keratinocyte | The keratinocyte is the major cell type of the epidermis, making up about 90% of epidermal

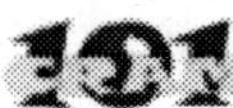

	cells. They are shed and replaced continuously from the stratum corneum.
Papilla	A papilla can be a small projection, such as a nipplelike projection on the skin, at the base of a hair or the root of a feather; the base of a new tooth.
Stratum **lucidum**	The stratum lucidum is a layer of the epidermis. It is a thin, clear layer of dead skin cells found beneath the stratum corneum of thick skin. contain eosinophilic cells with keratiniztion and no organels.
Stratum **corneum**	The stratum corneum ("the horny layer") is the outermost layer of the epidermis, and comprises the surface of the skin. It is composed mainly of dead cells that lack nuclei. As these dead cells slough off, they are continuously replaced by new cells from the stratum germinativum.
Desmosome	A desmosome (also known as macula adherens) is a cell structure specialized for cell-to-cell adhesion. It is a type of junctional complex.
Keratin	Keratin is a family of fibrous structural proteins; tough and insoluble, they form the hard but nonmineralized structures found in reptiles, birds and mammals.
Stratum **germinativum**	Stratum germinativum is the layer of keratinocytes that lies at the base of the epidermis immediately above the dermis. It consists of a single layer of tall cells lying on a basement membrane. These cells undergo rapid cell division to replenish the regular loss of skin by shedding from the surface.
Stratum **basale**	The deepest layer of the epidermis in which the cells divide is referred to as the stratum basale.
Lamina	A thin layer, such as the lamina of a vertebra or the lamina propria of a mucous membrane is referred to as lamina.
Constant	A behavior or characteristic that does not vary from one observation to another is referred to as a constant.
Protein	A protein is a complex, high-molecular-weight organic compound that consists of amino acids joined by peptide bonds. They are essential to the structure and function of all living cells and viruses. Many are enzymes or subunits of enzymes.
Cytoplasm	Cytoplasm refers to the contents of a cell excluding the nucleus and cell membrane. Cytoplasm is a homogeneous, generally clear jelly-like material that fills cells.
Stratum **spinosum**	In the skin, the stratum spinosum is a multi-layered arrangement of cuboidal cells that sits beneath the stratum granulosum. Adjacent cells are joined by desmosomes giving them the spiny appearance from which their name is derived.
Cohesion	The tendency of the molecules of a substance to stick together is referred to as cohesion.
Malpighian layer	Malpighian layer is a thin 1,88 mm thick basal and the deepest layer of the epidermis composed of dividing stem cells and anchoring cells, and the prickle cell layer considered as one unit. Skin originates at the bottom of the layer and grows outward.
Stratum granulosum	Stratum granulosum contains 3 to 5 rows of flattened cells whose cytoplasm contains small granules. The granules are proteins that are in the process of transforming into the waterproofing protein keratin.
Histidine	Histidine is one of the 20 most common natural amino acids present in proteins. In the nutritional sense, in humans, histidine is considered an essential amino acid, but mostly only in children.
Phosphate	A phosphate is a polyatomic ion or radical consisting of one phosphorus atom and four oxygen. In the ionic form, it carries a -3 formal charge, and is denoted PO_4^{3-}.

Phosphate group	The functional group -0P0$_3$H$_2$; the transfer of energy from one compound to another is often accomplished by the transfer of a phosphate group.
Microscope	A microscope is an instrument for viewing objects that are too small to be seen by the naked or unaided eye.
Lipid	Lipid is one class of aliphatic hydrocarbon-containing organic compounds essential for the structure and function of living cells. They are characterized by being water-insoluble but soluble in nonpolar organic solvents.
Granular layer	The innermost layer contains the cell bodies of two types of cells: the numerous and tiny granule cells, and the larger Golgi cells. Mossy fibers enter the granular layer from their main point of origin, the pontine nuclei.
Lipid bilayer	A lipid bilayer is a membrane or zone of a membrane composed of lipid molecules (usually phospholipids). The lipid bilayer is a critical component of all biological membranes, including cell membranes, and is a prerequisite for cell-based organisms.
Organelle	Organelle refers to any structure within a cell that carries out one of its metabolic roles, such as mitochondria, centrioles, endoplasmic reticulum, and the nucleus.
Scleroprotein	A scleroprotein is a long filamentous protein molecule that forms one of the two main classes of tertiary structure protein (the other being globular proteins). They are only found in animals and are practically water-insoluble.
Polypeptide	Polypeptide refers to polymer of many amino acids linked by peptide bonds.
Molecular weight	The molecular mass of a substance, called molecular weight and abbreviated as MW, is the mass of one molecule of that substance, relative to the unified atomic mass unit u (equal to 1/12 the mass of one atom of carbon-12).
Plasma	Fluid portion of circulating blood is called plasma.
Plasma membrane	The unit membrane that encloses a cell and controls the traffic of molecules in and out of the cell is the plasma membrane.
Enzyme	An enzyme is a protein that catalyzes, or speeds up, a chemical reaction. They are essential to sustain life because most chemical reactions in biological cells would occur too slowly, or would lead to different products, without them.
Hydrolytic enzyme	A hydrolytic enzyme breaks down proteins, carbohydrates, and fat molecules into their simplest units. The hydrolysis of polymers by hydrolytic enzymes results in free monomers.
Carotene	Carotene is an orange photosynthetic pigment important for photosynthesis. It is responsible for the orange color of the carrot and many other fruits and vegetables. It contributes to photosynthesis by transmitting the light energy it absorbs to chlorophyll.
Follicle	Follicle refers to a cluster of cells surrounding, protecting, and nourishing a developing egg cell in the ovary; also secretes estrogen. In botany, a follicle is a type of simple dry fruit produced by certain flowering plants. It is regarded as one the most primitive types of fruits, and derives from a simple pistil or carpel.
Hair follicle	A hair follicle is part of the skin that grows hair by packing old cells together. Attached to the follicle is a sebaceous gland, a tiny sebum-producing gland found everywhere except on the palms and soles of the feet.
Cysteine	Cysteine is a naturally occurring hydrophobic amino acid which has a thiol group and is found in most proteins, though only in small quantities.
Invagination	Infolding of one part of a structure into another is invagination.
Extension	Movement increasing the angle between parts at a joint is referred to as extension.

Mitochondria	Cytoplasmic organelles responsible for ATP generation for cellular activities are referred to as mitochondria.
Interstice	A interstice is a small structural space between tissues or parts of an organ.
Tyrosinase	Tyrosinase (Catechol Oxidase) is an enzyme that catalyses the oxidation of phenols (such as tyrosine) and is widespread in plants and animals. When a person has a mutated tyrosinase gene they have albinism.
Vesicle	Membranous, cytoplasmic sac formed by an infolding of the cell membrane is called a vesicle.
Light microscope	An optical instrument with lenses that refract visible light to magnify images and project them into a viewer's eye or onto photographic film is referred to as light microscope.
Micrograph	A micrograph is a photograph or similar image taken through a microscope or similar device to show a magnified image of an item.
Collagen	Collagen is the main protein of connective tissue in animals and the most abundant protein in mammals, making up about 1/4 of the total. It is one of the long, fibrous structural proteins whose functions are quite different from those of globular proteins such as enzymes.
Ratio	In number and more generally in algebra, a ratio is the linear relationship between two quantities.
Lysosome	Organelle that contains enzymes that degrade worn cell parts is called a lysosome.
DNA	Deoxyribonucleic acid (DNA) is a nucleic acid —usually in the form of a double helix— that contains the genetic instructions specifying the biological development of all cellular forms of life, and most viruses.
Albinism	Albinism is a lack of pigmentation in the eyes, skin and hair. Albinism is an inherited condition resulting from the combination of recessive alleles passed from both parents of an individual. This condition is known to affect mammals, fish, birds, reptiles, and amphibians.
Tyrosine	Tyrosine is one of the 20 amino acids that are used by cells to synthesize proteins. It plays a key role in signal transduction, since it can be tagged (phosphorylated) with a phosphate group by protein kinases to alter the functionality and activity of certain enzymes.
Antigen	An antigen is a substance that stimulates an immune response, especially the production of antibodies. They are usually proteins or polysaccharides, but can be any type of molecule, including small molecules (haptens) coupled to a protein (carrier).
Nerve	A nerve is an enclosed, cable-like bundle of nerve fibers or axons, which includes the glia that ensheath the axons in myelin.
Base	The common definition of a base is a chemical compound that absorbs hydronium ions when dissolved in water (a proton acceptor). An alkali is a special example of a base, where in an aqueous environment, hydroxide ions are donated.
Free nerve ending	A free nerve ending is an unspecialized, afferent nerve ending, meaning it brings information from the body's periphery to the brain. They are unencapsulated and have no complex sensory structures, unlike those found in Meissner's or Pacinian corpuscles.
Lymphocyte	A lymphocyte is a type of white blood cell involved in the human body's immune system. There are two broad categories, namely T cells and B cells.
Fiber	Fibers used by man come from a wide variety of sources: Natural fiber include those made out of plants, animal and mineral sources. Natural fibers can be classified according to their origin.
Pemphigus	Pemphigus is an autoimmune disorder that causes blistering and raw sores on skin and mucous membranes. As with other autoimmune disorders, it is caused when the body's defenses mistake

	its own tissues as foreign, and attack the cells.
Lead	Lead is a chemical element in the periodic table that has the symbol Pb and atomic number 82. A soft, heavy, toxic and malleable poor metal, lead is bluish white when freshly cut but tarnishes to dull gray when exposed to air. Lead is used in building construction, lead-acid batteries, bullets and shot, and is part of solder, pewter, and fusible alloys.
Dense connective tissue	Dense connective tissue has collagen fibers as its main matrix element. Crowded between the collagen fibers are rows of fibroblasts, fiber-forming cells, that manufacture the fibers. Dense connective tissue forms strong, rope-like structures such as tendons and ligaments. Tendons attach skeletal muscles to bones; ligaments connect bones to bones at joints.
Collagen fibril	Collagen fibril refers to extracellular structure formed by self-assembly of secreted fibrillar collagen subunits. An abundant constituent of the extracellular matrix in many animal tissues.
Glycosaminog-ycan	Glycosaminoglycan is a long unbranched polysaccharide, made up of repeating disaccharides that may be sulphated (e.g. glucuronic acid, iduronic acid, galactose, galactosamine, glucosamine).
Elastin	Elastin, is a protein in connective tissue that is elastic and allows many tissues in the body to resume their shape after stretching or contracting. Elastin helps skin to return to its original position when it is poked or pinched.
Collagen fiber	White fiber in the matrix of connective tissue, giving flexibility and strength is called collagen fiber.
Elastic fiber	Elastic fiber is a bundles of proteins (elastin) found in connective tissue and produced by fibroblasts and smooth muscle cells in arteries.
Sebaceous gland	The sebaceous gland is found in the skin of mammals. They secrete an oily substance called sebum that is made of fat and the debris of dead fat-producing cells. These glands exist in humans througout the skin except in the palms and soles.
Sympathetic	The sympathetic nervous system activates what is often termed the "fight or flight response". It is an automatic regulation system, that is, one that operates without the intervention of conscious thought.
Afferent nerve	Axons that carry information inward to the central nervous system from the periphery of the body is called an afferent nerve.
Veins	Blood vessels that return blood toward the heart from the circulation are referred to as veins.
Vein	Vein in animals, is a vessel that returns blood to the heart. In plants, a vascular bundle in a leaf, composed of xylem and phloem.
Sensory receptor	A sensory receptor is a structure that recognizes a stimulus in the internal or external environment of an organism. In response to stimuli the sensory receptor initiates sensory transduction by creating graded potentials or action potentials in the same cell or in an adjacent one.
Tactile	Tactile refers to the sense of touch.
Pain	Pain is an unpleasant sensation which may be associated with actual or potential tissue damage and which may have physical and emotional components.
Histology	Histology is the study of tissue sectioned as a thin slice, using a microscope. It can be described as microscopic anatomy.
Labia minora	The labia minora are two soft folds of skin within the labia majora and to either side of the

	opening of the vagina.
Glans penis	The glans penis is the sensitive erectile tip of the penis. It is wholly or partially covered by the foreskin, except when the foreskin is retracted, such as during sexual intercourse while the penis is erect, or when the foreskin has been removed by circumcision.
Clitoris	The clitoris is a sexual organ in the body of female mammals. The visible knob-like portion is located near the anterior junction of the labia minora, above the opening of the vagina. Unlike its male counterpart, the penis,the clitoris has no urethra, is not involved in urination, and its sole function is to induce sexual pleasure.
Penis	The penis is the male reproductive organ and for mammals additionally serves as the external male organ of urination.
Glan	A glan is a structure internally composed of corpus spongiosum in males or of corpus cavernosa and vestibular tissue in females that is located at the tip of homologous genital structures involved in sexual arousal.
Androgen	Androgen is the generic term for any natural or synthetic compound, usually a steroid hormone, that stimulates or controls the development and maintenance of masculine characteristics in vertebrates by binding to androgen receptors.
Thyroid	The thyroid is one of the larger endocrine glands in the body. It is located in the neck and produces hormones, principally thyroxine and triiodothyronine, that regulate the rate of metabolism and affect the growth and rate of function of many other systems in the body.
Hormone	A hormone is a chemical messenger from one cell to another. All multicellular organisms produce hormones. The best known hormones are those produced by endocrine glands of vertebrate animals, but hormones are produced by nearly every organ system and tissue type in a human or animal body. Hormone molecules are secreted directly into the bloodstream, they move by circulation or diffusion to their target cells, which may be nearby cells in the same tissue or cells of a distant organ of the body.
Adrenal	In mammals, the adrenal glands are the triangle-shaped endocrine glands that sit atop the kidneys. They are chiefly responsible for regulating the stress response through the synthesis of corticosteroids and catecholamines, including cortisol and adrenaline.
Pubis	The pubis, the anterior part of the hip bone, is divisible into a body, a superior and an inferior ramus.
Thyroid hormones	The thyroid hormones, thyroxine (T4) and triiodothyronine (T3), are tyrosine-based hormones produced by the thyroid gland. An important component in the synthesis is iodine. They act on the body to increase the basal metabolic rate, affect protein synthesis and increase the body's sensitivity to catecholamines.
Capillary	A capillary is the smallest of a body's blood vessels, measuring 5-10 micro meters. They connect arteries and veins, and most closely interact with tissues. Their walls are composed of a single layer of cells, the endothelium. This layer is so thin that molecules such as oxygen, water and lipids can pass through them by diffusion and enter the tissues.
Medulla	Medulla in general means the inner part, and derives from the Latin word for 'marrow'. In medicine it is contrasted to the cortex.
Cortex	In anatomy and zoology the cortex is the outermost or superficial layer of an organ or the outer portion of the stem or root of a plant.
Capillaries	Capillaries refer to the smallest of the blood vessels and the sites of exchange between the blood and tissue cells.
Muscle	Muscle is a contractile form of tissue. It is one of the four major tissue types, the other

	three being epithelium, connective tissue and nervous tissue. Muscle contraction is used to move parts of the body, as well as to move substances within the body.
Smooth muscle	Smooth muscle is a type of non-striated muscle, found within the "walls" of hollow organs; such as blood vessels, the bladder, the uterus, and the gastrointestinal tract. Smooth muscle is used to move matter within the body, via contraction; it generally operates "involuntarily", without nerve stimulation.
Depression	In everyday language depression refers to any downturn in mood, which may be relatively transitory and perhaps due to something trivial. This is differentiated from Clinical depression which is marked by symptoms that last two weeks or more and are so severe that they interfere with daily living.
Inductive	Characteristic of disciplinary methods, such as reasoning, that attempt to foster an understanding of the principles behind parental demands is referred to as inductive.
Dorsal	In anatomy, the dorsal is the side in which the backbone is located. This is usually the top of an animal, although in humans it refers to the back.
Dorsal surface	The dorsal surface is arched from above downward, and is subdivided into two unequal parts by the spine; the portion above the spine is called the supraspinatous fossa, and that below it the infraspinous fossa.
Oxygen	Oxygen is a chemical element in the periodic table. It has the symbol O and atomic number 8. Oxygen is the second most common element on Earth, composing around 46% of the mass of Earth's crust and 28% of the mass of Earth as a whole, and is the third most common element in the universe.
Sebum	Oily secretion of the sebaceous glands is sebum.
Pyramidal cell	A pyramidal cell is a multipolar neuron located in the hippocampus and cerebral cortex. These cells have a triangular-shaped soma, or cell body, with both apical dendrites and basal dendrites.
Testosterone	Testosterone is a steroid hormone from the androgen group. Testosterone is secreted in the testes of men and the ovaries of women. It is the principal male sex hormone and the "original" anabolic steroid. In both males and females, it plays key roles in health and well-being.
Inflammation	Inflammation is the first response of the immune system to infection or irritation and may be referred to as the innate cascade.
Cholinergic	A synapse is cholinergic if it uses acetylcholine as its neurotransmitter. The parasympathetic nervous system is entirely cholinergic.
Adrenergic	Pertaining to epinephrine or norepinephrine, as in adrenergic neurons that secrete one of these chemicals or adrenergic effects on a target organ is called adrenegic.
Eye	An eye is an organ that detects light. Different kinds of light-sensitive organs are found in a variety of creatures. The simplest eyes do nothing but detect whether the surroundings are light or dark, while more complex eyes can distinguish shapes and colors.
Tumor	An abnormal mass of cells that forms within otherwise normal tissue is a tumor. This growth can be either malignant or benign
Myoepithelial cell	Myoepithelial cell refers to type of unstriated muscle cell found in epithelia, e.g. In the iris of the eye and in glandular tissue.
Salt	Salt is a term used for ionic compounds composed of positively charged cations and negatively charged anions, so that the product is neutral and without a net charge.

Uric acid	An insoluble precipitate of nitrogenous waste excreted by land snails, insects, birds, and some reptiles is called uric acid.
Ammonia	Ammonia is a compound of nitrogen and hydrogen with the formula NH_3. At standard temperature and pressure ammonia is a gas. It is toxic and corrosive to some materials, and has a characteristic pungent odor.
Sodium	Sodium is the chemical element in the periodic table that has the symbol Na (Natrium in Latin) and atomic number 11. Sodium is a soft, waxy, silvery reactive metal belonging to the alkali metals that is abundant in natural compounds (especially halite). It is highly reactive.
Acid	An acid is a water-soluble, sour-tasting chemical compound that when dissolved in water, gives a solution with a pH of less than 7.
Urea	Urea is an organic compound of carbon, nitrogen, oxygen and hydrogen, CON_2H_4 or $(NH_2)_2CO$. Urea is essentially a waste product: it has no physiological function. It is dissolved in blood and excreted by the kidney.
Absorption	Absorption is a physical or chemical phenomenon or a process in which atoms, molecules, or ions enter some bulk phase - gas, liquid or solid material. In nutrition, amino acids are broken down through digestion, which begins in the stomach.
Ion	Ion refers to an atom or molecule that has gained or lost one or more electrons, thus acquiring an electrical charge.
Blood plasma	Blood plasma is the liquid component of blood, in which the blood cells are suspended. Serum is the same as blood plasma except that clotting factors (such as fibrin) have been removed.
Incidence	In epidemiological studies of a particular disorder, the rate at which new cases occur in a given place at a given time is called incidence.
Melanoma	Melanoma is a malignant tumor of melanocytes. Melanocytes predominantly occur in the skin but can be found elsewhere, especially the eye. The vast majority of melanomas originate in the skin.
Distribution	Distribution in pharmacology is a branch of pharmacokinetics describing reversible transfer of drug from one location to another within the body.
Biochemistry	Biochemistry studies how complex chemical reactions give rise to life. It is a hybrid branch of chemistry which specialises in the chemical processes in living organisms.
Physiology	The study of the function of cells, tissues, and organs is referred to as physiology.

Urine	Concentrated filtrate produced by the kidneys and excreted via the bladder is called urine.
Urethra	In anatomy, the urethra is a tube which connects the urinary bladder to the outside of the body. The urethra has an excretory function in both sexes, to pass urine to the outside, and also a reproductive function in the male, as a passage for sperm.
Bladder	A hollow muscular storage organ for storing urine is a bladder.
Ureter	A ureter is a duct that carries urine from the kidneys to the urinary bladder. They are muscular tubes that can propel urine along by the motions of peristalsis.
Organ	Organ refers to a structure consisting of several tissues adapted as a group to perform specific functions.
Electrolyte	An electrolyte is a substance that dissociates into free ions when dissolved (or molten), to produce an electrically conductive medium. Because they generally consist of ions in solution, they are also known as ionic solutions.
Renin	Renin is a circulating enzyme released mainly by juxtaglomerular cells of the kidneys in response to low blood volume or low body NaCl content.
Blood	Blood is a circulating tissue composed of fluid plasma and cells. The main function of blood is to supply nutrients (oxygen, glucose) and constitutional elements to tissues and to remove waste products.
Blood pressure	Blood pressure is the pressure exerted by the blood on the walls of the blood vessels.
Erythrocyte	Red blood cells are the most common type of blood cell and are the vertebrate body's principal means of delivering oxygen from the lungs or gills to body tissues via the blood. Red blood cells are also known as erythrocyte.
Erythropoietin	Erythropoietin is a glycoprotein hormone that is a growth factor for erythrocyte (red blood cell) precursors in the bone marrow. It increases the number of red blood cells in the blood.
Prohormone	A prohormone is a chemical compound that is a precursor to a hormone, usually with minimal hormonal effect by itself.
Steroid	A steroid is a lipid characterized by a carbon skeleton with four fused rings. Different steroids vary in the functional groups attached to these rings. Hundreds of distinct steroids have been identified in plants and animals. Their most important role in most living systems is as hormones.
Renal pelvis	The renal pelvis represents the funnel-like dilated proximal part of the ureter. The major function of the renal pelvis is to act as a funnel for urine flowing to the ureter.
Lymph vessel	Lymph vessel refers to one of the system of vessels carrying lymph from the lymph capillaries to the veins.
Kidney	The kidney is a bean-shaped excretory organ in vertebrates. Part of the urinary system, the kidneys filter wastes (especially urea) from the blood and excrete them, along with water, as urine.
Medial	In anatomical terms of location toward or near the midline is called medial.
Pelvis	The pelvis is the bony structure located at the base of the spine (properly known as the caudal end). The pelvis incorporates the socket portion of the hip joint for each leg (in bipeds) or hind leg (in quadrupeds). It forms the lower limb (or hind-limb) girdle of the skeleton.
Nerve	A nerve is an enclosed, cable-like bundle of nerve fibers or axons, which includes the glia that ensheath the axons in myelin.

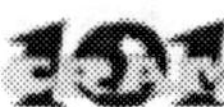

Lymph	Lymph originates as blood plasma lost from the circulatory system, which leaks out into the surrounding tissues. The lymphatic system collects this fluid by diffusion into lymph capillaries, and returns it to the circulatory system.
Renal	Pertaining to the kidney is referred to as renal.
Medulla	Medulla in general means the inner part, and derives from the Latin word for 'marrow'. In medicine it is contrasted to the cortex.
Cortex	In anatomy and zoology the cortex is the outermost or superficial layer of an organ or the outer portion of the stem or root of a plant.
Renal medulla	The renal medulla is the innermost part of the kidney. The renal medulla is split up into a number of sections, known as the renal pyramids.
Nephron	A nephron is the basic structural and functional unit of the kidney. Its chief function is to regulate water and soluble substances by filtering the blood, reabsorbing what is needed and excreting the rest as urine. They eliminate wastes from the body, regulate blood volume and pressure, control levels of electrolytes and metabolites, and regulate blood pH.
Base	The common definition of a base is a chemical compound that absorbs hydronium ions when dissolved in water (a proton acceptor). An alkali is a special example of a base, where in an aqueous environment, hydroxide ions are donated.
Proximal convoluted tubule	Highly coiled region of a nephron near the glomerular capsule, where tubular reabsorption takes place is called the proximal convoluted tubule.
Distal convoluted tubule	The distal convoluted tubule is a portion of kidney nephron between the loop of Henle and the collecting duct system. It is partly responsible for the regulation of potassium, sodium, calcium, and pH.
Renal corpuscle	A renal corpuscle is the initial filtering component of a nephron. It consists of a glomerulus, a small network of capillaries, enclosed in a Bowman's capsule, a sac-like structure.
Capillaries	Capillaries refer to the smallest of the blood vessels and the sites of exchange between the blood and tissue cells.
Filtration	Filtration involved in passive transport is the movement of water and solute molecules across the cell membrane due to hydrostatic pressure by the cardiovascular system.
Glomerulus	A glomerulus is a capillary tuft surrounded by Bowman's capsule in nephrons of the vertebrate kidney. It receives its blood supply from an afferent arteriole of the renal circulation, and empties into an efferent arteriole.
Capillary	A capillary is the smallest of a body's blood vessels, measuring 5-10 micro meters. They connect arteries and veins, and most closely interact with tissues. Their walls are composed of a single layer of cells, the endothelium. This layer is so thin that molecules such as oxygen, water and lipids can pass through them by diffusion and enter the tissues.
Visceral	Visceral refers to the internal organs of an animal.
Parietal	When speaking of inner organs, visceral means close to or attached to the organ, while parietal is more distant. For example, the visceral pleura is attached to the lung and the parietal pleura is attached to the chest wall.
Arteriole	An arteriole is a blood vessel that extends and branches out from an artery and leads to capillaries. They have thick muscular walls and are the primary site of vascular resistance.
Afferent	The afferent arteriole is a blood vessel that supply the nephrons in many excretory systems.

arteriole	They branch from the renal artery which supplies blood to the kidneys, and later diverge into the capillaries of the glomerulus.
Epithelium	Epithelium is a tissue composed of a layer of cells. Epithelium can be found lining internal (e.g. endothelium, which lines the inside of blood vessels) or external (e.g. skin) free surfaces of the body. Functions include secretion, absorption and protection.
Lamina	A thin layer, such as the lamina of a vertebra or the lamina propria of a mucous membrane is referred to as lamina.
Fiber	Fibers used by man come from a wide variety of sources: Natural fiber include those made out of plants, animal and mineral sources. Natural fibers can be classified according to their origin.
Squamous epithelium	The squamous epithelium is epithelium consisting of one or more cell layers, the most superficial of which is composed of flat, scalelike or platelike cells.
Proximal tubule	The proximal tubule is a segment of a nephron that starts at Bowman's capsule and extends to the renal medulla.
Podocytes	Podocytes are cells of the visceral epithelium in the kidneys and form a crucial component of the glomerular filtration barrier, contributing size selectivity and maintaining a massive filtration surface.
Diaphragm	The diaphragm is a shelf of muscle extending across the bottom of the ribcage. It is critically important in respiration: in order to draw air into the lungs, the diaphragm contracts, thus enlarging the thoracic cavity and reducing intra-thoracic pressure.
Cytoplasm	Cytoplasm refers to the contents of a cell excluding the nucleus and cell membrane. Cytoplasm is a homogeneous, generally clear jelly-like material that fills cells.
Actin	A protein in a muscle fiber that, together with myosin, is responsible for contraction and relaxation is actin.
Endothelial cell	A endothelial cell also controls the passage of materials — and the transit of white blood cells — into and out of the bloodstream. In some organs, there are highly differentiated endothelial cells to perform specialized 'filtering' functions.
Actin filament	An actin filament is a helical protein filament formed by the polymerization of globular actin molecules. They provide mechanical support for the cell, determine the cell shape, enable cell movements; and participate in certain cell junctions.
Fusion	Fusion refers to the combination of two atoms into a single atom as a result of a collision, usually accompanied by the release of energy.
Microscope	A microscope is an instrument for viewing objects that are too small to be seen by the naked or unaided eye.
Fibronectin	Fibronectin is a high molecular weight glycoprotein containing about 5% carbohydrate that bind to receptor proteins spanning the cell membrane called integrins. In addition to integrins, they also bind extracellular matrix components such as collagen, fibrin and heparin.
Juxtamedullary nephron	A nephron with long loops of Henle that extends into the medulla and creates a concentrated interstitium through the countercurrent mechanism is a juxtamedullary nephron.
Proteoglycan	Molecule consisting of one or more glycosaminoglycan chains attached to a core protein is referred to as proteoglycan.
Protein	A protein is a complex, high-molecular-weight organic compound that consists of amino acids joined by peptide bonds. They are essential to the structure and function of all living cells

	and viruses. Many are enzymes or subunits of enzymes.
Albumin	Albumin refers generally to any protein with water solubility, which is moderately soluble in concentrated salt solutions, and experiences heat coagulation (protein denaturation).
Glomeruli	Glomeruli are important waystations in the pathway from the nose to the olfactory cortex. Each receives input from olfactory receptor neurons expressing only one type of olfactory receptor. There are tens of millions of olfactory receptor cells, but only about two thousand glomeruli. By combining so much input, the olfactory system is able to detect even very faint odors.
Hydrostatic pressure	Hydrostatic pressure refers to pressure exerted by fluids, such as blood pressure.
Colloid	Colloid refers to a mixture that contains dispersed particles larger than molecules but small enough so that they do not settle out.
Plasma	Fluid portion of circulating blood is called plasma.
Glomerular filtrate	Filtered portion of blood contained within the glomerular capsule is glomerular filtrate.
Net filtration	In most vascular beds of the body, filtration occurs across the arteriolar end of the capillary and reabsorption occurs across the venular end. In general, there is net filtration across capillary beds (i.e., filtration > reabsorption) that is picked up by the lymphatics.
Blood plasma	Blood plasma is the liquid component of blood, in which the blood cells are suspended. Serum is the same as blood plasma except that clotting factors (such as fibrin) have been removed.
Macromolecule	A macromolecule is a molecule with a large molecular mass, but generally the use of the term is restricted to polymers and molecules which structurally include polymers.
Artery	Vessel that takes blood away from the heart to the tissues and organs of the body is called an artery.
Vein	Vein in animals, is a vessel that returns blood to the heart. In plants, a vascular bundle in a leaf, composed of xylem and phloem.
Veins	Blood vessels that return blood toward the heart from the circulation are referred to as veins.
Angiotensin II	Angiotensin II is formed by the action of renin on angiotensinogen. Renin, produced in the kidneys in response to decreased blood pressure, cleaves the peptide bond between the leucine and the valine residues on angiotensinogen.
Angiotensin	Angiotensin is a polypeptide in the blood that causes vasoconstriction, increased blood pressure, and aldosterone release from the adrenal cortex. Angiotensin is produced in the liver from precursor angiotensinogen, a serum globulin. It plays an important role in the renin-angiotensin system.
Receptor	A receptor is a protein on the cell membrane or within the cytoplasm or cell nucleus that binds to a specific molecule (a ligand), such as a neurotransmitter, hormone, or other substance, and initiates the cellular response to the ligand. Receptor, in immunology, the region of an antibody which shows recognition of an antigen.
Cytokine	A type of protein secreted by a T lymphocyte that attacks viruses, virally infected cells, and cancer cells is referred to as cytokine.
Prostaglandin	A prostaglandin is any member of a group of lipid compounds that are derived from fatty acids and have important functions in the animal body.
Extracellular	Outside the cell is called extracellular.

Mitochondria	Cytoplasmic organelles responsible for ATP generation for cellular activities are referred to as mitochondria.
Brush border	Brush border refers to dense covering of microvilli on the apical surface of epithelial cells in the intestine and kidney. The microvilli aid absorption by increasing the surface area of the cell.
Transverse	A transverse (also known as axial or horizontal) plane is an X-Y plane, parallel to the ground, which (in humans) separates the superior from the inferior, or put another way, the head from the feet.
Peritubular capillaries	The network of tiny blood vessels that surrounds the proximal and distal tubules in the kidney are called peritubular capillaries.
Canaliculi	Canaliculi are small, microscopic canals between the various lacunae of ocified bone. The radiating processes of the osteocytes project into these canals. In cartilage, the lacunae and hence, the chondrocytes, are isolated from each other. Materials picked up by osteocytes adjacent to blood vessels, are distributed throughout the bone matrix via the canaliculi.
Vesicle	Membranous, cytoplasmic sac formed by an infolding of the cell membrane is called a vesicle.
Muscle	Muscle is a contractile form of tissue. It is one of the four major tissue types, the other three being epithelium, connective tissue and nervous tissue. Muscle contraction is used to move parts of the body, as well as to move substances within the body.
Juxtaglomerular cell	The juxtaglomerular cell synthesizes, stores, and secretes the enzyme renin. They are specialized smooth muscle cells in the wall of the afferent arteriole that drains blood from the glomerulus.
Smooth muscle	Smooth muscle is a type of non-striated muscle, found within the "walls" of hollow organs; such as blood vessels, the bladder, the uterus, and the gastrointestinal tract. Smooth muscle is used to move matter within the body, via contraction; it generally operates "involuntarily", without nerve stimulation.
Distal tubule	In the vertebrate kidney, the portion of a nephron that helps refine filtrate and empty it into a collecting duct is called the distal tubule.
Macula	The macula is an oval yellow spot near the center of the retina of the human eye. Near its center is the fovea, a small pit that contains the largest concentration of cone cells in the eye and is responsible for central vision.
Lysosome	Organelle that contains enzymes that degrade worn cell parts is called a lysosome.
Monomer	In chemistry, a monomer is a small molecule that may become chemically bonded to other monomers to form a polymer.
Invagination	Infolding of one part of a structure into another is invagination.
Sodium	Sodium is the chemical element in the periodic table that has the symbol Na (Natrium in Latin) and atomic number 11. Sodium is a soft, waxy, silvery reactive metal belonging to the alkali metals that is abundant in natural compounds (especially halite). It is highly reactive.
Ion	Ion refers to an atom or molecule that has gained or lost one or more electrons, thus acquiring an electrical charge.
Absorption	Absorption is a physical or chemical phenomenon or a process in which atoms, molecules, or ions enter some bulk phase - gas, liquid or solid material. In nutrition, amino acids are broken down through digestion, which begins in the stomach.
Excretion	Excretion is the biological process by which an organism chemically separates waste products

from its body. The waste products are then usually expelled from the body by elimination.

Amino acid | An amino acid is any molecule that contains both amino and carboxylic acid functional groups. They are the basic structural building units of proteins. They form short polymer chains called peptides or polypeptides which in turn form structures called proteins.

Phosphate | A phosphate is a polyatomic ion or radical consisting of one phosphorus atom and four oxygen. In the ionic form, it carries a -3 formal charge, and is denoted PO_4^{3-}.

Glucose | Glucose, a simple monosaccharide sugar, is one of the most important carbohydrates and is used as a source of energy in animals and plants. Glucose is one of the main products of photosynthesis and starts respiration.

Calcium | Calcium is the chemical element in the periodic table that has the symbol Ca and atomic number 20. Calcium is a soft grey alkaline earth metal that is used as a reducing agent in the extraction of thorium, zirconium and uranium. Calcium is also the fifth most abundant element in the Earth's crust.

Acid | An acid is a water-soluble, sour-tasting chemical compound that when dissolved in water, gives a solution with a pH of less than 7.

Creatinine | Creatinine is a nitrogenous organic acid that helps supply energy to muscle cells. Creatinine is a breakdown product of creatine phosphate in muscle, and is usually produced at a fairly constant rate by the body.

Penicillin | Penicillin refers to a group of β-lactam antibiotics used in the treatment of bacterial infections caused by susceptible, usually Gram-positive, organisms.

Urinary system | The urinary system is the organ system that produces, stores, and carries urine. In humans it includes two kidneys, two ureters, the urinary bladder, two sphincter muscles, and the urethra.

Histology | Histology is the study of tissue sectioned as a thin slice, using a microscope. It can be described as microscopic anatomy.

Hypertonic | A hypertonic cell environment has a higher concentration of solutes than in cytoplasm. In a hypertonic environment, osmosis causes water to flow out of the cell. If enough water is removed in this way, the cytoplasm will have such a small concentration of water that the cell has difficulty functioning.

Osmolarity | Osmolarity is a measure of the osmoles of solute per litre of solution, while the osmolality is a measure of the osmoles of solute per kilogram of solvent.

Micrograph | A micrograph is a photograph or similar image taken through a microscope or similar device to show a magnified image of an item.

Aldosterone | Aldosterone is a steroid hormone synthesized from cholesterol by the enzyme aldosterone synthase. It helps regulate the body's electrolyte balance by acting on the mineralocorticoid receptor. It diminishes the secretion of sodium ions and therefore, water and stimulates the secretion of potassium ions through the kidneys.

Potassium | Potassium is a chemical element in the periodic table. It has the symbol K (L. kalium) and atomic number 19. Potassium is a soft silvery-white metallic alkali metal that occurs naturally bound to other elements in seawater and many minerals.

Ammonium | The ammonium cation is a positively charged polyatomic ion of the chemical formula NH_4+ and a molecular mass of 18.04, resulting from protonation of ammonia (NH_3).

Hydrogen | Hydrogen is a chemical element in the periodic table that has the symbol H and atomic number 1. At standard temperature and pressure it is a colorless, odorless, nonmetallic, univalent, tasteless, highly flammable diatomic gas.

Collagen	Collagen is the main protein of connective tissue in animals and the most abundant protein in mammals, making up about 1/4 of the total. It is one of the long, fibrous structural proteins whose functions are quite different from those of globular proteins such as enzymes.
Leukocyte	A white blood cell is a leukocyte. They help to defend the body against infectious disease and foreign materials as part of the immune system.
Cortical collecting duct	The cortical collecting duct receives filtrate from multiple connecting tubules and descend into the renal medulla to form medullary collecting ducts in the collecting duct system of the kidney.
Light microscope	An optical instrument with lenses that refract visible light to magnify images and project them into a viewer's eye or onto photographic film is referred to as light microscope.
Hormone	A hormone is a chemical messenger from one cell to another. All multicellular organisms produce hormones. The best known hormones are those produced by endocrine glands of vertebrate animals, but hormones are produced by nearly every organ system and tissue type in a human or animal body. Hormone molecules are secreted directly into the bloodstream, they move by circulation or diffusion to their target cells, which may be nearby cells in the same tissue or cells of a distant organ of the body.
Antidiuretic hormone	Antidiuretic hormone is a hormone that is mainly released when the body is low on water; it causes the kidneys to save water by concentrating the urine and is also involved in the creation of thirst. It is a peptide hormone produced by the hypothalamus, and stored in the posterior part of the pituitary gland.
Channel	Channel, in communications (sometimes called communications channel), refers to the medium used to convey information from a sender (or transmitter) to a receiver.
Juxtaglomerular apparatus	The juxtaglomerular apparatus is a renal structure consisting of the macula densa and juxtaglomerular cells. Juxtaglomerular cells (JG cells) are the site of renin secretion.
Tunica media	The tunica media is the middle layer of an artery. It is made up of smooth muscle cells and elastic tissue. It lays between the tunica intima on the inside and the tunica adventitia on the outside.
Hemorrhage	Loss of blood from the circulatory system is referred to as a hemorrhage.
Enzyme	An enzyme is a protein that catalyzes, or speeds up, a chemical reaction. They are essential to sustain life because most chemical reactions in biological cells would occur too slowly, or would lead to different products, without them.
Dehydration	Dehydration is the removal of water from an object. Medically, dehydration is a serious and potentially life-threatening condition in which the body contains an insufficient volume of water for normal functioning.
Renal artery	The renal artery normally arise off the abdominal aorta and supply the kidneys with blood. The arterial supply of the kidneys is variable and there may be one or more supplying each kidney.
Course	Pattern of development and change of a disorder over time is a course.
Renal cortex	The renal cortex is the outer portion of the kidney between the renal capsule and the renal medulla. It forms a continuous smooth outer zone in the adult which extends down between the pyramids.
Endothelium	The endothelium is the layer of thin, flat cells that lines the interior surface of blood vessels, forming an interface between circulating blood in the lumen and the rest of the vessel wall.
Tissue	A collection of interconnected cells that perform a similar function within an organism is

	called tissue.
Muscle fiber	Cell with myofibrils containing actin and myosin filaments arranged within sarcomeres is a muscle fiber.
Parenchyma	The parenchyma are the functional parts of an organ in the body (i.e. the nephrons of the kidney, the alveoli of the lungs). In plants parenchyma cells are thin-walled cells of the ground tissue that make up the bulk of most nonwoody structures, although sometimes their cell walls can be lignified.
Sphincter	Muscle that surrounds a tube and closes or opens the tube by contracting and relaxing is referred to as sphincter.
Prostate	The prostate is a gland that is part of male mammalian sex organs. Its main function is to secrete and store a clear, slightly basic fluid that is part of semen. The prostate differs considerably between species anatomically, chemically and physiologically.
Urethral meatus	The urethral meatus is the external opening of the urethra on the body surface through which urine is discharged.
Sperm	Sperm refers to the male sex cell with three distinct parts at maturity: head, middle piece, and tail.
Elevation	Elevation refers to upward movement of a part of the body.
Dorsal	In anatomy, the dorsal is the side in which the backbone is located. This is usually the top of an animal, although in humans it refers to the back.
Utricle	A fluid-filled inner ear chamber containing hair cells that detect the position of the head relative to gravity is an utricle.
Ejaculatory duct	The Ejaculatory duct is a part of the human male anatomy, which causes the reflex action of ejaculation. Each male has two of them. They begin at the vas deferens, pass through the prostate, and empty into the urethra at the Colliculus seminalis.
Seminal fluid	Semen is composed of sperm and seminal fluid. About 10-30% of the seminal fluid is produced by the prostate gland, the rest is produced by the two seminal vesicles.
Striated muscle	Striated muscle refers to contractile tissue characterized by multinucleated cells containing highly ordered arrangements of actin and myosin microfilaments. Also known as skeletal muscle.
Connective tissue	Connective tissue is any type of biological tissue with an extensive extracellular matrix and often serves to support, bind together, and protect organs.
Penis	The penis is the male reproductive organ and for mammals additionally serves as the external male organ of urination.
Fossa navicularis	The fossa navicularis is the enlargement of the distal penile urethra just proximal to the urethral meatus (the external urethral orifice). It can also refer to a structure present in both men and women.
Gland	A gland is an organ in an animal's body that synthesizes a substance for release such as hormones, often into the bloodstream or into cavities inside the body or its outer surface.
Endocytosis	Endocytosis is a process where cells absorb material (molecules or other cells) from outside by engulfing it with their cell membranes.
Exocytosis	Exocytosis is the process by which a cell is able to get rid of large molecules or materials including wastes through its membrane. The process involves a [vacuole], containing the material, fusing with the membrane.

Urinary bladder

In the anatomy of mammals, the urinary bladder is the organ that collects urine excreted by the kidneys prior to disposal by urination. Urine enters the bladder via the ureters and exits via the urethra.

Plasma membrane

The unit membrane that encloses a cell and controls the traffic of molecules in and out of the cell is the plasma membrane.

Gland	A gland is an organ in an animal's body that synthesizes a substance for release such as hormones, often into the bloodstream or into cavities inside the body or its outer surface.
Endocrine gland	An endocrine gland is one of a set of internal organs involved in the secretion of hormones into the blood. These glands are known as ductless, which means they do not have tubes inside them.
Microsphere	A microsphere is a protein protocell, small spherical units postulated by some scientists as a key stage in the origin of life. They do not reproduce or pass on any type of genetic material.
Follicle	Follicle refers to a cluster of cells surrounding, protecting, and nourishing a developing egg cell in the ovary; also secretes estrogen. In botany, a follicle is a type of simple dry fruit produced by certain flowering plants. It is regarded as one the most primitive types of fruits, and derives from a simple pistil or carpel.
Thyroid	The thyroid is one of the larger endocrine glands in the body. It is located in the neck and produces hormones, principally thyroxine and triiodothyronine, that regulate the rate of metabolism and affect the growth and rate of function of many other systems in the body.
Atrial natriuretic factor	Atrial natriuretic factor is a peptide hormone involved in the homeostatic control of body water and sodium. It is released by atrial monocytes, cells in the atria of the heart, in response to signals of raized blood pressure and acts to reduce this.
Placenta	The placenta is an organ present only in female placental mammals during gestation. It is composed of two parts, one genetically and biologically part of the fetus, the other part of the mother. It is implanted in the wall of the uterus, where it receives nutrients and oxygen from the mother's blood and passes out waste.
Kidney	The kidney is a bean-shaped excretory organ in vertebrates. Part of the urinary system, the kidneys filter wastes (especially urea) from the blood and excrete them, along with water, as urine.
Juxtaglomerular cell	The juxtaglomerular cell synthesizes, stores, and secretes the enzyme renin. They are specialized smooth muscle cells in the wall of the afferent arteriole that drains blood from the glomerulus.
Digestive tract	The digestive tract is the system of organs within multicellular animals which takes in food, digests it to extract energy and nutrients, and expels the remaining waste.
Hormone	A hormone is a chemical messenger from one cell to another. All multicellular organisms produce hormones. The best known hormones are those produced by endocrine glands of vertebrate animals, but hormones are produced by nearly every organ system and tissue type in a human or animal body. Hormone molecules are secreted directly into the bloodstream, they move by circulation or diffusion to their target cells, which may be nearby cells in the same tissue or cells of a distant organ of the body.
Cytokine	A type of protein secreted by a T lymphocyte that attacks viruses, virally infected cells, and cancer cells is referred to as cytokine.
Extracellular	Outside the cell is called extracellular.
Somatostatin	Somatostatin is hormone secreted not only by cells of the hypothalamus but also by so called delta cells of stomach, intestine and pancreas. It binds to somatostatin receptors. All actions of the hormone are inhibitory.
Insulin	Insulin is a polypeptide hormone that regulates carbohydrate metabolism. Apart from being the primary effector in carbohydrate homeostasis, it also has a substantial effect on small vessel muscle tone, controls storage and release of fat (triglycerides) and cellular uptake of both amino acids and some electrolytes.

Islets of Langerhans	The endocrine (i.e., hormone-producing) cells of the pancreas are grouped in the Islets of Langerhans.
Receptor	A receptor is a protein on the cell membrane or within the cytoplasm or cell nucleus that binds to a specific molecule (a ligand), such as a neurotransmitter, hormone, or other substance, and initiates the cellular response to the ligand. Receptor, in immunology, the region of an antibody which shows recognition of an antigen.
Tissue	A collection of interconnected cells that perform a similar function within an organism is called tissue.
Organ	Organ refers to a structure consisting of several tissues adapted as a group to perform specific functions.
Target cell	Specific cell on which a hormone exerts its effect is a target cell.
Blood	Blood is a circulating tissue composed of fluid plasma and cells. The main function of blood is to supply nutrients (oxygen, glucose) and constitutional elements to tissues and to remove waste products.
Endocrine system	The endocrine system is a set of internal organs involved in the secretion of hormones into the blood. These glands are known as ductless, which means they do not have tubes inside them.
Central nervous system	The central nervous system comprized of the brain and spinal cord, represents the largest part of the nervous system. Together with the peripheral nervous system, it has a fundamental role in the control of behavior.
Adenohypophysis	The adenohypophysis comprises the anterior lobe of the pituitary gland and is part of the endocrine system. Under the influence of the hypothalamus, the anterior pituitary produces and secretes several peptide hormones that regulate many physiological processes including stress, growth, and reproduction.
Nervous system	The nervous system of an animal coordinates the activity of the muscles, monitors the organs, constructs and processes input from the senses, and initiates actions.
Immune system	The immune system is the system of specialized cells and organs that protect an organism from outside biological influences. When the immune system is functioning properly, it protects the body against bacteria and viral infections, destroying cancer cells and foreign substances.
Affect	Affect is the scientific term used to describe a subject's externally displayed mood. This can be assesed by the nurse by observing facial expression, tone of voice, and body language.
Immune response	The body's defensive reaction to invasion by bacteria, viral agents, or other foreign substances is called immune response.
Pituitary gland	The pituitary gland or hypophysis is an endocrine gland about the size of a pea that sits in the small, bony cavity (sella turcica) at the base of the brain. Its posterior lobe is connected to a part of the brain called the hypothalamus via the infundibulum (or stalk), giving rise to the tuberoinfundibular pathway.
Sphenoid bone	The sphenoid bone is a bone situated at the base of the skull in front of the temporals and basilar part of the occipital. It somewhat resembles a butterfly with its wings extended, and is divided into a median portion or body, two great wings and two small wings extending outward from the sides of the body, and two pterygoid processes which project from it below.
Nerve tissue	Nerve tissue refers the specialized tissue making up the central and peripheral nervous systems; consists of neurons and glial cells.
Hypophysis	The pituitary gland, or hypophysis, is an endocrine gland about the size of a pea that sits

	in the small, bony cavity (sella turcica) at the base of the brain.
Ectoderm	Ectoderm refers to the outer layer of three embryonic cell layers in a gastrula; forms the skin of the gastrula and gives rise to the epidermis and nervous system in the adult.
Nerve	A nerve is an enclosed, cable-like bundle of nerve fibers or axons, which includes the glia that ensheath the axons in myelin.
Embryogenesis	Embryogenesis is the process by which the embryo is formed and develops. It starts with the fertilization of the ovum, which is then called a zygote.
Diencephalon	The diencephalon is the region of the brain that includes the epithalamus, thalamus, and hypothalamus. It is located above the mesencephalon of the brain stem. Sensory information is relayed between the brain stem and the rest of the brain regions.
Brain	The part of the central nervous system involved in regulating and controlling body activity and interpreting information from the senses transmitted through the nervous system is referred to as the brain.
Embryo	A prenatal stage of development after germ layers form but before the rudiments of all organs are present is referred to as an embryo.
Oral cavity	The mouth, also known as the buccal cavity or the oral cavity, is the opening through which an animal or human takes in food and water. It is usually located in the head, but not always; the mouth of a planarium is in the middle of its belly.
Base	The common definition of a base is a chemical compound that absorbs hydronium ions when dissolved in water (a proton acceptor). An alkali is a special example of a base, where in an aqueous environment, hydroxide ions are donated.
Median	The median is a number that separates the higher half of a sample, a population, or a probability distribution from the lower half. It is the middle value in a distribution, above and below which lie an equal number of values.
Neurohypophysis	The neurohypophysis comprises the posterior lobe of the pituitary gland and is part of the endocrine system. Despite its name, the posterior pituitary gland is not a gland, rather, it is largely a collection of axonal projections from the hypothalamus that terminate behind the anterior pituitary gland.
Median eminence	The median eminence is part of the inferior boundary for the hypothalamus. It is integral to the hypophyseal portal system which connects the Hypothalamus with the Anterior lobe of the pituatary gland.
Cranial	In the limbs of most animals, the terms cranial and caudal are used in the regions proximal to the carpus (the wrist, in the forelimb) and the tarsus (the ankle in the hindlimb). Objects and surfaces closer to or facing towards the head are cranial; those facing away or further from the head are caudal.
Internal carotid artery	In human anatomy, the internal carotid artery is a major artery of the head and neck. It arises from the common carotid artery when it bifurcates into an internal and external branch. It has no branches in the neck. It ascends and enters the skull through the carotid canal. Inside the cranium, it gives off the ophthalmic artery .
Artery	Vessel that takes blood away from the heart to the tissues and organs of the body is called an artery.
Carotid artery	In human anatomy, the carotid artery refers to a number of major arteries in the head and neck.
Capillaries	Capillaries refer to the smallest of the blood vessels and the sites of exchange between the blood and tissue cells.

Capillary — A capillary is the smallest of a body's blood vessels, measuring 5-10 micro meters. They connect arteries and veins, and most closely interact with tissues. Their walls are composed of a single layer of cells, the endothelium. This layer is so thin that molecules such as oxygen, water and lipids can pass through them by diffusion and enter the tissues.

Irrigate — To gently flush a canal with fluid is to irrigate the area.

Plexus — A plexus is also a network of blood vessels, with the choroid plexuses of the brain being the most commonly mentioned example. A choroid plexus is very thin and vascular roof plates of the most anterior and most posterior cavities of the brain which expand into the interiors of the cavities.

Hypothalamus — Located below the thalamus, the hypothalamus links the nervous system to the endocrine system by synthesizing and secreting neurohormones often called releasing hormones because they function by stimulating the secretion of hormones from the anterior pituitary gland.

Peptide — Peptide is the family of molecules formed from the linking, in a defined order, of various amino acids. The link between one amino acid residue and the next is an amide bond, and is sometimes referred to as a peptide bond.

Neuron — The neuron is a major class of cells in the nervous system. In vertebrates, they are found in the brain, the spinal cord and in the nerves and ganglia of the peripheral nervous system, and their primary role is to process and transmit neural information.

Axon — An axon is a long slender projection of a nerve cell, or neuron, which conducts electrical impulses away from the neuron's cell body or soma. They are in effect the primary transmission lines of the nervous system, and as bundles they help make up nerves.

Hypophyseal portal system — The hypophyseal portal system is the system of blood vessels that supplies blood to part of the hypothalamus and the anterior pituitary and allows endocrine communication between the two structures. It is one of only a few portal systems of circulation in the body; that is, it involves two capillary beds connected by venules rather than arterioles.

Protein — A protein is a complex, high-molecular-weight organic compound that consists of amino acids joined by peptide bonds. They are essential to the structure and function of all living cells and viruses. Many are enzymes or subunits of enzymes.

Blood vessel — A blood vessel is a part of the circulatory system and function to transport blood throughout the body. The most important types, arteries and veins, are so termed because they carry blood away from or towards the heart, respectively.

Gonadotropin — A hormone that stimulates the gonads is gonadotropin. They are protein hormones secreted by gonadotrope cells of the pituitary gland of vertebrates.

Infundibulum — An infundibulum is a funnel-shape cavity or organ.

Luteinizing hormone — Luteinizing hormone is a hormone synthesized and secreted by gonadotropes in the anterior lobe of the pituitary gland. In both males and females, it stimulates the production of sex steroids from the gonads.

Intermediate zone — The intermediate zone receives input from the corticopontocerebellar fibers that originate from the motor cortex. These fibers carry a duplicate of the information that was sent from the motor cortex to the spine in order to effect a movement.

Action potential — The sequence of electrical changes occurring when a nerve cell membrane is exposed to a stimulus that exceeds its threshold is called action potential.

Microscope — A microscope is an instrument for viewing objects that are too small to be seen by the naked or unaided eye.

Light microscope — An optical instrument with lenses that refract visible light to magnify images and project

	them into a viewer's eye or onto photographic film is referred to as light microscope.
Amino acid	An amino acid is any molecule that contains both amino and carboxylic acid functional groups. They are the basic structural building units of proteins. They form short polymer chains called peptides or polypeptides which in turn form structures called proteins.
Acid	An acid is a water-soluble, sour-tasting chemical compound that when dissolved in water, gives a solution with a pH of less than 7.
Proteolysis	Degradation of a protein by cellular enzymes called proteases or by intramolecular digestion at one or more of its peptide bonds is referred to as proteolysis.
Vasopressin	Vasopressin is a human hormone that is mainly released when the body is low on water; it causes the kidneys to conserve water by concentrating the urine. It has also various functions in the brain.
Oxytocin	Oxytocin is a hormone, found in humans and other mammals, which is involved in the facilitation of birth and breastfeeding as well as in bonding and the formation of trust between people.
Fiber	Fibers used by man come from a wide variety of sources: Natural fiber include those made out of plants, animal and mineral sources. Natural fibers can be classified according to their origin.
Osmoreceptor	A neuron that converts changes in the osmotic potential of interstial fluids into action potentials is an osmoreceptor.
Arginine	Arginine is an α-amino acid. The L-form is one of the 20 most common natural amino acids. In mammals, arginine is classified as a semiessential or conditionally essential amino acid, depending on the developmental stage and health status of the individual.
Salt	Salt is a term used for ionic compounds composed of positively charged cations and negatively charged anions, so that the product is neutral and without a net charge.
Arteriole	An arteriole is a blood vessel that extends and branches out from an artery and leads to capillaries. They have thick muscular walls and are the primary site of vascular resistance.
Muscle	Muscle is a contractile form of tissue. It is one of the four major tissue types, the other three being epithelium, connective tissue and nervous tissue. Muscle contraction is used to move parts of the body, as well as to move substances within the body.
Smooth muscle	Smooth muscle is a type of non-striated muscle, found within the "walls" of hollow organs; such as blood vessels, the bladder, the uterus, and the gastrointestinal tract. Smooth muscle is used to move matter within the body, via contraction; it generally operates "involuntarily", without nerve stimulation.
Endogenous	Originating internally, such as the endogenous cholesterol synthesized in the body in contrast to the exogenous cholesterol coming from the diet is referred to as endogenous. Compare with exogenous.
Blood pressure	Blood pressure is the pressure exerted by the blood on the walls of the blood vessels.
Childbirth	Childbirth (also called labour, birth, partus or parturition) is the culmination of a human pregnancy with the emergence of a newborn infant from its mother's uterus.
Alveoli	Alveoli are anatomical structures that have the form of a hollow cavity. In the lung, the pulmonary alveoli are spherical outcroppings of the respiratory bronchioles and are the primary sites of gas exchange with the blood.
Myoepithelial cell	Myoepithelial cell refers to type of unstriated muscle cell found in epithelia, e.g. In the iris of the eye and in glandular tissue.

Mammary gland — The mammary gland is the organ in the female mammal that produces milk for the sustenance of the young. These exocrine glands are enlarged and modified sweat glands and are the characteristic of mammals which gave the class its name.

Cervix — The cervix is actually the lower, narrow portion of the uterus where it joins with the top end of the vagina. It is cylindrical or conical in shape and protrudes through the upper anterior vaginal wall.

Vagina — The vagina is the tubular tract leading from the uterus to the exterior of the body in female placental mammals and marsupials, or to the cloaca in female birds, monotremes, and some reptiles. Female insects and other invertebrates also have a vagina, which is the terminal part of the oviduct.

Ovary — The primary reproductive organ of a female is called an ovary.

Growth hormone — Growth hormone is a polypeptide hormone synthesised and secreted by the anterior pituitary gland which stimulates growth and cell reproduction in humans and other vertebrate animals.

Polyuria — Excessive output of urine is called polyuria.

Lesion — A lesion is a non-specific term referring to abnormal tissue in the body. It can be caused by any disease process including trauma (physical, chemical, electrical), infection, neoplasm, metabolic and autoimmune.

Urine — Concentrated filtrate produced by the kidneys and excreted via the bladder is called urine.

Optic nerve — The optic nerve is the nerve that transmits visual information from the retina to the brain. The blind spot of the eye is produced by the absence of retina where the optic nerve leaves the eye. This is because there are no photoreceptors in this area.

Tumor — An abnormal mass of cells that forms within otherwise normal tissue is a tumor. This growth can be either malignant or benign

Vascular smooth muscle — Vascular smooth muscle refers to the particular type of smooth muscle found within, and composing the majority of the wall of blood vessels.

Diagnosis — In medicine, diagnosis is the process of identifying a medical condition or disease by its signs, symptoms, and from the results of various diagnostic procedures.

Inhibition — The ability to prevent from making some cognitive or behavioral response is called inhibition.

Medulla — Medulla in general means the inner part, and derives from the Latin word for 'marrow'. In medicine it is contrasted to the cortex.

Adrenal — In mammals, the adrenal glands are the triangle-shaped endocrine glands that sit atop the kidneys. They are chiefly responsible for regulating the stress response through the synthesis of corticosteroids and catecholamines, including cortisol and adrenaline.

Cortex — In anatomy and zoology the cortex is the outermost or superficial layer of an organ or the outer portion of the stem or root of a plant.

Adrenal medulla — Composed mainly of hormone-producing chromaffin cells, the adrenal medulla is the principal site of the conversion of the amino acid tyrosine into the catecholamines epinephrine and norepinephrine.

Adrenal cortex — Situated along the perimeter of the adrenal gland, the adrenal cortex mediates the stress response through the production of mineralocorticoids and glucocorticoids, including aldosterone and cortisol respectively. It is also a secondary site of androgen synthesis.

Adrenal gland — In mammals, the adrenal gland (also known as suprarenal glands or colloquially as kidney hats) are the triangle-shaped endocrine glands that sit atop the kidneys; their name

	indicates that position.
Sympathetic	The sympathetic nervous system activates what is often termed the "fight or flight response". It is an automatic regulation system, that is, one that operates without the intervention of conscious thought.
Epithelium	Epithelium is a tissue composed of a layer of cells. Epithelium can be found lining internal (e.g. endothelium, which lines the inside of blood vessels) or external (e.g. skin) free surfaces of the body. Functions include secretion, absorption and protection.
Ganglion	In vertebrate anatomy, a ganglion is a tissue mass that contains the dendrites and cell bodies (or "somata") of nerve cells, in most case ones belonging to the peripheral nervous system.
Ganglion cell	A ganglion cell is a type of neuron located in the retina of the eye that receives visual information from photoreceptors via various intermediate cells such as bipolar cells, amacrine cells, and horizontal cells. The axons are myelinated.
Septa	Septa are thin walls or partitions between the internal chambers (camerae) of the shell of a cephalopod, namely nautiloids or ammonoids.
Dense connective tissue	Dense connective tissue has collagen fibers as its main matrix element. Crowded between the collagen fibers are rows of fibroblasts, fiber-forming cells, that manufacture the fibers. Dense connective tissue forms strong, rope-like structures such as tendons and ligaments. Tendons attach skeletal muscles to bones; ligaments connect bones to bones at joints.
Connective tissue	Connective tissue is any type of biological tissue with an extensive extracellular matrix and often serves to support, bind together, and protect organs.
Adrenal glands	The adrenal glands are the triangle-shaped endocrine glands that sit atop the kidneys; their name indicates that position. They are chiefly responsible for regulating the stress response through the synthesis of corticosteroids and catecholamines, including cortisol and adrenaline.
Erythrocyte	Red blood cells are the most common type of blood cell and are the vertebrate body's principal means of delivering oxygen from the lungs or gills to body tissues via the blood. Red blood cells are also known as erythrocyte.
Venous blood	In the circulatory system, venous blood or peripheral blood is blood returning to the heart. With one exception (the pulmonary vein) this blood is deoxygenated and high in carbon dioxide, having released oxygen and absorbed CO_2 in the tissues.
Endothelium	The endothelium is the layer of thin, flat cells that lines the interior surface of blood vessels, forming an interface between circulating blood in the lumen and the rest of the vessel wall.
Diaphragm	The diaphragm is a shelf of muscle extending across the bottom of the ribcage. It is critically important in respiration: in order to draw air into the lungs, the diaphragm contracts, thus enlarging the thoracic cavity and reducing intra-thoracic pressure.
Lamina	A thin layer, such as the lamina of a vertebra or the lamina propria of a mucous membrane is referred to as lamina.
Steroid	A steroid is a lipid characterized by a carbon skeleton with four fused rings. Different steroids vary in the functional groups attached to these rings. Hundreds of distinct steroids have been identified in plants and animals. Their most important role in most living systems is as hormones.
Veins	Blood vessels that return blood toward the heart from the circulation are referred to as veins.

Vein
Vein in animals, is a vessel that returns blood to the heart. In plants, a vascular bundle in a leaf, composed of xylem and phloem.

Steroid hormones
Steroid hormones are steroids which act as hormones. They can be grouped into five groups by the receptors to which they bind: glucocorticoids, mineralocorticoids, androgens, estrogens, and progestagens.

Exocytosis
Exocytosis is the process by which a cell is able to get rid of large molecules or materials including wastes through its membrane. The process involves a [vacuole], containing the material, fusing with the membrane.

Plasma
Fluid portion of circulating blood is called plasma.

Lipid
Lipid is one class of aliphatic hydrocarbon-containing organic compounds essential for the structure and function of living cells. They are characterized by being water-insoluble but soluble in nonpolar organic solvents.

Plasma membrane
The unit membrane that encloses a cell and controls the traffic of molecules in and out of the cell is the plasma membrane.

Zona glomerulosa
The zona glomerulosa is the most superficial layer of the adrenal cortex, lying directly beneath the adrenal gland's capsule. In response to increased potassium levels or decreased blood flow to the kidneys, it secretes aldosterone into the blood as part of the renin-angiotensin system.

Zona reticularis
The innermost layer of the adrenal cortex, the zona reticularis sits beneath the zona fasciculata and atop the adrenal medulla. Its cells are arranged in a network of cords and has the same functions as cells of the zona fasciculata.

Cholesterol
Cholesterol is a steroid, a lipid, and an alcohol, found in the cell membranes of all body tissues, and transported in the blood plasma of all animals. It is an important component of the membranes of cells, providing stability; it makes the membrane's fluidity stable over a bigger temperature interval.

Esters
Esters are organic compounds in which an organic group replaces a hydrogen atom in an oxygen acid. An oxygen acid is an acid whose molecule has an -OH group from which the hydrogen (H) can dissociate as an H^+ ion.

Cytoplasm
Cytoplasm refers to the contents of a cell excluding the nucleus and cell membrane. Cytoplasm is a homogeneous, generally clear jelly-like material that fills cells.

Pyramidal cell
A pyramidal cell is a multipolar neuron located in the hippocampus and cerebral cortex. These cells have a triangular-shaped soma, or cell body, with both apical dendrites and basal dendrites.

Epinephrine
Epinephrine is a hormone and a neurotransmitter. Epinephrine plays a central role in the short-term stress reaction—the physiological response to threatening or exciting conditions (fight-or-flight response). It is secreted by the adrenal medulla.

Enkephalins
Opiate-like brain chemicals that regulate reactions to pain and stress are enkephalins.

Adenosine
Adenosine is a nucleoside comprized of adenine attached to a ribose (ribofuranose) moiety via a β-N_9-glycosidic bond. Adenosine plays an important role in biochemical processes, such as energy transfer - as adenosine triphosphate (ATP) and adenosine diphosphate (ADP) - as well as in signal transduction as cyclic adenosine monophosphate, cAMP.

Dopamine
Dopamine is a chemical naturally produced in the body. In the brain, dopamine functions as a neurotransmitter, activating dopamine receptors. Dopamine is also a neurohormone released by the hypothalamus. Its main function as a hormone is to inhibit the release of prolactin from the anterior lobe of the pituitary.

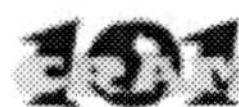

Adenosine triphosphate	Organic molecule that stores energy and releases energy for use in cellular processes is adenosine triphosphate.
Catecholamines	A class of compounds, including epinephrine and norepinephrine, that are synthesized from the amino acid tyrosine are called catecholamines.
Norepinephrine	Norepinephrine is a catecholamine and a phenethylamine with chemical formula $C_8H_{11}NO_3$. It is released from the adrenal glands as a hormone into the blood, but it is also a neurotransmitter in the nervous system where it is released from noradrenergic neurons during synaptic transmission.
Catecholamine	Catecholamine is a chemical compound derived from the amino acid tyrosine that acts as a hormone or neurotransmitter. They are examples of phenethylamines.
Cholinergic	A synapse is cholinergic if it uses acetylcholine as its neurotransmitter. The parasympathetic nervous system is entirely cholinergic.
Glucocorticoid	Glucocorticoid is a class of steroid hormones characterized by the ability to bind with the cortisol receptor and trigger similar effects. They are distinguished from mineralocorticoids and sex steroids by the specific receptors, target cells, and effects.
Alarm reaction	The first stage of the general adaptation syndrome, which is triggered by the impact of a stressor and characterized by sympathetic activity is called the alarm reaction.
Hypertension	Hypertension is a medical condition where the blood pressure in the arteries is chronically elevated. Persistent hypertension is one of the risk factors for strokes, heart attacks, heart failure and arterial aneurysm, and is a leading cause of chronic renal failure.
Heart rate	Heart rate is a term used to describe the frequency of the cardiac cycle. It is considered one of the four vital signs. Usually it is calculated as the number of contractions of the heart in one minute and expressed as "beats per minute".
Glucose	Glucose, a simple monosaccharide sugar, is one of the most important carbohydrates and is used as a source of energy in animals and plants. Glucose is one of the main products of photosynthesis and starts respiration.
Vasoconstriction	Vasoconstriction refers to a decrease in the diameter of a blood vessel.
Tyrosine	Tyrosine is one of the 20 amino acids that are used by cells to synthesize proteins. It plays a key role in signal transduction, since it can be tagged (phosphorylated) with a phosphate group by protein kinases to alter the functionality and activity of certain enzymes.
Conversion	Conversion syndrome describes a condition in which physical symptoms arise for which there is no clear explanation.
Autonomic ganglia	Autonomic ganglia are clusters of neuronal cell bodies and their dendrites and are essentially a junction between autonomic nerves originating from the central nervous system and autonomic nerves innervating their target organs in the periphery.
Elevation	Elevation refers to upward movement of a part of the body.
Androgen	Androgen is the generic term for any natural or synthetic compound, usually a steroid hormone, that stimulates or controls the development and maintenance of masculine characteristics in vertebrates by binding to androgen receptors.
Addison disease	Addison disease (also known as chronic adrenal insufficiency, or hypocortisolism) is a rare endocrine disorder which results in the body not producing sufficient amounts of certain adrenal hormones. This disease refers specifically to primary adrenal insufficiency, in which the adrenal glands themselves malfunction; secondary adrenal insufficiency occurs when the anterior pituitary gland does not produce enough adrenocorticotropic hormone (ACTH) to adequately stimulate the adrenal glands.

Mineralocort-coids	Hormones the adrenal cortex secretes that influence the concentrations of electrolytes in body fluids are called mineralocorticoids.
Mineralocort-coid	Mineralocorticoid is a class of steroids characterized by their similarity to aldosterone and their influence on salt and water metabolism.
Carcinoma	Cancer that originates in the coverings of the body, such as the skin or the lining of the intestinal tract is a carcinoma.
Pancreas	The pancreas is a retroperitoneal organ that serves two functions: exocrine - it produces pancreatic juice containing digestive enzymes, and endocrine - it produces several important hormones, namely insulin.
Glucagon	A peptide hormone secreted by islet cells in the pancreas that raises the level of glucose in the blood is referred to as glucagon. Glucagon is a 29 amino acid polypeptide acting as an important hormone in carbohydrate metabolism.
Polypeptide	Polypeptide refers to polymer of many amino acids linked by peptide bonds.
Crystal	Crystal is a solid in which the constituent atoms, molecules, or ions are packed in a regularly ordered, repeating pattern extending in all three spatial dimensions.
Zinc	Zinc is a chemical element in the periodic table that has the symbol Zn and atomic number 30.
Gold	Gold is a chemical element in the periodic table that has the symbol Au and atomic number 79. A soft, shiny, yellow, dense, malleable, ductile (trivalent and univalent) transition metal, gold does not react with most chemicals but is attacked by chlorine, fluorine and aqua regia.
Autoimmune	Autoimmune refers to immune reactions against normal body cells; self against self.
Diabetes	Diabetes is a medical disorder characterized by varying or persistent elevated blood sugar levels, especially after eating. All types of diabetes share similar symptoms and complications at advanced stages: dehydration and ketoacidosis, cardiovascular disease, chronic renal failure, retinal damage which can lead to blindness, nerve damage which can lead to erectile dysfunction, gangrene with risk of amputation of toes, feet, and even legs.
Genes	Genes are the units of heredity in living organisms. They are encoded in the organism's genetic material (usually DNA or RNA), and control the development and behavior of the organism.
Autoimmune disease	Disease that results when the immune system mistakenly attacks the body's own tissues is referred to as autoimmune disease.
Susceptibility	The degree of resistance of a host to a pathogen is susceptibility.
Obesity	The state of being more than 20 percent above the average weight for a person of one's height is called obesity.
Endoderm	Cells migrating inward along the archenteron form the inner layer of the gastrula, which develops into the endoderm.
Isthmus	An isthmus is a narrow strip of land that is bordered on two sides by water and connects two larger land masses. It is the inverse of a strait (which lies between two land masses and connects two larger bodies of water).
Larynx	The larynx is an organ in the neck of mammals involved in protection of the trachea and sound production. The larynx houses the vocal cords, and is situated at the point where the upper tract splits into the trachea and the esophagus.
Anatomy	Anatomy is the branch of biology that deals with the structure and organization of living things. It can be divided into animal anatomy (zootomy) and plant anatomy (phytonomy).

Physiology	The study of the function of cells, tissues, and organs is referred to as physiology.
Thyroxine	The thyroid hormone thyroxine is a tyrosine-based hormone produced by the thyroid gland. An important component in the synthesis is iodine. It acts on the body to increase the basal metabolic rate, affect protein synthesis and increase the body's sensitivity to catecholamines.
Oxygen	Oxygen is a chemical element in the periodic table. It has the symbol O and atomic number 8. Oxygen is the second most common element on Earth, composing around 46% of the mass of Earth's crust and 28% of the mass of Earth as a whole, and is the third most common element in the universe.
Basal metabolic rate	Basal metabolic rate, is the rate of metabolism that occurs when an individual is at rest in a warm environment and is in the post absorptive state, and has not eaten for at least 12 hours.
Triiodothyronine	A hormone produced by the thyroid gland that speeds up the metabolic rate is called triiodothyronine.
Metabolic rate	Energy expended by the body per unit time is called metabolic rate.
Carbohydrate	Carbohydrate is a chemical compound that contains oxygen, hydrogen, and carbon atoms. They consist of monosaccharide sugars of varying chain lengths and that have the general chemical formula $C_n(H_2O)_n$ or are derivatives of such.
Metabolism	Metabolism is the biochemical modification of chemical compounds in living organisms and cells. This includes the biosynthesis of complex organic molecules (anabolism) and their breakdown (catabolism).
Thyroid hormones	The thyroid hormones, thyroxine (T4) and triiodothyronine (T3), are tyrosine-based hormones produced by the thyroid gland. An important component in the synthesis is iodine. They act on the body to increase the basal metabolic rate, affect protein synthesis and increase the body's sensitivity to catecholamines.
Colloid	Colloid refers to a mixture that contains dispersed particles larger than molecules but small enough so that they do not settle out.
Variable	A characteristic or aspect in which people, objects, events, or conditions vary is called variable.
Loose connective tissue	Loose connective tissue or Areolar connective tissue holds organs and epithelia in place, and has a variety of proteinaceous fibers, including collagen and elastin. It is also important in inflammation.
Parenchyma	The parenchyma are the functional parts of an organ in the body (i.e. the nephrons of the kidney, the alveoli of the lungs). In plants parenchyma cells are thin-walled cells of the ground tissue that make up the bulk of most nonwoody structures, although sometimes their cell walls can be lignified.
Endothelial cell	A endothelial cell also controls the passage of materials — and the transit of white blood cells — into and out of the bloodstream. In some organs, there are highly differentiated endothelial cells to perform specialized 'filtering' functions.
Squamous epithelium	The squamous epithelium is epithelium consisting of one or more cell layers, the most superficial of which is composed of flat, scalelike or platelike cells.
Lysosome	Organelle that contains enzymes that degrade worn cell parts is called a lysosome.
Mitochondria	Cytoplasmic organelles responsible for ATP generation for cellular activities are referred to as mitochondria.

Staining — Staining is a biochemical technique of adding a class-specific (DNA, proteins, lipids, carbohydrates) dye to a substrate to qualify or quantify the presence of a specific compound. They are frequently used to highlight structures in tissues for viewing, often with the aid of different microscopes.

Sugar — A sugar is the simplest molecule that can be identified as a carbohydrate. These include monosaccharides and disaccharides, trisaccharides and the oligosaccharides. The term "glyco-" indicates the presence of a sugar in an otherwise non-carbohydrate substance.

Calcitonin — Calcitonin is a a 32 amino acid polypeptide hormone that is produced in humans primarily by the C cells of the thyroid, and in many other animals in the ultimobranchial body.

Calcium — Calcium is the chemical element in the periodic table that has the symbol Ca and atomic number 20. Calcium is a soft grey alkaline earth metal that is used as a reducing agent in the extraction of thorium, zirconium and uranium. Calcium is also the fifth most abundant element in the Earth's crust.

Symporter — A symporter, also known as a coporter, is an integral membrane protein that is involved in secondary active transport. It works by binding to two molecules at a time and using the gradient of one solutes concentration (S1) to force the other molecule against its gradient (S2).

Anterior pituitary — The anterior pituitary comprises the anterior lobe of the pituitary gland and is part of the endocrine system. Under the influence of the hypothalamus, the anterior pituitary produces and secretes several peptide hormones that regulate many physiological processes including stress, growth, and reproduction.

Activation — As reflected by facial expressions, the degree of arousal a person is experiencing is referred to as activation.

Residue — A residue refers to a portion of a larger molecule, a specific monomer of a polysaccharide, protein or nucleic acid.

Transport protein — A transport protein is a protein involved in facilitated diffusion. Changes in the conformation move the binding site to the opposite side of the protein.

Iodine — Iodine is a chemical element in the periodic table that has the symbol I and atomic number 53. It is required as a trace element for most living organisms. Chemically, iodine is the least reactive of the halogens, and the most electropositive halogen. Iodine is primarily used in medicine, photography and in dyes.

Serum — Serum is the same as blood plasma except that clotting factors (such as fibrin) have been removed. Blood plasma contains fibrinogen.

Anion — A negatively-charged ion, which has more electrons in its electron shell than it has protons in its nucleus, is known as an anion, for it is attracted to anodes; a positively-charged ion, which has fewer electrons than protons, is known as a cation, for it is attracted to cathodes.

Osteoblast — An osteoblast is a mononucleate cell that produces a protein that produces osteoid.

Parathyroid hormone — Parathyroid hormone is secreted by the parathyroid glands as a polypeptide containing 84 amino acids. It acts to increase the concentration of calcium in the blood, whereas calcitonin (a hormone produced by the thyroid gland) acts to decrease calcium concentration.

Phosphate — A phosphate is a polyatomic ion or radical consisting of one phosphorus atom and four oxygen. In the ionic form, it carries a -3 formal charge, and is denoted PO_4^{3-}.

Absorption — Absorption is a physical or chemical phenomenon or a process in which atoms, molecules, or ions enter some bulk phase - gas, liquid or solid material. In nutrition, amino acids are

	broken down through digestion, which begins in the stomach.
Gastrointestinal tract	The gastrointestinal tract is the system of organs within multicellular animals which takes in food, digests it to extract energy and nutrients, and expels the remaining waste.
Vitamin	An organic compound other than a carbohydrate, lipid, or protein that is needed for normal metabolism but that the body cannot synthesize in adequate amounts is called a vitamin.
Parathyroid gland	One of four endocrine glands embedded in the surface of the thyroid gland that secrete parathyroid hormone is called a parathyroid gland.
Pineal gland	The pineal gland is a small endocrine gland in the brain. It is located near the center of the brain, between the two hemispheres, tucked in a groove where the two rounded thalamic bodies join.
Epiphysis	Epiphysis refers to the end of a long bone.
Pia mater	The pia mater is the delicate innermost layer of the meninges - the membranes surrounding the brain and spinal cord.
Astrocyte	An astrocyte is a characteristic star-shaped cell in the brain. They are the biggest cells found in brain tissue and outnumber the neurons ten to one. A commonly accepted function is to structure physically the brain. A second function is to provide neurons with nutrients such as glucose. They regulate the flow of nutrients provided by capillaries by forming the blood-brain barrier.
Silver	Silver is a chemical element with the symbol Ag. A soft white lustrous transition metal, it has the highest electrical and thermal conductivity of any metal and occurs in minerals and in free form.
Synapse	A junction, or relay point, between two neurons, or between a neuron and an effector cell. Electrical and chemical signals are relayed from one cell to another at a synapse.
Myelin	Myelin is an electrically insulating fatty layer that surrounds the axons of many neurons, especially those in the peripheral nervous system. It is an outgrowth of glial cells: Schwann cells supply the myelin for peripheral neurons while oligodendrocytes supply it to those of the central nervous system.
Vesicle	Membranous, cytoplasmic sac formed by an infolding of the cell membrane is called a vesicle.
Melatonin	Melatonin, 5-methoxy-N-acetyltryptamine, is a hormone produced by pinealocytes in the pineal gland (located in the brain) and also by the retina and GI tract. Production of melatonin by the pineal gland is stimulated by darkness and inhibited by light.
Serotonin	Serotonin is a monoamine neurotransmitter synthesized in serotonergic neurons in the central nervous system and enterochromaffin cells in the gastrointestinal tract. It is believed to play an important part of the biochemistry of depression, migraine, bipolar disorder and anxiety.
Enzyme	An enzyme is a protein that catalyzes, or speeds up, a chemical reaction. They are essential to sustain life because most chemical reactions in biological cells would occur too slowly, or would lead to different products, without them.
Lead	Lead is a chemical element in the periodic table that has the symbol Pb and atomic number 82. A soft, heavy, toxic and malleable poor metal, lead is bluish white when freshly cut but tarnishes to dull gray when exposed to air. Lead is used in building construction, lead-acid batteries, bullets and shot, and is part of solder, pewter, and fusible alloys.
Noradrenaline	Noradrenaline is released from the adrenal glands as a hormone into the blood, but it is also a neurotransmitter in the nervous system. As a stress hormone, it affects parts of the human brain where attention and impulsivity are controlled.

Neuroendocrine system	The network of neurons and glands that make and secrete hormones is referred to as the neuroendocrine system.
Medicine	Medicine is the branch of health science and the sector of public life concerned with maintaining or restoring human health through the study, diagnosis and treatment of disease and injury.
Internal medicine	Doctors of internal medicine ("internists") focus on adult medicine and have had special study and training focusing on the prevention and treatment of adult diseases. At least three of their seven or more years of medical school and postgraduate training are dedicated to learning how to prevent, diagnose, and treat diseases that affect adults.
Posterior pituitary	The posterior pituitary gland comprises the posterior lobe of the pituitary gland and is part of the endocrine system. Despite its name, the posterior pituitary gland is not a gland, rather, it is largely a collection of axonal projections from the hypothalamus that terminate behind the anterior pituitary gland.
Carboxypeptidase	An enzyme found within the small intestine that splits off one amino acid at a time, beginning at the end of the polypeptide that has a free carboxyl group is called carboxypeptidase.
Endocrinology	Endocrinology is a branch of medicine dealing with disorders of the endocrine system and its specific secretions called hormones.
Stress	Stress refers to a condition that is a response to factors that change the human systems normal state.
Releasing hormone	A releasing hormone is a hormone whose main purpose is to stimulate the release of another hormone.

Spermatozoa	A sperm cell, spermatozooa (pl. spermatozoa), or spermatozoan, is the haploid cell that is the male gamete. It is carried in fluid called semen, and is capable of fertilising an egg cell to form a zygote.
Muscle	Muscle is a contractile form of tissue. It is one of the four major tissue types, the other three being epithelium, connective tissue and nervous tissue. Muscle contraction is used to move parts of the body, as well as to move substances within the body.
Gland	A gland is an organ in an animal's body that synthesizes a substance for release such as hormones, often into the bloodstream or into cavities inside the body or its outer surface.
Muscle contraction	A muscle contraction occurs when a muscle cell (called a muscle fiber) shortens. There are three general types: skeletal, heart, and smooth.
Smooth muscle	Smooth muscle is a type of non-striated muscle, found within the "walls" of hollow organs; such as blood vessels, the bladder, the uterus, and the gastrointestinal tract. Smooth muscle is used to move matter within the body, via contraction; it generally operates "involuntarily", without nerve stimulation.
Penis	The penis is the male reproductive organ and for mammals additionally serves as the external male organ of urination.
Semen	Semen is a fluid that contains spermatozoa. It is secreted by the gonads (sexual glands) of male or hermaphroditic animals including humans for fertilization of female ova. Semen discharged by an animal or human is known as ejaculate, and the process of discharge is called ejaculation.
Testosterone	Testosterone is a steroid hormone from the androgen group. Testosterone is secreted in the testes of men and the ovaries of women. It is the principal male sex hormone and the "original" anabolic steroid. In both males and females, it plays key roles in health and well-being.
Metabolite	The term metabolite is usually restricted to small molecules. They are the intermediates and products of metabolism. A primary metabolite is directly involved in the normal growth, development, and reproduction. A secondary metabolite is not directly involved in those processes, but usually has important ecological function.
Physiology	The study of the function of cells, tissues, and organs is referred to as physiology.
Hormone	A hormone is a chemical messenger from one cell to another. All multicellular organisms produce hormones. The best known hormones are those produced by endocrine glands of vertebrate animals, but hormones are produced by nearly every organ system and tissue type in a human or animal body. Hormone molecules are secreted directly into the bloodstream, they move by circulation or diffusion to their target cells, which may be nearby cells in the same tissue or cells of a distant organ of the body.
Testes	The testes are the male generative glands in animals. Male mammals have two testes, which are often contained within an extension of the abdomen called the scrotum.
Dihydrotesto-terone	Dihydrotestosterone is a biologically active metabolite of the hormone testosterone, formed primarily in the prostate gland, testes, hair follicles, and adrenal glands by the enzyme 5á-reductase by means of reducing the Ä4,5 double-bond. Dihydrotestosterone belongs to the class of compounds called androgens, also commonly called androgenic hormones or testoids. It is thought to be approximately 30 times more potent than testosterone because of increased affinity to the androgen receptor.
Albuginea	The anatomical term albuginea refers to a layer of white, fibrous tissue.
Tissue	A collection of interconnected cells that perform a similar function within an organism is called tissue.

Dense connective tissue	Dense connective tissue has collagen fibers as its main matrix element. Crowded between the collagen fibers are rows of fibroblasts, fiber-forming cells, that manufacture the fibers. Dense connective tissue forms strong, rope-like structures such as tendons and ligaments. Tendons attach skeletal muscles to bones; ligaments connect bones to bones at joints.
Connective tissue	Connective tissue is any type of biological tissue with an extensive extracellular matrix and often serves to support, bind together, and protect organs.
Glans penis	The glans penis is the sensitive erectile tip of the penis. It is wholly or partially covered by the foreskin, except when the foreskin is retracted, such as during sexual intercourse while the penis is erect, or when the foreskin has been removed by circumcision.
Epididymis	The epididymis is part of the human male reproductive system and is present in all male mammals. It is a narrow, tightly-coiled tube connecting the efferent ducts from the rear of each testicle to its vas deferens.
Prostate	The prostate is a gland that is part of male mammalian sex organs. Its main function is to secrete and store a clear, slightly basic fluid that is part of semen. The prostate differs considerably between species anatomically, chemically and physiologically.
Prepuce	The prepuce is a retractable piece of skin which covers part of the genitals of primates and other mammals. On a male, this covers the head of the penis (the glans penis). On a female, it surrounds and protects the clitoris.
Urethra	In anatomy, the urethra is a tube which connects the urinary bladder to the outside of the body. The urethra has an excretory function in both sexes, to pass urine to the outside, and also a reproductive function in the male, as a passage for sperm.
Vesicle	Membranous, cytoplasmic sac formed by an infolding of the cell membrane is called a vesicle.
Bladder	A hollow muscular storage organ for storing urine is a bladder.
Ampulla	Base of a semicircular canal in the inner ear is called ampulla. The Ampulla also refers to a dilated segment in a tubular structure, and they are also the bulb-like structures above the tube feet in echinoderms.
Septa	Septa are thin walls or partitions between the internal chambers (camerae) of the shell of a cephalopod, namely nautiloids or ammonoids.
Glan	A glan is a structure internally composed of corpus spongiosum in males or of corpus cavernosa and vestibular tissue in females that is located at the tip of homologous genital structures involved in sexual arousal.
Bulbourethral gland	The bulbourethral gland is a small, rounded, and somewhat lobulated body, of a yellow color, about the size of a pea, placed behind and lateral to the membranous portion of the urethra, between the two layers of the fascia of the urogenital diaphragm. They secrete a clear fluid known as pre-ejaculate.
Ejaculatory duct	The Ejaculatory duct is a part of the human male anatomy, which causes the reflex action of ejaculation. Each male has two of them. They begin at the vas deferens, pass through the prostate, and empty into the urethra at the Colliculus seminalis.
Tunica albuginea	Tunica albuginea is an anatomy term that literaly means "white covering." It is used to refer to several structures.
Ductus deferens	The ductus deferens is part of the human male anatomy. There are two of them; they are muscular tubes (surrounded by smooth muscle) connecting the left and right epididymis to the ejaculatory ducts in order to move sperm.
Reproductive system	A reproductive system is the ensembles and interactions of organs and or substances within an organism that stricly pertain to reproduction. As an example, this would include in the case

	of female mammals, the hormone estrogen, the womb and eggs but not the breast.
Seminiferous tubule	Highly coiled duct within the male testes that produces and transports sperm is the seminiferous tubule.
Loose connective tissue	Loose connective tissue or Areolar connective tissue holds organs and epithelia in place, and has a variety of proteinaceous fibers, including collagen and elastin. It is also important in inflammation.
Leydig **cell**	The Leydig cell is found adjacent to the seminiferous tubules in the testes.
Leydig	A Leydig cell is found adjacent to the seminiferous tubules in the testes. They can synthesize testosterone and are often closely related to nerves. They also have round vesicular nuclei and a granular eosinophilic cytoplasm.
Nerve	A nerve is an enclosed, cable-like bundle of nerve fibers or axons, which includes the glia that ensheath the axons in myelin.
Blood	Blood is a circulating tissue composed of fluid plasma and cells. The main function of blood is to supply nutrients (oxygen, glucose) and constitutional elements to tissues and to remove waste products.
Interstitial cell	An interstitial cell are those present in the ovary, which secrete androgens.
Androgen	Androgen is the generic term for any natural or synthetic compound, usually a steroid hormone, that stimulates or controls the development and maintenance of masculine characteristics in vertebrates by binding to androgen receptors.
Dorsal	In anatomy, the dorsal is the side in which the backbone is located. This is usually the top of an animal, although in humans it refers to the back.
Visceral	Visceral refers to the internal organs of an animal.
Parietal	When speaking of inner organs, visceral means close to or attached to the organ, while parietal is more distant. For example, the visceral pleura is attached to the lung and the parietal pleura is attached to the chest wall.
Epithelium	Epithelium is a tissue composed of a layer of cells. Epithelium can be found lining internal (e.g. endothelium, which lines the inside of blood vessels) or external (e.g. skin) free surfaces of the body. Functions include secretion, absorption and protection.
Labyrinth	The labyrinth is a system of fluid passages in the inner ear, comprising the vestibular system and the auditory system, which provides the sense of balance.
Channel	Channel, in communications (sometimes called communications channel), refers to the medium used to convey information from a sender (or transmitter) to a receiver.
Meiosis	In biology, meiosis is the process that transforms one diploid cell into four haploid cells in eukaryotes in order to redistribute the diploid's cell's genome.
Spermatogenesis	Spermatogenesis refers to the creation, or genesis, of spermatozoa, which occurs in the male gonads.
Cell **division**	Cell division (or local doubling) is the process by which a cell, called the parent cell divides into two cells, called daughter cells. Cell division is usually a small segment of a larger cell cycle.
Lamina	A thin layer, such as the lamina of a vertebra or the lamina propria of a mucous membrane is referred to as lamina.
Chromo**somes**	Physical structures in the cell's nucleus that house the genes. Each human cell has 23 pairs

	of chromosomes.
Haploid	The single set of chromosomes in a gamete (sperm or egg) is called a haploid set of chromosomes. In humans a haploid set of chromosomes contains 23 chromosomes.
DNA	Deoxyribonucleic acid (DNA) is a nucleic acid —usually in the form of a double helix— that contains the genetic instructions specifying the biological development of all cellular forms of life, and most viruses.
Population	Population refers to all members of a well-defined group of organisms, events, or things.
Sperm	Sperm refers to the male sex cell with three distinct parts at maturity: head, middle piece, and tail.
Diploid	Body cell with two full sets of chromosomes, in humans is referred to as diploid.
Fertilization	Fertilization is fusion of gametes to form a new organism. In animals, the process involves a sperm fusing with an ovum, which eventually leads to the development of an embryo.
Ovum	An ovum is a female sex cell or gamete. It is a mature egg cell released during ovulation from an ovary.
Condensation	Combining several people, objects, or events into a single dream image is referred to as condensation.
Cytoplasm	Cytoplasm refers to the contents of a cell excluding the nucleus and cell membrane. Cytoplasm is a homogeneous, generally clear jelly-like material that fills cells.
Soma	The soma is the bulbous end of a neuron, containing the nucleus. The cell nucleus is a key feature of the soma. The nucleus is the source of most of the RNA that is produced in neurons and most proteins are produced from mRNAs that do not travel far from the nucleus.
Spermatozoon	Spermatozoon is the haploid cell that is the male gamete. It is carried in fluid called semen, and is capable of fertilizing an egg cell to form a zygote.
Mitochondria	Cytoplasmic organelles responsible for ATP generation for cellular activities are referred to as mitochondria.
Centriole	A cellular structure built of microtubules that organizes the mitotic spindle is called a centriole.
Acid	An acid is a water-soluble, sour-tasting chemical compound that when dissolved in water, gives a solution with a pH of less than 7.
Genome	In biology the genome of an organism is the whole hereditary information of an organism that is encoded in the DNA (or, for some viruses, RNA). This includes both the genes and the non-coding sequences.
Egg	An egg is the zygote, resulting from fertilization of the ovum. It nourishes and protects the embryo.
Motility	Motility is the ability to move spontaneously and independently. The term can apply to single cells, or to multicellular organisms.
Phosphatase	A phosphatase is an enzyme that hydrolyses phosphoric acid monoesters into a phosphate ion and a molecule with a free hydroxyl group.
Acrosome	Cap on the head of the spermatozoon, with hydrolytic enzymes that help the spermatozoon to penetrate the ovum is an acrosome.
Protease	Protease refers to an enzyme that breaks peptide bonds between amino acids of proteins.
Trypsin	The enzyme trypsin is produced in the pancreas in the form of trypsinogen, and is then

	transported to the small intestine, where begins the digestion of proteins to polypeptides and amino acids.
Enzyme	An enzyme is a protein that catalyzes, or speeds up, a chemical reaction. They are essential to sustain life because most chemical reactions in biological cells would occur too slowly, or would lead to different products, without them.
Hydrolytic enzyme	A hydrolytic enzyme breaks down proteins, carbohydrates, and fat molecules into their simplest units. The hydrolysis of polymers by hydrolytic enzymes results in free monomers.
Acrosomal vesicle	The region at the head end of a sperm cell that contains a sac of hydrolytic enzymes used to digest the protective coating of the egg is called the acrosomal vesicle.
Neuraminidase	Neuraminidase is an antigenic glycoprotein enzyme found on the surface of the Influenza virus.
Hyaluronidase	Hyaluronidase refers to an enzyme that digests proteoglycans. Found in sperm cells, it helps digest the coatings surrounding an egg so the sperm can penetrate the egg cell membrane.
Micrograph	A micrograph is a photograph or similar image taken through a microscope or similar device to show a magnified image of an item.
Microtubule	A hollow rod of the protein tubulin in the cytoplasm is referred to as the microtubule.
Lysosome	Organelle that contains enzymes that degrade worn cell parts is called a lysosome.
Plasma	Fluid portion of circulating blood is called plasma.
Plasma membrane	The unit membrane that encloses a cell and controls the traffic of molecules in and out of the cell is the plasma membrane.
Extracellular	Outside the cell is called extracellular.
Base	The common definition of a base is a chemical compound that absorbs hydronium ions when dissolved in water (a proton acceptor). An alkali is a special example of a base, where in an aqueous environment, hydroxide ions are donated.
Organelle	Organelle refers to any structure within a cell that carries out one of its metabolic roles, such as mitochondria, centrioles, endoplasmic reticulum, and the nucleus.
Protein	A protein is a complex, high-molecular-weight organic compound that consists of amino acids joined by peptide bonds. They are essential to the structure and function of all living cells and viruses. Many are enzymes or subunits of enzymes.
Microscopy	Microscopy is any technique for producing visible images of structures or details too small to otherwise be seen by the human eye, using a microscope or other magnification tool.
Injection	A method of rapid drug delivery that puts the substance directly in the bloodstream, in a muscle, or under the skin is called injection.
Microscope	A microscope is an instrument for viewing objects that are too small to be seen by the naked or unaided eye.
Invagination	Infolding of one part of a structure into another is invagination.
Occluding junction	Type of cell junction that seals cells together in an epithelium, forming a barrier through which even small molecules cannot pass, is referred to as occluding junction.
Interstitial space	The space between the endothelial cells and target cells, such as the liver or the smooth muscle cells that line the vascular bed is interstitial space.
Phagocytosis	Phagocytosis (literally, "cell eating") is a form of endocytosis where large particles are enveloped by the cell membrane of a (usually larger) cell and internalized to form a

	phagosome, or "food vacuole."
Immune system	The immune system is the system of specialized cells and organs that protect an organism from outside biological influences. When the immune system is functioning properly, it protects the body against bacteria and viral infections, destroying cancer cells and foreign substances.
Autoimmune	Autoimmune refers to immune reactions against normal body cells; self against self.
Scrotum	In some male mammals the scrotum is an external bag of skin and muscle containing the testicles. It is an extension of the abdomen, and is located between the penis and anus.
Malnutrition	Malnutrition is a general term for the medical condition in a person or animal caused by an unbalanced diet—either too little or too much food, or a diet missing one or more important nutrients.
Alcoholism	A disorder that involves long-term, repeated, uncontrolled, compulsive, and excessive use of alcoholic beverages and that impairs the drinker's health and work and social relationships is called alcoholism.
Lead	Lead is a chemical element in the periodic table that has the symbol Pb and atomic number 82. A soft, heavy, toxic and malleable poor metal, lead is bluish white when freshly cut but tarnishes to dull gray when exposed to air. Lead is used in building construction, lead-acid batteries, bullets and shot, and is part of solder, pewter, and fusible alloys.
Cadmium	Cadmium is a chemical element in the periodic table that has the symbol Cd and atomic number 48. A relatively rare, soft, bluish-white, toxic transition metal, cadmium occurs with zinc ores and is used largely in batteries.
Salt	Salt is a term used for ionic compounds composed of positively charged cations and negatively charged anions, so that the product is neutral and without a net charge.
Infection	The invasion and multiplication of microorganisms in body tissues is called an infection.
Follicle	Follicle refers to a cluster of cells surrounding, protecting, and nourishing a developing egg cell in the ovary; also secretes estrogen. In botany, a follicle is a type of simple dry fruit produced by certain flowering plants. It is regarded as one the most primitive types of fruits, and derives from a simple pistil or carpel.
Estradiol	Estradiol is a sex hormone. Labelled the "female" hormone but also present in males it represents the major estrogen in humans. Critical for sexual functioning estradiol also supports bone growth.
Regression	Return to a form of behavior characteristic of an earlier stage of development is a regression.
Fetus	Fetus refers to a developing human from the ninth week of gestation until birth; has all the major structures of an adult.
Capillaries	Capillaries refer to the smallest of the blood vessels and the sites of exchange between the blood and tissue cells.
Capillary	A capillary is the smallest of a body's blood vessels, measuring 5-10 micro meters. They connect arteries and veins, and most closely interact with tissues. Their walls are composed of a single layer of cells, the endothelium. This layer is so thin that molecules such as oxygen, water and lipids can pass through them by diffusion and enter the tissues.
Hypophysis	The pituitary gland, or hypophysis, is an endocrine gland about the size of a pea that sits in the small, bony cavity (sella turcica) at the base of the brain.
Immune response	The body's defensive reaction to invasion by bacteria, viral agents, or other foreign

	substances is called immune response.
Gonadotropin	A hormone that stimulates the gonads is gonadotropin. They are protein hormones secreted by gonadotrope cells of the pituitary gland of vertebrates.
Puberty	A time in the life of a developing individual characterized by the increasing production of sex hormones, which cause it to reach sexual maturity is called puberty.
Organ	Organ refers to a structure consisting of several tissues adapted as a group to perform specific functions.
Tumor	An abnormal mass of cells that forms within otherwise normal tissue is a tumor. This growth can be either malignant or benign
Precocious puberty	Precocious puberty means early puberty.
Gonadotropic hormone	Substance secreted by anterior pituitary that regulates the activity of the ovaries and testes is referred to as gonadotropic hormone.
Genitalia	The Latin term genitalia is used to describe the sex organs, and in the English language this term and genital area are most often used to describe the externally visible sex organs or external genitalia: in males the penis and scrotum, in females the vulva.
Gestation	Gestation refers to pregnancy; the state of carrying developing young within the female reproductive tract.
Estrogen	Estrogen is a steroid that functions as the primary female sex hormone. While present in both men and women, they are found in women in significantly higher quantities.
Activin	Activin is a peptide that enhances FSH synthesis and secretion and participates in the regulation of the menstrual cycle. It does the opposite as inhibin.
Adenohypophysis	The adenohypophysis comprises the anterior lobe of the pituitary gland and is part of the endocrine system. Under the influence of the hypothalamus, the anterior pituitary produces and secretes several peptide hormones that regulate many physiological processes including stress, growth, and reproduction.
Artery	Vessel that takes blood away from the heart to the tissues and organs of the body is called an artery.
Plexus	A plexus is also a network of blood vessels, with the choroid plexuses of the brain being the most commonly mentioned example. A choroid plexus is very thin and vascular roof plates of the most anterior and most posterior cavities of the brain which expand into the interiors of the cavities.
Blood vessel	A blood vessel is a part of the circulatory system and function to transport blood throughout the body. The most important types, arteries and veins, are so termed because they carry blood away from or towards the heart, respectively.
Reproduction	Biological reproduction is the biological process by which new individual organisms are produced. Reproduction is a fundamental feature of all known life; each individual organism exists as the result of reproduction by an antecedent.
Luteinizing hormone	Luteinizing hormone is a hormone synthesized and secreted by gonadotropes in the anterior lobe of the pituitary gland. In both males and females, it stimulates the production of sex steroids from the gonads.
Histology	Histology is the study of tissue sectioned as a thin slice, using a microscope. It can be described as microscopic anatomy.
Digestion	Digestion refers to the mechanical and chemical breakdown of food into molecules small enough

	for the body to absorb; the second main stage of food processing, following ingestion.
Stereocilia	Stereocilia are mechanosensing organelles of hair cells, which respond to fluid motion or fluid pressure changes in numerous types of animals for numerous functions. As acoustic sensors in mammals, they are lined up in the Organ of Corti in the cochlea of the inner ear.
Mucosa	The mucosa is a lining of ectodermic origin, covered in epithelium, and involved in absorption and secretion. They line various body cavities that are exposed to the external environment and internal organs.
Fiber	Fibers used by man come from a wide variety of sources: Natural fiber include those made out of plants, animal and mineral sources. Natural fibers can be classified according to their origin.
Elastic fiber	Elastic fiber is a bundles of proteins (elastin) found in connective tissue and produced by fibroblasts and smooth muscle cells in arteries.
Spermatic cord	The spermatic cord is the name given to the cord-like structure formed by the vas deferens and surrounding tissue (veins, arteries, nerves, and lymphatic vessels) that run from the abdomen down to each testicle.
Seminal vesicles	The seminal vesicles are a pair of glands on the posterior surface of the urinary bladder of males. They secrete a significant proportion of the fluid that ultimately becomes semen.
Carbohydrate	Carbohydrate is a chemical compound that contains oxygen, hydrogen, and carbon atoms. They consist of monosaccharide sugars of varying chain lengths and that have the general chemical formula $C_n(H_2O)_n$ or are derivatives of such.
Fructose	Fructose is a simple sugar (monosaccharide) found in many foods and one of the three most important blood sugars along with glucose and galactose.
Cancer	Cancer is a class of diseases or disorders characterized by uncontrolled division of cells and the ability of these cells to invade other tissues, either by direct growth into adjacent tissue through invasion or by implantation into distant sites by metastasis.
Hyperplasia	Hyperplasia is a general term for an increase in the number of the cells of an organ or tissue causing it to increase in size.
Collagen	Collagen is the main protein of connective tissue in animals and the most abundant protein in mammals, making up about 1/4 of the total. It is one of the long, fibrous structural proteins whose functions are quite different from those of globular proteins such as enzymes.
Collagen fiber	White fiber in the matrix of connective tissue, giving flexibility and strength is called collagen fiber.
Hypertrophy	Hypertrophy is the increase of the size of an organ. It should be distinguished from hyperplasia which occurs due to cell division; hypertrophy occurs due to an increase in cell size rather than division. It is most commonly seen in muscle that has been actively stimulated, the most well-known method being exercise.
Antigen	An antigen is a substance that stimulates an immune response, especially the production of antibodies. They are usually proteins or polysaccharides, but can be any type of molecule, including small molecules (haptens) coupled to a protein (carrier).
Diagnosis	In medicine, diagnosis is the process of identifying a medical condition or disease by its signs, symptoms, and from the results of various diagnostic procedures.
Serum	Serum is the same as blood plasma except that clotting factors (such as fibrin) have been removed. Blood plasma contains fibrinogen.
Glandular	Columnar epithelium with goblet cells is called glandular epithelium. Some parts of the

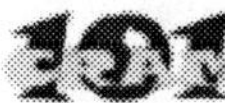

epithelium	glandular epithelium consist of such a large number of goblet cells that there are only a few normal epithelial cells left. Columnar and cuboidal epithelial cells often become specialized as gland cells which are capable of synthesising and secreting certain substances such as enzymes, hormones, milk, mucus, sweat, wax and saliva.
Mucus	Mucus is a slippery secretion of the lining of various membranes in the body (mucous membranes). Mucus aids in the protection of the lungs by trapping foreign particles that enter the nose during normal breathing. Additionally, it prevents tissues from drying out.
Skin	Skin is an organ of the integumentary system composed of a layer of tissues that protect underlying muscles and organs.
Squamous epithelium	The squamous epithelium is epithelium consisting of one or more cell layers, the most superficial of which is composed of flat, scalelike or platelike cells.
Sebaceous	The sebaceous glands are glands found in the skin of mammals. They secrete an oily substance called sebum that is made of fat (lipids) and the debris of dead fat-producing cells.
Sebaceous gland	The sebaceous gland is found in the skin of mammals. They secrete an oily substance called sebum that is made of fat and the debris of dead fat-producing cells. These glands exist in humans througout the skin except in the palms and soles.
Oxygen	Oxygen is a chemical element in the periodic table. It has the symbol O and atomic number 8. Oxygen is the second most common element on Earth, composing around 46% of the mass of Earth's crust and 28% of the mass of Earth as a whole, and is the third most common element in the universe.
Shunt	In medicine, a shunt is a hole or passage which moves, or allows movement of, fluid from one part of the body to another. The term may describe either congenital or acquired shunts; and acquired shunts may be either biological or mechanical.
Vein	Vein in animals, is a vessel that returns blood to the heart. In plants, a vascular bundle in a leaf, composed of xylem and phloem.
Sympathetic	The sympathetic nervous system activates what is often termed the "fight or flight response". It is an automatic regulation system, that is, one that operates without the intervention of conscious thought.
Vasodilator	A vasodilator is a substance that causes blood vessels in the body to become wider by relaxing the smooth muscle in the vessel wall. This will reduce blood pressure (since there is more room for the blood) and might allow blood to flow around a clot.
Inhibition	The ability to prevent from making some cognitive or behavioral response is called inhibition.
Vasoconstrictor	A vasoconstrictor is any substance that acts to constrict blood vessels. Many act on specific receptors, such as vasopressin receptors or adrenoreceptors. They are are also used clinically to increase blood pressure or to reduce local blood flow.
Calcium	Calcium is the chemical element in the periodic table that has the symbol Ca and atomic number 20. Calcium is a soft grey alkaline earth metal that is used as a reducing agent in the extraction of thorium, zirconium and uranium. Calcium is also the fifth most abundant element in the Earth's crust.
Intracellular	Intracellular refers to having to do with the interior of a cell.
Orgasm	Orgasm refers to rhythmic contractions of the reproductive structures, accompanied by extreme pleasure, at the peak of sexual excitement in both sexes; includes ejaculation by the male.
Nucleotide	A building block of a nucleic acid molecule, consisting of a sugar, a nitrogenous base, and a phosphate group is called a nucleotide.

Erectile dysfunction | Erectile dysfunction is the inability to develop or maintain an erection of the penis for satisfactory sexual intercourse regardless of the capability of ejaculation. There are various underlying causes, many of which are medically reversible.

Transverse | A transverse (also known as axial or horizontal) plane is an X-Y plane, parallel to the ground, which (in humans) separates the superior from the inferior, or put another way, the head from the feet.

Brain | The part of the central nervous system involved in regulating and controlling body activity and interpreting information from the senses transmitted through the nervous system is referred to as the brain.

Anatomy | Anatomy is the branch of biology that deals with the structure and organization of living things. It can be divided into animal anatomy (zootomy) and plant anatomy (phytonomy).

Biochemistry | Biochemistry studies how complex chemical reactions give rise to life. It is a hybrid branch of chemistry which specialises in the chemical processes in living organisms.

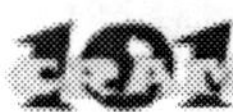

Hormone	A hormone is a chemical messenger from one cell to another. All multicellular organisms produce hormones. The best known hormones are those produced by endocrine glands of vertebrate animals, but hormones are produced by nearly every organ system and tissue type in a human or animal body. Hormone molecules are secreted directly into the bloodstream, they move by circulation or diffusion to their target cells, which may be nearby cells in the same tissue or cells of a distant organ of the body.
Organ	Organ refers to a structure consisting of several tissues adapted as a group to perform specific functions.
Reproductive system	A reproductive system is the ensembles and interactions of organs and or substances within an organism that stricly pertain to reproduction. As an example, this would include in the case of female mammals, the hormone estrogen, the womb and eggs but not the breast.
Menarche	Menarche is the first menstrual period as a girl's body progresses through the changes of puberty. Menarche usually occurs about two years after the first changes of breast development.
Menopause	Menopause is the physiological cessation of menstrual cycles associated with advancing age in species that experience such cycles. Menopause is sometimes referred to as change of life or climacteric.
Variable	A characteristic or aspect in which people, objects, events, or conditions vary is called variable.
Involution	Shrinkage of a tissue or organ by autolysis, such as involution of the thymus after childhood and of the uterus after pregnancy is referred to as involution.
Gland	A gland is an organ in an animal's body that synthesizes a substance for release such as hormones, often into the bloodstream or into cavities inside the body or its outer surface.
Mammary gland	The mammary gland is the organ in the female mammal that produces milk for the sustenance of the young. These exocrine glands are enlarged and modified sweat glands and are the characteristic of mammals which gave the class its name.
Ovaries	Ovaries are egg-producing reproductive organs found in female organisms.
Ovary	The primary reproductive organ of a female is called an ovary.
Epithelium	Epithelium is a tissue composed of a layer of cells. Epithelium can be found lining internal (e.g. endothelium, which lines the inside of blood vessels) or external (e.g. skin) free surfaces of the body. Functions include secretion, absorption and protection.
Albuginea	The anatomical term albuginea refers to a layer of white, fibrous tissue.
Tissue	A collection of interconnected cells that perform a similar function within an organism is called tissue.
Dense connective tissue	Dense connective tissue has collagen fibers as its main matrix element. Crowded between the collagen fibers are rows of fibroblasts, fiber-forming cells, that manufacture the fibers. Dense connective tissue forms strong, rope-like structures such as tendons and ligaments. Tendons attach skeletal muscles to bones; ligaments connect bones to bones at joints.
Connective tissue	Connective tissue is any type of biological tissue with an extensive extracellular matrix and often serves to support, bind together, and protect organs.
Follicle	Follicle refers to a cluster of cells surrounding, protecting, and nourishing a developing egg cell in the ovary; also secretes estrogen. In botany, a follicle is a type of simple dry fruit produced by certain flowering plants. It is regarded as one the most primitive types of fruits, and derives from a simple pistil or carpel.

Tunica albuginea	Tunica albuginea is an anatomy term that literaly means "white covering." It is used to refer to several structures.
Ovarian follicle	Ovarian follicle is the roughly spherical cell aggregation in the ovary containing an ovum and from which the egg is released during ovulation.
Loose connective tissue	Loose connective tissue or Areolar connective tissue holds organs and epithelia in place, and has a variety of proteinaceous fibers, including collagen and elastin. It is also important in inflammation.
Population	Population refers to all members of a well-defined group of organisms, events, or things.
Yolk sac	The yolk sac is the first element seen in the gestational sac during pregnancy, usually at 5 weeks gestation. It is filled with fluid, the vitelline fluid, which possibly may be utilized for the nourishment of the embryo during the earlier stages of its existence.
Yolk	Dense nutrient material that is present in the egg of a bird or reptile is referred to as yolk.
Gonad	Gonad refers to a sex organ in an animal; an ovary or a testis. It is the organ that makes gametes.
Meiosis	In biology, meiosis is the process that transforms one diploid cell into four haploid cells in eukaryotes in order to redistribute the diploid's cell's genome.
Egg	An egg is the zygote, resulting from fertilization of the ovum. It nourishes and protects the embryo.
Atresia	Atresia is a condition in which a body orifice or passage in the body is abnormally closed or absent. Examples of atresia include biliary atresia.
Endometrium	The endometrium is the inner uterine membrane in mammals which is developed in preparation for the implantation of a fertilized egg upon its arrival into the uterus.
Ligament	A ligament is a short band of tough fibrous connective tissue composed mainly of long, stringy collagen fibres. They connect bones to other bones to form a joint. (They do not connect muscles to bones.)
Cervix	The cervix is actually the lower, narrow portion of the uterus where it joins with the top end of the vagina. It is cylindrical or conical in shape and protrudes through the upper anterior vaginal wall.
Menstrual cycle	The menstrual cycle is the set of recurring physiological changes in a female's body that are under the control of the reproductive hormone system and necessary for reproduction. Besides humans, only other great apes exhibit menstrual cycles, in contrast to the estrus cycle of most mammalian species.
Lamina	A thin layer, such as the lamina of a vertebra or the lamina propria of a mucous membrane is referred to as lamina.
Chromosomes	Physical structures in the cell's nucleus that house the genes. Each human cell has 23 pairs of chromosomes.
Organelle	Organelle refers to any structure within a cell that carries out one of its metabolic roles, such as mitochondria, centrioles, endoplasmic reticulum, and the nucleus.
Cytoplasm	Cytoplasm refers to the contents of a cell excluding the nucleus and cell membrane. Cytoplasm is a homogeneous, generally clear jelly-like material that fills cells.
Mitochondria	Cytoplasmic organelles responsible for ATP generation for cellular activities are referred to as mitochondria.

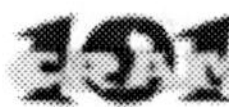

Puberty — A time in the life of a developing individual characterized by the increasing production of sex hormones, which cause it to reach sexual maturity is called puberty.

Hypophysis — The pituitary gland, or hypophysis, is an endocrine gland about the size of a pea that sits in the small, bony cavity (sella turcica) at the base of the brain.

Hypertrophy — Hypertrophy is the increase of the size of an organ. It should be distinguished from hyperplasia which occurs due to cell division; hypertrophy occurs due to an increase in cell size rather than division. It is most commonly seen in muscle that has been actively stimulated, the most well-known method being exercise.

Zona pellucida — The zona pellucida is a glycoprotein matrix surrounding the plasma membrane of an oocyte. This structure binds spermatozoa, and is required to initiate the acrosome reaction.

Plasma — Fluid portion of circulating blood is called plasma.

Progesterone — Progesterone is a C-21 steroid hormone involved in the female menstrual cycle, pregnancy (supports gestation) and embryogenesis of humans and other species.

Androgen — Androgen is the generic term for any natural or synthetic compound, usually a steroid hormone, that stimulates or controls the development and maintenance of masculine characteristics in vertebrates by binding to androgen receptors.

Estrogen — Estrogen is a steroid that functions as the primary female sex hormone. While present in both men and women, they are found in women in significantly higher quantities.

Protein — A protein is a complex, high-molecular-weight organic compound that consists of amino acids joined by peptide bonds. They are essential to the structure and function of all living cells and viruses. Many are enzymes or subunits of enzymes.

Steroid — A steroid is a lipid characterized by a carbon skeleton with four fused rings. Different steroids vary in the functional groups attached to these rings. Hundreds of distinct steroids have been identified in plants and animals. Their most important role in most living systems is as hormones.

Glycosaminog-ycan — Glycosaminoglycan is a long unbranched polysaccharide, made up of repeating disaccharides that may be sulphated (e.g. glucuronic acid, iduronic acid, galactose, galactosamine, glucosamine).

Enzyme — An enzyme is a protein that catalyzes, or speeds up, a chemical reaction. They are essential to sustain life because most chemical reactions in biological cells would occur too slowly, or would lead to different products, without them.

Androstenedione — Androstenedione is a 19-carbon steroid hormone produced in the adrenal glands and the gonads as an intermediate step in the biochemical pathway that produces the androgen testosterone and the estrogens estrone and estradiol. It is the common precursor of male and female sex hormones. Some androstenedione is also secreted into the plasma, and may be converted in peripheral tissues to testosterone and estrogens.

Blood vessel — A blood vessel is a part of the circulatory system and function to transport blood throughout the body. The most important types, arteries and veins, are so termed because they carry blood away from or towards the heart, respectively.

Blood — Blood is a circulating tissue composed of fluid plasma and cells. The main function of blood is to supply nutrients (oxygen, glucose) and constitutional elements to tissues and to remove waste products.

Collagen — Collagen is the main protein of connective tissue in animals and the most abundant protein in mammals, making up about 1/4 of the total. It is one of the long, fibrous structural proteins whose functions are quite different from those of globular proteins such as enzymes.

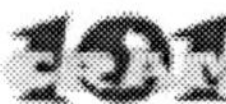

Scar	A scar results from the biologic process of wound repair in the skin and other tissues of the body. It is a connective tissue that fills the wound.
Ovulation	Ovulation is the process in the menstrual cycle by which a mature ovarian follicle ruptures and discharges an ovum (also known as an oocyte, female gamete, or casually, an egg) that participates in reproduction.
Oviduct	In oviparous animals (those that lay eggs), the passage from the ovaries to the outside of the body is known as the oviduct. The eggs travel along the oviduct.
Anovulatory cycle	The anovulatory cycle is a menstrual cycle characterized by varying degrees of menstrual intervals and the absence of ovulation and a luteal phase. In the absence of ovulation, there will be infertility.
Stimulus	Stimulus in a nervous system, a factor that triggers sensory transduction.
Luteinizing hormone	Luteinizing hormone is a hormone synthesized and secreted by gonadotropes in the anterior lobe of the pituitary gland. In both males and females, it stimulates the production of sex steroids from the gonads.
Anterior pituitary	The anterior pituitary comprises the anterior lobe of the pituitary gland and is part of the endocrine system. Under the influence of the hypothalamus, the anterior pituitary produces and secretes several peptide hormones that regulate many physiological processes including stress, growth, and reproduction.
Pituitary gland	The pituitary gland or hypophysis is an endocrine gland about the size of a pea that sits in the small, bony cavity (sella turcica) at the base of the brain. Its posterior lobe is connected to a part of the brain called the hypothalamus via the infundibulum (or stalk), giving rise to the tuberoinfundibular pathway.
Capillaries	Capillaries refer to the smallest of the blood vessels and the sites of exchange between the blood and tissue cells.
Capillary	A capillary is the smallest of a body's blood vessels, measuring 5-10 micro meters. They connect arteries and veins, and most closely interact with tissues. Their walls are composed of a single layer of cells, the endothelium. This layer is so thin that molecules such as oxygen, water and lipids can pass through them by diffusion and enter the tissues.
Venule	A vessel that conveys blood between a capillary bed and a vein is a venule.
Edema	Edema is swelling of any organ or tissue due to accumulation of excess fluid. Edema has many root causes, but its common mechanism is accumulation of fluid into the tissues.
Vasopressin	Vasopressin is a human hormone that is mainly released when the body is low on water; it causes the kidneys to conserve water by concentrating the urine. It has also various functions in the brain.
Prostaglandin	A prostaglandin is any member of a group of lipid compounds that are derived from fatty acids and have important functions in the animal body.
Acid	An acid is a water-soluble, sour-tasting chemical compound that when dissolved in water, gives a solution with a pH of less than 7.
Ischemia	Narrowing of arteries caused by plaque buildup within the arteries is called ischemia.
Stigma	Stigma refers to a personal characteristic that at least some other individuals perceive negatively because that characteristic is different than those of the general population.
Uterine tube	Also called the oviduct, the tube leading out of the ovary to the uterus, into which the secondary oocyte is released is referred to as uterine tube.
Corona radiata	The layer of cells surrounding an egg after ovulation is a corona radiata.

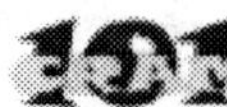

Endocrine gland	An endocrine gland is one of a set of internal organs involved in the secretion of hormones into the blood. These glands are known as ductless, which means they do not have tubes inside them.
Corpus luteum	The corpus luteum is a small, temporary endocrine structure in animals. It develops from an ovarian follicle during the luteal phase of the estrous cycle, following the release of a mature egg from the follicle during ovulation. While the egg traverses the Fallopian tube into the uterus, the corpus luteum remains in the ovary.
Parenchyma	The parenchyma are the functional parts of an organ in the body (i.e. the nephrons of the kidney, the alveoli of the lungs). In plants parenchyma cells are thin-walled cells of the ground tissue that make up the bulk of most nonwoody structures, although sometimes their cell walls can be lignified.
Apoptosis	In biology, apoptosis is one of the main types of programmed cell death (PCD). As such, it is a process of deliberate life relinquishment by an unwanted cell in a multicellular organism.
Menstruation	Loss of blood and tissue from the uterine lining at the end of a female reproductive cycle are referred to as menstruation.
Mucosa	The mucosa is a lining of ectodermic origin, covered in epithelium, and involved in absorption and secretion. They line various body cavities that are exposed to the external environment and internal organs.
Embryo	A prenatal stage of development after germ layers form but before the rudiments of all organs are present is referred to as an embryo.
Placenta	The placenta is an organ present only in female placental mammals during gestation. It is composed of two parts, one genetically and biologically part of the fetus, the other part of the mother. It is implanted in the wall of the uterus, where it receives nutrients and oxygen from the mother's blood and passes out waste.
Isolation	Isolation refers to the degree to which groups do not live in the same communities.
Interstitial cell	An interstitial cell are those present in the ovary, which secrete androgens.
Lipid	Lipid is one class of aliphatic hydrocarbon-containing organic compounds essential for the structure and function of living cells. They are characterized by being water-insoluble but soluble in nonpolar organic solvents.
Infundibulum	An infundibulum is a funnel-shape cavity or organ.
Muscle	Muscle is a contractile form of tissue. It is one of the four major tissue types, the other three being epithelium, connective tissue and nervous tissue. Muscle contraction is used to move parts of the body, as well as to move substances within the body.
Muscle contraction	A muscle contraction occurs when a muscle cell (called a muscle fiber) shortens. There are three general types: skeletal, heart, and smooth.
Capacitation	Capacitation is the final step in the maturation of mammalian spermatozoa and is required to render them competent to fertilize an oocyte. The sperm move normally and look mature prior to capacitation. In vivo this final step typically occurs after ejaculation, in the female reproductive tract.
Spermatozoa	A sperm cell, spermatozooa (pl. spermatozoa), or spermatozoan, is the haploid cell that is the male gamete. It is carried in fluid called semen, and is capable of fertilising an egg cell to form a zygote.
Activation	As reflected by facial expressions, the degree of arousal a person is experiencing is referred to as activation.

Diploid | Body cell with two full sets of chromosomes, in humans is referred to as diploid.

Ampulla | Base of a semicircular canal in the inner ear is called ampulla. The Ampulla also refers to a dilated segment in a tubular structure, and they are also the bulb-like structures above the tube feet in echinoderms.

Fertilization | Fertilization is fusion of gametes to form a new organism. In animals, the process involves a sperm fusing with an ovum, which eventually leads to the development of an embryo.

Spermatozoon | Spermatozoon is the haploid cell that is the male gamete. It is carried in fluid called semen, and is capable of fertilizing an egg cell to form a zygote.

Zygote | A zygote is a cell that is the result of fertilization. That is, two haploid cells—usually (but not always) an ovum from a female and a sperm cell from a male—merge into a single diploid cell called the zygote.

Uterus | The uterus is the major female reproductive organ of most mammals. One end, the cervix, opens into the vagina; the other is connected on both sides to the fallopian tubes. The main function is to accept a fertilized ovum which becomes implanted into the endometrium, and derives nourishment from blood vessels which develop exclusively for this purpose.

Cell division | Cell division (or local doubling) is the process by which a cell, called the parent cell divides into two cells, called daughter cells. Cell division is usually a small segment of a larger cell cycle.

Extension | Movement increasing the angle between parts at a joint is referred to as extension.

Peritoneum | In higher vertebrates, the peritoneum is the serous membrane that forms the lining of the abdominal cavity - it covers most of the intra-abdominal organs. The peritoneum both supports the abdominal organs and serves as a conduit for their blood and lymph vessels and nerves.

Visceral | Visceral refers to the internal organs of an animal.

Serosa | A serosa is a smooth membrane consisting of a thin layer of cells that excrete a fluid, known as serous fluid. Two-layered serous membranes line the cavities that contain the heart (part of the pericardium), lungs (the pleura) and intestines (the peritoneum), enclosing their contents.

Smooth muscle | Smooth muscle is a type of non-striated muscle, found within the "walls" of hollow organs; such as blood vessels, the bladder, the uterus, and the gastrointestinal tract. Smooth muscle is used to move matter within the body, via contraction; it generally operates "involuntarily", without nerve stimulation.

Labyrinth | The labyrinth is a system of fluid passages in the inner ear, comprising the vestibular system and the auditory system, which provides the sense of balance.

Cilia | Microscopic, hairlike processes on the exposed surfaces of certain epithelial cells are cilia.

Gonadotropin | A hormone that stimulates the gonads is gonadotropin. They are protein hormones secreted by gonadotrope cells of the pituitary gland of vertebrates.

Adenohypophysis | The adenohypophysis comprises the anterior lobe of the pituitary gland and is part of the endocrine system. Under the influence of the hypothalamus, the anterior pituitary produces and secretes several peptide hormones that regulate many physiological processes including stress, growth, and reproduction.

Activin | Activin is a peptide that enhances FSH synthesis and secretion and participates in the regulation of the menstrual cycle. It does the opposite as inhibin.

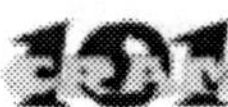

Follicular phase	The follicular phase is the beginning phase of the estrous cycle in animals. It begins with the regression of the corpus luteum (called luteolysis) and ends with ovulation. The main hormone controlling this stage is estradiol.
Luteal phase	The luteal phase is the latter phase of the estrous cycle in animals. It begins with the formation of the corpus luteum and ends in either pregnancy or luteolysis. The main hormone controlling this stage is progesterone.
Syndrome	Syndrome is the association of several clinically recognizable features, signs, symptoms, phenomena or characteristics which often occur together, so that the presence of one feature alerts the physician to the presence of the others
Ectopic pregnancy	An ectopic pregnancy is one in which the fertilized ovum is implanted in any tissue other than the uterine wall.
Hemorrhage	Loss of blood from the circulatory system is referred to as a hemorrhage.
Internal Os	The endocervical canal terminates at the internal os which is the opening of the cervix inside the uterine cavity.
Adventitia	Adventitia is the outermost connective tissue covering of any organ, vessel, or other structure. For example, the connective tissue that surrounds an artery is called the adventitia because it is considered extraneous to the artery.
Myometrium	The myometrium is the middle layer of the uterine wall consisting of smooth muscle cells and supporting stromal and vascular tissue.
Muscle fiber	Cell with myofibrils containing actin and myosin filaments arranged within sarcomeres is a muscle fiber.
Fiber	Fibers used by man come from a wide variety of sources: Natural fiber include those made out of plants, animal and mineral sources. Natural fibers can be classified according to their origin.
Hyperplasia	Hyperplasia is a general term for an increase in the number of the cells of an organ or tissue causing it to increase in size.
Staining	Staining is a biochemical technique of adding a class-specific (DNA, proteins, lipids, carbohydrates) dye to a substrate to qualify or quantify the presence of a specific compound. They are frequently used to highlight structures in tissues for viewing, often with the aid of different microscopes.
Artery	Vessel that takes blood away from the heart to the tissues and organs of the body is called an artery.
Micrograph	A micrograph is a photograph or similar image taken through a microscope or similar device to show a magnified image of an item.
Secretory phase	The phase of development of the endometrium during which, after the proliferative phase, the endometrium stops growing but starts producing secretions under the influence of progesterone, so it corresponds with the luteal phase in the ovarian cycle is called the secretory phase.
Proliferative phase	About two or three days after a wound occurs, fibroblasts begin to enter the wound site, marking the onset of the proliferative phase even before the inflammatory phase has ended. As in the other phases of wound healing, steps in the proliferative phase do not occur in a series but rather partially overlap in time.
Glycogen	Glycogen refers to a complex, extensively branched polysaccharide of many glucose monomers; serves as an energy-storage molecule in liver and muscle cells.

Implantation — Implantation refers to attachment and penetration of the embryo into the lining of the uterus.

Cytokine — A type of protein secreted by a T lymphocyte that attacks viruses, virally infected cells, and cancer cells is referred to as cytokine.

Vagina — The vagina is the tubular tract leading from the uterus to the exterior of the body in female placental mammals and marsupials, or to the cloaca in female birds, monotremes, and some reptiles. Female insects and other invertebrates also have a vagina, which is the terminal part of the oviduct.

Decidua — Decidua is the term for the uterine lining (endometrium) during a pregnancy. It is formed under the influence of progesterone and serves to support and interact with the gestation. The decidua represents the maternal portion of the placenta.

Morula — A morula is an embryo at an early stage of embryonic development, consisting of approximately 4-16 cells (called blastomeres). The morula is produced by embryonic cleavage, the rapid cell division of the zygote.

Segmentation — Segmentation in biology refers to the division of some metazoan bodies and plant body plans into a series of semi-repetitive segments, and the question of the benefits and costs of doing so.

Blastomere — A blastomere is a type of cell produced by division of the egg after fertilization.

Trophoblast — The outer membrane surrounding the embryo in mammals is called the trophoblast.

Blastocyst — An early stage of prenatal development that consists of a hollow ball of cells is a blastocyst.

Attachment — Attachment refers to the psychological tendency to seek closeness to another person, to feel secure when that person is present, and to feel anxious when that person is absent.

Fetus — Fetus refers to a developing human from the ninth week of gestation until birth; has all the major structures of an adult.

Chorion — In animals, the outermost extraembryonic membrane, which becomes the mammalian embryo's part of the placenta is referred to as the chorion.

Venous blood — In the circulatory system, venous blood or peripheral blood is blood returning to the heart. With one exception (the pulmonary vein) this blood is deoxygenated and high in carbon dioxide, having released oxygen and absorbed CO_2 in the tissues.

Prolactin — Prolactin is a hormone synthesised and secreted by lactotrope cells in the anterior pituitary gland. It is made up of 199 amino acids, and has a molecular weight of about 23,000 daltons and has many effects, the most significant of which is to stimulate the mammary glands to produce milk (lactation).

Embryology — Embryology is the branch of developmental biology that studies embryos and their development

Cesarean — A caesarean section (cesarean section AE), or C-section, is a form of childbirth in which a surgical incision is made through a mother's abdomen (laparotomy) and uterus (hysterotomy) to deliver one or more babies. It is usually performed when a vaginal delivery would lead to medical complications.

Cesarean section — A cesarean section is a form of childbirth in which a surgical incision is made through a mother's abdomen and uterus to deliver one or more babies. It is usually performed when a vaginal delivery would lead to medical complications.

Placenta previa — The placenta growing partly or all the way over the opening to the cervix, usually causing abruptio placentae is a placenta previa.

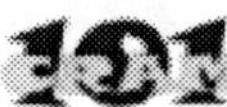

Chorionic villi	The chorion develops chorionic villi, which are finger-like projections on its surface. The chorionic villi extend downward through the uterine lining into the maternal blood supply to help supply the developing embryo with oxygen and nutrients.
Mucus	Mucus is a slippery secretion of the lining of various membranes in the body (mucous membranes). Mucus aids in the protection of the lungs by trapping foreign particles that enter the nose during normal breathing. Additionally, it prevents tissues from drying out.
Squamous epithelium	The squamous epithelium is epithelium consisting of one or more cell layers, the most superficial of which is composed of flat, scalelike or platelike cells.
Sperm	Sperm refers to the male sex cell with three distinct parts at maturity: head, middle piece, and tail.
Microorganism	A microorganism or microbe is an organism that is so small that it is microscopic (invisible to the naked eye).
Parturition	Processes that lead to and include birth and the expulsion of the afterbirth are called parturition.
Carcinoma	Cancer that originates in the coverings of the body, such as the skin or the lining of the intestinal tract is a carcinoma.
Cancer	Cancer is a class of diseases or disorders characterized by uncontrolled division of cells and the ability of these cells to invade other tissues, either by direct growth into adjacent tissue through invasion or by implantation into distant sites by metastasis.
Mortality	The incidence of death in a population is mortality.
Mortality rate	Mortality rate is the number of deaths (from a disease or in general) per 1000 people and typically reported on an annual basis.
Keratin	Keratin is a family of fibrous structural proteins; tough and insoluble, they form the hard but nonmineralized structures found in reptiles, birds and mammals.
Lactic acid	Lactic acid accumulates in skeletal muscles during extensive anaerobic exercise, causing temporary muscle pain. Lactic acid is quickly removed from muscles when they resume aerobic metabolism.
Bacteria	The domain that contains procaryotic cells with primarily diacyl glycerol diesters in their membranes and with bacterial rRNA. Bacteria also is a general term for organisms that are composed of procaryotic cells and are not multicellular.
Elastic fiber	Elastic fiber is a bundles of proteins (elastin) found in connective tissue and produced by fibroblasts and smooth muscle cells in arteries.
Lymphocyte	A lymphocyte is a type of white blood cell involved in the human body's immune system. There are two broad categories, namely T cells and B cells.
Neutrophil	Neutrophil refers to a type of phagocytic leukocyte.
Leukocyte	A white blood cell is a leukocyte. They help to defend the body against infectious disease and foreign materials as part of the immune system.
Nerve	A nerve is an enclosed, cable-like bundle of nerve fibers or axons, which includes the glia that ensheath the axons in myelin.
Pain	Pain is an unpleasant sensation which may be associated with actual or potential tissue damage and which may have physical and emotional components.
Cervical cancer	Cervical cancer is a malignancy of the cervix. Worldwide, it is the second most common cancer of women.

Adipose tissue	Adipose tissue is an anatomical term for loose connective tissue composed of adipocytes. Its main role is to store energy in the form of fat, although it also cushions and insulates the body. It has an important endocrine function in producing recently-discovered hormones such as leptin, resistin and TNFalpha.
Labia majora	A pair of outer thickened folds of skin that protect the female genital region is the labia majora.
Labia minora	The labia minora are two soft folds of skin within the labia majora and to either side of the opening of the vagina.
Genitalia	The Latin term genitalia is used to describe the sex organs, and in the English language this term and genital area are most often used to describe the externally visible sex organs or external genitalia: in males the penis and scrotum, in females the vulva.
Clitoris	The clitoris is a sexual organ in the body of female mammals. The visible knob-like portion is located near the anterior junction of the labia minora, above the opening of the vagina. Unlike its male counterpart, the penis,the clitoris has no urethra, is not involved in urination, and its sole function is to induce sexual pleasure.
Vulva	The outer features of the female reproductive anatomy is referred to as vulva.
Urethra	In anatomy, the urethra is a tube which connects the urinary bladder to the outside of the body. The urethra has an excretory function in both sexes, to pass urine to the outside, and also a reproductive function in the male, as a passage for sperm.
Inflammation	Inflammation is the first response of the immune system to infection or irritation and may be referred to as the innate cascade.
Cyst	A cyst is a closed sac having a distinct membrane and developing abnormally in a cavity or structure of the body. They may occur as a result of a developmental error in the embryo during pregnancy or they may be caused by infections.
Homologous	Homologous refers to structures that have the same embryonic or evolutionary origin but not necessarily the same function, such as the scrotum and labia majora. Also refers to two chromosomes with identical structures and gene loci but not necessarily identical alleles.
Penis	The penis is the male reproductive organ and for mammals additionally serves as the external male organ of urination.
Prepuce	The prepuce is a retractable piece of skin which covers part of the genitals of primates and other mammals. On a male, this covers the head of the penis (the glans penis). On a female, it surrounds and protects the clitoris.
Glan	A glan is a structure internally composed of corpus spongiosum in males or of corpus cavernosa and vestibular tissue in females that is located at the tip of homologous genital structures involved in sexual arousal.
Skin	Skin is an organ of the integumentary system composed of a layer of tissues that protect underlying muscles and organs.
Sweat gland	Gland responsible for the loss of a watery fluid, consisting mainly of sodium chloride (commonly known as salt) and urea in solution, that is secreted through the skin is a sweat gland.
Sebaceous	The sebaceous glands are glands found in the skin of mammals. They secrete an oily substance called sebum that is made of fat (lipids) and the debris of dead fat-producing cells.
Physiology	The study of the function of cells, tissues, and organs is referred to as physiology.
Tactile	Tactile refers to the sense of touch.

Arousal	Arousal is a physiological and psychological state involving the activation of the reticular activating system in the brain stem, the autonomic nervous system and the endocrine system, leading to increased heart rate and blood pressure and a condition of alertness and readiness to respond.
Pacinian corpuscle	Pacinian corpuscle refers to a sensory neuron surrounded by sheaths of connective tissue. Found in the deep layers of the skin, where it senses touch and vibration. It is one of the four major types of mechanoreceptor.
Myoepithelial cell	Myoepithelial cell refers to type of unstriated muscle cell found in epithelia, e.g. In the iris of the eye and in glandular tissue.
Alveoli	Alveoli are anatomical structures that have the form of a hollow cavity. In the lung, the pulmonary alveoli are spherical outcroppings of the respiratory bronchioles and are the primary sites of gas exchange with the blood.
Immunity	Resistance to the effects of specific disease-causing agents is called immunity.
Passive immunity	Passive immunity refers to temporary immunity obtained by acquiring ready-made antibodies or immune cells; lasts only a few weeks or months because the immune system has not been stimulated by antigens.
Secretory IgA	Secretory IgA is the primary immunoglobulin of the secretory immune system. It correlates inversely with self-reported levels of stress and is regarded by some as a potential biomarker for stress.
Hydration	Hydration can create a hydrate from which water can be reextracted. When hydration occurs in a chemical reaction it is called a hydration reaction, in which water is permanently and chemically combined with a reactant in a way that it can no longer be reextracted.
Areola	In anatomy, the term areola is used to describe any small circular area such as the colored skin surrounding the nipple.
Melanin	Broadly, melanin is any of the polyacetylene, polyaniline, and polypyrrole "blacks" or their mixed copolymers. The most common form of biological melanin is a polymer of either or both of two monomer molecules: indolequinone, and dihydroxyindole carboxylic acid.
Human placental lactogen	Human placental lactogen is a polypeptide placental hormone. Its structure is related to that of human growth hormone. It modifies the metabolic state of the mother during pregnancy to facilitate the energy supply of the fetus.
Lactation	Lactation describes the secretion of milk from the mammary glands, the process of providing that milk to the young, and the period of time that a mother lactates to feed her young. The process occurs in all female mammals, and in humans it is called breastfeeding.
Vacuole	Vacuole refers to a space or cavity within the cytoplasm of a cell.
Triglyceride	Triglyceride is a glyceride in which the glycerol is esterified with three fatty acids. They are the main constituent of vegetable oil and animal fats and play an important role in metabolism as energy sources. They contain a bit more than twice as much energy as carbohydrates and proteins.
Triglycerides	Triglycerides refer to fats and oils composed of fatty acids and glycerol; are the body's most concentrated source of energy fuel; also known as neutral fats.
Galactose	Galactose is a type of sugar found in dairy products, in sugar beets and other gums and mucilages. It is also synthesized by the body, where it forms part of glycolipids and glycoproteins in several tissues.
Lactose	Lactose is a disaccharide that makes up around 2-8% of the solids in milk. Lactose is a disaccharide consisting of two subunits, a galactose and a glucose linked together.

Glucose	Glucose, a simple monosaccharide sugar, is one of the most important carbohydrates and is used as a source of energy in animals and plants. Glucose is one of the main products of photosynthesis and starts respiration.
Sugar	A sugar is the simplest molecule that can be identified as a carbohydrate. These include monosaccharides and disaccharides, trisaccharides and the oligosaccharides. The term "glyco-" indicates the presence of a sugar in an otherwise non-carbohydrate substance.
Colostrum	Thin, milky fluid rich in proteins, including antibodies, that is secreted by the mammary glands a few days prior to or after delivery before true milk is secreted is called colostrum.
Receptor	A receptor is a protein on the cell membrane or within the cytoplasm or cell nucleus that binds to a specific molecule (a ligand), such as a neurotransmitter, hormone, or other substance, and initiates the cellular response to the ligand. Receptor, in immunology, the region of an antibody which shows recognition of an antigen.
Oxytocin	Oxytocin is a hormone, found in humans and other mammals, which is involved in the facilitation of birth and breastfeeding as well as in bonding and the formation of trust between people.
Posterior pituitary	The posterior pituitary gland comprises the posterior lobe of the pituitary gland and is part of the endocrine system. Despite its name, the posterior pituitary gland is not a gland, rather, it is largely a collection of axonal projections from the hypothalamus that terminate behind the anterior pituitary gland.
Absorption	Absorption is a physical or chemical phenomenon or a process in which atoms, molecules, or ions enter some bulk phase - gas, liquid or solid material. In nutrition, amino acids are broken down through digestion, which begins in the stomach.
Cellular component	The cellular component involves the movement of white blood cells from blood vessels into the inflamed tissue. The white blood cells, or leukocytes, take on an important role in inflammation; they extravasate (filter out) from the capillaries into tissue, and act as phagocytes, picking up bacteria and cellular debris. They may also aid by walling off an infection and preventing its spread.
Atrophy	Atrophy is the partial or complete wasting away of a part of the body. Causes of atrophy include poor nourishment, poor circulation, loss of hormonal support, loss of nerve supply to the target organ, disuse or lack of exercise, or disease intrinsic to the tissue itself.
Lungs	Lungs are the essential organs of respiration in air-breathing vertebrates. Their principal function is to transport oxygen from the atmosphere into the bloodstream, and to excrete carbon dioxide from the bloodstream into the atmosphere.
Brain	The part of the central nervous system involved in regulating and controlling body activity and interpreting information from the senses transmitted through the nervous system is referred to as the brain.
Mammography	Mammography is the process of using low-dose X-rays (usually around 0.7 mSv) to examine the human breast. It is used to look for different types of tumors and cysts.
Ultrasound	Ultrasound is sound with a frequency greater than the upper limit of human hearing, approximately 20 kilohertz. Medical use can visualise muscle and soft tissue, making them useful for scanning the organs, and obstetric ultrasonography is commonly used during pregnancy.
Induction	A discipline technique in which a parent uses reason and explanation of the consequences for others of a child's actions is called induction.
Pancreas	The pancreas is a retroperitoneal organ that serves two functions: exocrine - it produces

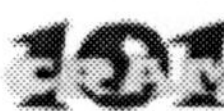

	pancreatic juice containing digestive enzymes, and endocrine - it produces several important hormones, namely insulin.
Neuroendocri-ology	Neuroendocrinology is the study of the interactions between the nervous system and the endocrine system. The concept arose from the recognition that the secretion of hormones from the pituitary gland was closely controlled by the brain, and especially by the hypothalamus.
Contraception	A behavior or device that prevents fertilization is called contraception.
Correlation	A statistical technique for determining the degree of association between two or more variables is referred to as correlation.
Reproduction	Biological reproduction is the biological process by which new individual organisms are produced. Reproduction is a fundamental feature of all known life; each individual organism exists as the result of reproduction by an antecedent.
Morphology	The scientific study of organic form, including both its development and function is morphology.

Photoreceptor	A photoreceptor is a specialized type of neuron that is capable of phototransduction. More specifically, the photoreceptor sends signals to other neurons by a change in its membrane potential when it absorbs photons.
Organ	Organ refers to a structure consisting of several tissues adapted as a group to perform specific functions.
Eye	An eye is an organ that detects light. Different kinds of light-sensitive organs are found in a variety of creatures. The simplest eyes do nothing but detect whether the surroundings are light or dark, while more complex eyes can distinguish shapes and colors.
Photosensitive	People that are photosensitive experience discomfort or get easily sunburned when exposed to UV light, which may come from sunlight or other sources including sunbeds. This is often caused by an allergy or a medication.
Skull	Skull refers to a bony protective encasement of the brain and the organs of hearing and equilibrium; includes the facial bones. Also called the cranium.
Nerve	A nerve is an enclosed, cable-like bundle of nerve fibers or axons, which includes the glia that ensheath the axons in myelin.
Brain	The part of the central nervous system involved in regulating and controlling body activity and interpreting information from the senses transmitted through the nervous system is referred to as the brain.
Lens	The lens or crystalline lens is a transparent, biconvex structure in the eye that, along with the cornea, helps to refract light to focus on the retina. Its function is thus similar to a man-made optical lens.
Ciliary body	The ciliary body is the part of the eye containing the ciliary muscle and ciliary processes. When the ciliary muscle relaxes, it flattens the lens which generally improves the focus for farther objects. When it contracts, the lens becomes more convex which generally improves the focus for closer objects.
Nerve tissue	Nerve tissue refers the specialized tissue making up the central and peripheral nervous systems; consists of neurons and glial cells.
Epithelium	Epithelium is a tissue composed of a layer of cells. Epithelium can be found lining internal (e.g. endothelium, which lines the inside of blood vessels) or external (e.g. skin) free surfaces of the body. Functions include secretion, absorption and protection.
Choroid	The choroid is the vascular layer of the eye lying between the retina and the sclera. The choroid provides oxygen and nourishment to the outer layers of the retina.
Cornea	The cornea is the transparent front part of the eye that covers the iris, pupil, and anterior chamber and provides most of an eye's optical power.
Tissue	A collection of interconnected cells that perform a similar function within an organism is called tissue.
Sclera	The sclera is the (usually) white outer coating of the eye made of tough fibrin connective tissue which gives the eye its shape and helps to protect the delicate inner parts.
Retina	The retina is a thin layer of cells at the back of the eyeball of vertebrates and some cephalopods; it is the part of the eye which converts light into nervous signals.
Iris	The colored part of the vertebrate eye, formed by the anterior portion of the choroid is called the iris.
Optic nerve	The optic nerve is the nerve that transmits visual information from the retina to the brain. The blind spot of the eye is produced by the absence of retina where the optic nerve leaves

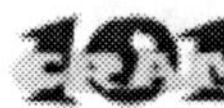

	the eye. This is because there are no photoreceptors in this area.
Ora serrata	The ora serrata is the junction between the retina and the ciliary body.
Cerebrum	Cerebrum refers to the largest, most sophisticated, and most dominant part of the vertebrate forebrain, made up of right and left cerebral hemispheres.
Central nervous system	The central nervous system comprized of the brain and spinal cord, represents the largest part of the nervous system. Together with the peripheral nervous system, it has a fundamental role in the control of behavior.
Nervous system	The nervous system of an animal coordinates the activity of the muscles, monitors the organs, constructs and processes input from the senses, and initiates actions.
Embryo	A prenatal stage of development after germ layers form but before the rudiments of all organs are present is referred to as an embryo.
Prosencephalon	The prosencephalon (or "forebrain") is the rostal-most portion of the brain. The prosencephalon, the mesencephalon, and rhombencephalon are the three primary portions of the brain during early development of the central nervous system.
Myelin	Myelin is an electrically insulating fatty layer that surrounds the axons of many neurons, especially those in the peripheral nervous system. It is an outgrowth of glial cells: Schwann cells supply the myelin for peripheral neurons while oligodendrocytes supply it to those of the central nervous system.
Fiber	Fibers used by man come from a wide variety of sources: Natural fiber include those made out of plants, animal and mineral sources. Natural fibers can be classified according to their origin.
Oligodendrocyte	Oligodendrocyte refers to type of glial cell in the vertebrate central nervous system that forms a myelin sheath around axons.
Anterior surface	The anterior surface of the body presents, in the middle line, a vertical crest, the sphenoidal crest, which articulates with the perpendicular plate of the ethmoid, and forms part of the septum of the nose.
Attachment	Attachment refers to the psychological tendency to seek closeness to another person, to feel secure when that person is present, and to feel anxious when that person is absent.
Protein	A protein is a complex, high-molecular-weight organic compound that consists of amino acids joined by peptide bonds. They are essential to the structure and function of all living cells and viruses. Many are enzymes or subunits of enzymes.
Pupil	Pupil refers to the opening in the iris that admits light into the interior of the vertebrate eye. Muscles in the iris regulate its size.
Humor	In traditional medicine practiced before the advent of modern technology, the four humours (or four humors) were four fluids that were thought to permeate the body and influence its health. A humor is any fluid substance in the body.
Anterior chamber	The anterior chamber if the fluid-filled space inside the eye between the iris and the cornea's innermost surface, the endothelium.
Aqueous humor	The aqueous humor is the clear, watery fluid that fills the complex space in the front of the eye which is bounded at the front by the cornea and at the rear by the front surface or face of the vitreous humor.
Collagen	Collagen is the main protein of connective tissue in animals and the most abundant protein in mammals, making up about 1/4 of the total. It is one of the long, fibrous structural proteins whose functions are quite different from those of globular proteins such as enzymes.

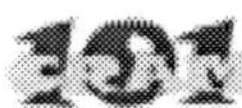

Dense connective tissue	Dense connective tissue has collagen fibers as its main matrix element. Crowded between the collagen fibers are rows of fibroblasts, fiber-forming cells, that manufacture the fibers. Dense connective tissue forms strong, rope-like structures such as tendons and ligaments. Tendons attach skeletal muscles to bones; ligaments connect bones to bones at joints.
Connective tissue	Connective tissue is any type of biological tissue with an extensive extracellular matrix and often serves to support, bind together, and protect organs.
Collagen fiber	White fiber in the matrix of connective tissue, giving flexibility and strength is called collagen fiber.
Loose connective tissue	Loose connective tissue or Areolar connective tissue holds organs and epithelia in place, and has a variety of proteinaceous fibers, including collagen and elastin. It is also important in inflammation.
Melanocyte	Melanocyte cells are located in the bottom layer of the skin's epidermis. With a process called melanogenesis, they produce melanin, a pigment in the skin, eyes, and hair.
Lamina	A thin layer, such as the lamina of a vertebra or the lamina propria of a mucous membrane is referred to as lamina.
Elastic fiber	Elastic fiber is a bundles of proteins (elastin) found in connective tissue and produced by fibroblasts and smooth muscle cells in arteries.
Endothelium	The endothelium is the layer of thin, flat cells that lines the interior surface of blood vessels, forming an interface between circulating blood in the lumen and the rest of the vessel wall.
Transverse	A transverse (also known as axial or horizontal) plane is an X-Y plane, parallel to the ground, which (in humans) separates the superior from the inferior, or put another way, the head from the feet.
Conjunctiva	Conjunctiva refers to a mucous membrane that helps keep the eye moist; lines the inner surface of the eyelids and covers the front of the eyeball, except the cornea.
Muscle	Muscle is a contractile form of tissue. It is one of the four major tissue types, the other three being epithelium, connective tissue and nervous tissue. Muscle contraction is used to move parts of the body, as well as to move substances within the body.
Medial	In anatomical terms of location toward or near the midline is called medial.
Artery	Vessel that takes blood away from the heart to the tissues and organs of the body is called an artery.
Long ciliary nerve	The long ciliary nerve usually arises from the nasociliary between the two heads of the Rectus lateralis. It passes forward on the lateral side of the optic nerve, and enters the postero-superior angle of the ciliary ganglion
Collagen fibril	Collagen fibril refers to extracellular structure formed by self-assembly of secreted fibrillar collagen subunits. An abundant constituent of the extracellular matrix in many animal tissues.
Extension	Movement increasing the angle between parts at a joint is referred to as extension.
Squamous epithelium	The squamous epithelium is epithelium consisting of one or more cell layers, the most superficial of which is composed of flat, scalelike or platelike cells.
Corneal endothelium	Corneal endothelium is the inner most layer of the cornea, the corneal endothelium is a monolayer of squamous epithelial cells lining the anterior chamber of the eye. The corneal endothelium engages in fluid transport, and is responsible for the hydration of the cornea.
Sodium	Sodium is the chemical element in the periodic table that has the symbol Na (Natrium in

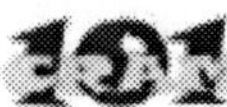

	Latin) and atomic number 11. Sodium is a soft, waxy, silvery reactive metal belonging to the alkali metals that is abundant in natural compounds (especially halite). It is highly reactive.
Ion	Ion refers to an atom or molecule that has gained or lost one or more electrons, thus acquiring an electrical charge.
Blood vessel	A blood vessel is a part of the circulatory system and function to transport blood throughout the body. The most important types, arteries and veins, are so termed because they carry blood away from or towards the heart, respectively.
Blood	Blood is a circulating tissue composed of fluid plasma and cells. The main function of blood is to supply nutrients (oxygen, glucose) and constitutional elements to tissues and to remove waste products.
Metabolite	The term metabolite is usually restricted to small molecules. They are the intermediates and products of metabolism. A primary metabolite is directly involved in the normal growth, development, and reproduction. A secondary metabolite is not directly involved in those processes, but usually has important ecological function.
Diffusion	Random movement of molecules from a region of higher concentration toward one of lower concentration is referred to as diffusion.
Channel	Channel, in communications (sometimes called communications channel), refers to the medium used to convey information from a sender (or transmitter) to a receiver.
Trabecular meshwork	The trabecular meshwork is an area of tissue located around the base of the cornea, near the ciliary body, and is responsible for draining the aqueous humour from the eye via the anterior chamber (the chamber on the front of the eye covered by the cornea).
Bipolar cell	The bipolar cell has a central body from which two sets of processes arise. At one end, they form synapses with either a single cone cell, or a number of rod cells. They also make sinapses with the Horizontal Cells. At the other end, they form synapses with ganglion cells, which fire action potentials along the optic nerve.
Ganglion	In vertebrate anatomy, a ganglion is a tissue mass that contains the dendrites and cell bodies (or "somata") of nerve cells, in most case ones belonging to the peripheral nervous system.
Fovea	The fovea, a part of the eye, is a spot located in the center of the macula. The fovea is responsible for sharp central vision. At the center of the fovea there is a pit with a diameter of about 0.2 mm. It has a high concentration of cone cells and virtually no rods.
Axon	An axon is a long slender projection of a nerve cell, or neuron, which conducts electrical impulses away from the neuron's cell body or soma. They are in effect the primary transmission lines of the nervous system, and as bundles they help make up nerves.
Rods	Rods, are photoreceptor cells in the retina of the eye that can function in less intense light than can the other type of photoreceptor, cone cells.
Ganglion cell	A ganglion cell is a type of neuron located in the retina of the eye that receives visual information from photoreceptors via various intermediate cells such as bipolar cells, amacrine cells, and horizontal cells. The axons are myelinated.
Histology	Histology is the study of tissue sectioned as a thin slice, using a microscope. It can be described as microscopic anatomy.
Lymphocyte	A lymphocyte is a type of white blood cell involved in the human body's immune system. There are two broad categories, namely T cells and B cells.
Plasma	Fluid portion of circulating blood is called plasma.

Papilla	A papilla can be a small projection, such as a nipplelike projection on the skin, at the base of a hair or the root of a feather; the base of a new tooth.
Projection	Attributing one's own undesirable thoughts, impulses, traits, or behaviors to others is referred to as projection.
Melanin	Broadly, melanin is any of the polyacetylene, polyaniline, and polypyrrole "blacks" or their mixed copolymers. The most common form of biological melanin is a polymer of either or both of two monomer molecules: indolequinone, and dihydroxyindole carboxylic acid.
Desmosome	A desmosome (also known as macula adherens) is a cell structure specialized for cell-to-cell adhesion. It is a type of junctional complex.
Veins	Blood vessels that return blood toward the heart from the circulation are referred to as veins.
Vein	Vein in animals, is a vessel that returns blood to the heart. In plants, a vascular bundle in a leaf, composed of xylem and phloem.
Endothelial cell	A endothelial cell also controls the passage of materials — and the transit of white blood cells — into and out of the bloodstream. In some organs, there are highly differentiated endothelial cells to perform specialized 'filtering' functions.
Intraocular	Intraocular describes anything of or related to the inside of the eyeball.
Glaucoma	Glaucoma is a group of diseases of the optic nerve involving loss of retinal ganglion cells in a characteristic pattern of optic neuropathy.
Intraocular pressure	Intraocular pressure s the fluid pressure inside the eye. It may become elevated due to anatomical problems, inflammation of the eye, genetic factors, or as a side-effect from medication.
Myofilaments	The thick and thin filaments that form the myofibrils are referred to as myofilaments.
Sphincter	Muscle that surrounds a tube and closes or opens the tube by contracting and relaxing is referred to as sphincter.
Smooth muscle	Smooth muscle is a type of non-striated muscle, found within the "walls" of hollow organs; such as blood vessels, the bladder, the uterus, and the gastrointestinal tract. Smooth muscle is used to move matter within the body, via contraction; it generally operates "involuntarily", without nerve stimulation.
Sympathetic	The sympathetic nervous system activates what is often termed the "fight or flight response". It is an automatic regulation system, that is, one that operates without the intervention of conscious thought.
Carbohydrate	Carbohydrate is a chemical compound that contains oxygen, hydrogen, and carbon atoms. They consist of monosaccharide sugars of varying chain lengths and that have the general chemical formula $C_n(H_2O)_n$ or are derivatives of such.
Organelle	Organelle refers to any structure within a cell that carries out one of its metabolic roles, such as mitochondria, centrioles, endoplasmic reticulum, and the nucleus.
Displacement	An unconscious defense mechanism in which the individual directs aggressive or sexual feelings away from the primary object to someone or something safe is referred to as displacement. Displacement in linguistics is simply the ability to talk about things not present.
Ciliary muscle	The ciliary muscle is a smooth muscle that affects zonules in the eye (fibers that suspend the lens in position during accommodation), enabling changes in lens shape for light focusing.

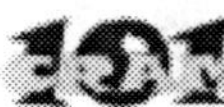

Accommodation	Accommodation is the process by which the eye increases optical power to maintain a clear image (focus) on the retina.
Radiation	The emission of electromagnetic waves by all objects warmer than absolute zero is referred to as radiation.
Cataract	Opaqueness of the lens of the eye, making the lens incapable of transmitting light is called a cataract.
Diabetes	Diabetes is a medical disorder characterized by varying or persistent elevated blood sugar levels, especially after eating. All types of diabetes share similar symptoms and complications at advanced stages: dehydration and ketoacidosis, cardiovascular disease, chronic renal failure, retinal damage which can lead to blindness, nerve damage which can lead to erectile dysfunction, gangrene with risk of amputation of toes, feet, and even legs.
Glucose	Glucose, a simple monosaccharide sugar, is one of the most important carbohydrates and is used as a source of energy in animals and plants. Glucose is one of the main products of photosynthesis and starts respiration.
Diabetes mellitus	Diabetes mellitus is a medical disorder characterized by varying or persistent hyperglycemia (elevated blood sugar levels), especially after eating. All types of diabetes mellitus share similar symptoms and complications at advanced stages.
Acid	An acid is a water-soluble, sour-tasting chemical compound that when dissolved in water, gives a solution with a pH of less than 7.
Laminin	Laminin is a family of heterotrimeric glycoproteins found in the basal lamina underlying epithelia. Their binding to type IV collagen contributes to the self-assembly of the basal lamina from components secreted by cells, and their recognition by growth cone integrins is important to the function of the basal lamina.
Vesicle	Membranous, cytoplasmic sac formed by an infolding of the cell membrane is called a vesicle.
Ectoderm	Ectoderm refers to the outer layer of three embryonic cell layers in a gastrula; forms the skin of the gastrula and gives rise to the epidermis and nervous system in the adult.
Invagination	Infolding of one part of a structure into another is invagination.
Mitochondria	Cytoplasmic organelles responsible for ATP generation for cellular activities are referred to as mitochondria.
Cytoplasm	Cytoplasm refers to the contents of a cell excluding the nucleus and cell membrane. Cytoplasm is a homogeneous, generally clear jelly-like material that fills cells.
Vitamin	An organic compound other than a carbohydrate, lipid, or protein that is needed for normal metabolism but that the body cannot synthesize in adequate amounts is called a vitamin.
Skin	Skin is an organ of the integumentary system composed of a layer of tissues that protect underlying muscles and organs.
Phagocytosis	Phagocytosis (literally, "cell eating") is a form of endocytosis where large particles are enveloped by the cell membrane of a (usually larger) cell and internalized to form a phagosome, or "food vacuole."
Digestion	Digestion refers to the mechanical and chemical breakdown of food into molecules small enough for the body to absorb; the second main stage of food processing, following ingestion.
Variable	A characteristic or aspect in which people, objects, events, or conditions vary is called variable.
Synapse	A junction, or relay point, between two neurons, or between a neuron and an effector cell. Electrical and chemical signals are relayed from one cell to another at a synapse.

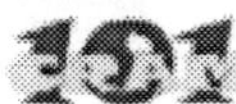

Neuron	The neuron is a major class of cells in the nervous system. In vertebrates, they are found in the brain, the spinal cord and in the nerves and ganglia of the peripheral nervous system, and their primary role is to process and transmit neural information.
Cone cell	The cone cell is a photoreceptor in the retina of the eye which functions only in relatively bright light. There are about 6 million in the human eye, concentrated at the fovea. They gradually become more sparse towards the outside of the retina. They are less sensitive to light than the rod cells, but allow the perception of color and detail.
Cilia	Microscopic, hairlike processes on the exposed surfaces of certain epithelial cells are cilia.
Microscopy	Microscopy is any technique for producing visible images of structures or details too small to otherwise be seen by the human eye, using a microscope or other magnification tool.
Saccule	One of the two fluid-filled sacs in the cochlea separated by the basilar membrane that senses vertical motion of the head is the saccule.
Rod cell	Rod cell refers to photoreceptor cells in the retina of the eye that can function in less intense light than can the other type of photoreceptor, cone cells. Since they are more light-sensitive, they are responsible for night vision. There are about 100 million of them in the human retina.
Plasma membrane	The unit membrane that encloses a cell and controls the traffic of molecules in and out of the cell is the plasma membrane.
Glycogen	Glycogen refers to a complex, extensively branched polysaccharide of many glucose monomers; serves as an energy-storage molecule in liver and muscle cells.
Rhodopsin	Rhodopsin is expressed in vertebrate photoreceptor cells. It is a pigment of the retina that is responsible for both the formation of the photoreceptor cells and the first events in the perception of light. Rhodopsins belong to the class of G-protein coupled receptors. It is the chemical that allows night-vision, and is extremely sensitive to light.
Stimulus	Stimulus in a nervous system, a factor that triggers sensory transduction.
Phospholipid	Phospholipid is a class of lipids formed from four components: fatty acids, a negatively-charged phosphate group, an alcohol and a backbone. Phospholipids with a glycerol backbone are known as glycerophospholipids or phosphoglycerides.
Astrocyte	An astrocyte is a characteristic star-shaped cell in the brain. They are the biggest cells found in brain tissue and outnumber the neurons ten to one. A commonly accepted function is to structure physically the brain. A second function is to provide neurons with nutrients such as glucose. They regulate the flow of nutrients provided by capillaries by forming the blood-brain barrier.
Visual acuity	The ability of the eyes to distinguish fine detail is visual acuity.
Blind spot	In anatomy, the blind spot is the region of the retina where the optic nerve and blood vessels pass through to connect to the back of the eye. Since there are no light receptors there, a part of the field of vision is not perceived.
Nerve cell	A cell specialized to originate or transmit nerve impulses is referred to as nerve cell.
Receptor	A receptor is a protein on the cell membrane or within the cytoplasm or cell nucleus that binds to a specific molecule (a ligand), such as a neurotransmitter, hormone, or other substance, and initiates the cellular response to the ligand. Receptor, in immunology, the region of an antibody which shows recognition of an antigen.
Aldehyde	An aldehyde is either a functional group consisting of a terminal carbonyl group or a compound containing a terminal carbonyl group.

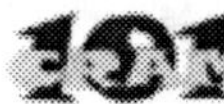

Opsin	Opsin is a group of light-sensitive, 7 pass transmembrane protein/pigment found in photoreceptor cells.
Color vision	Ability to detect the color of an object, dependent on three kinds of cone cells is called color vision.
Theory	Theory refers to an explanatory statement, or set of statements, that concisely summarizes the state of knowledge on a phenomenon and provides direction for further study.
Conductance	The capacity of heat, electricity, or a substance to pass through a particular material is a conductance.
Calcium	Calcium is the chemical element in the periodic table that has the symbol Ca and atomic number 20. Calcium is a soft grey alkaline earth metal that is used as a reducing agent in the extraction of thorium, zirconium and uranium. Calcium is also the fifth most abundant element in the Earth's crust.
Intracellular	Intracellular refers to having to do with the interior of a cell.
Action potential	The sequence of electrical changes occurring when a nerve cell membrane is exposed to a stimulus that exceeds its threshold is called action potential.
Depolarization	Depolarization is a decrease in the absolute value of a cell's membrane potential. Thus, changes in membrane voltage in which the membrane potential becomes less positive or less negative are both depolarizations.
Horizontal cell	The horizontal cell is a laterally interconnecting neuron in the outer plexiform layer of the retina.They help integrate information before it is sent to the brain.
Amacrine cell	The amacrine cell is an interneuron in the retina which operate at the Inner Plexiform Layer, the second synaptic retinal layer where bipolar cells and ganglion cells synapse. They are responsible for complex processing of the retinal image, adjusting image brightness and, for detecting motion.
Retinal	Retinal is fundamental in the transduction of light into visual signals in the photoreceptor level of the retina.
Ophthalmoscope	The ophthalmoscope, invented by Hermann von Helmholtz, is an instrument used to examine the eye. Its use is crucial in determining the health of the retina and the vitreous humor.
Depression	In everyday language depression refers to any downturn in mood, which may be relatively transitory and perhaps due to something trivial. This is differentiated from Clinical depression which is marked by symptoms that last two weeks or more and are so severe that they interfere with daily living.
Vacuole	Vacuole refers to a space or cavity within the cytoplasm of a cell.
Goblet cell	A goblet cell is a glandular simple columnar epithelial cell that is specifically designed to secrete mucus.
Gland	A gland is an organ in an animal's body that synthesizes a substance for release such as hormones, often into the bloodstream or into cavities inside the body or its outer surface.
Sebaceous	The sebaceous glands are glands found in the skin of mammals. They secrete an oily substance called sebum that is made of fat (lipids) and the debris of dead fat-producing cells.
Sebaceous gland	The sebaceous gland is found in the skin of mammals. They secrete an oily substance called sebum that is made of fat and the debris of dead fat-producing cells. These glands exist in humans througout the skin except in the palms and soles.
Golgi apparatus	Golgi apparatus refers to an organelle in eukaryotic cells consisting of stacks of membranous sacs that modify, store, and ship products of the endoplasmic reticulum.

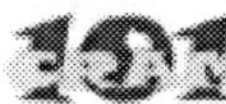

Lysosome	Organelle that contains enzymes that degrade worn cell parts is called a lysosome.
Enzyme	An enzyme is a protein that catalyzes, or speeds up, a chemical reaction. They are essential to sustain life because most chemical reactions in biological cells would occur too slowly, or would lead to different products, without them.
Follicle	Follicle refers to a cluster of cells surrounding, protecting, and nourishing a developing egg cell in the ovary; also secretes estrogen. In botany, a follicle is a type of simple dry fruit produced by certain flowering plants. It is regarded as one the most primitive types of fruits, and derives from a simple pistil or carpel.
Sweat gland	Gland responsible for the loss of a watery fluid, consisting mainly of sodium chloride (commonly known as salt) and urea in solution, that is secreted through the skin is a sweat gland.
Glomerulus	A glomerulus is a capillary tuft surrounded by Bowman's capsule in nephrons of the vertebrate kidney. It receives its blood supply from an afferent arteriole of the renal circulation, and empties into an efferent arteriole.
Canaliculi	Canaliculi are small, microscopic canals between the various lacunae of ocified bone. The radiating processes of the osteocytes project into these canals. In cartilage, the lacunae and hence, the chondrocytes, are isolated from each other. Materials picked up by osteocytes adjacent to blood vessels, are distributed throughout the bone matrix via the canaliculi.
Nasolacrimal duct	The nasolacrimal duct carries tears from the lacrimal sac into the nasal cavity. Excess tears flow through nasolacrimal duct which opens in the nose. This is the reason the nose starts to run when a person is crying.
Lacrimal gland	A gland above the eye that secretes tears is called the lacrimal gland.
Fornix	The fornix is a C-shaped bundle of fibres (axons) in the brain, and carries signals from the hippocampus to the mammillary bodies and septal nuclei.
Serous	The term serous fluid is used for various bodily fluids that are typically pale yellow and transparent, and of a benign nature.
Parotid	The parotid gland is the largest of the salivary glands. It is found in the subcutaneous tissue of the face, overlying the mandibular ramus and anterior and inferior to the external
Myoepithelial cell	Myoepithelial cell refers to type of unstriated muscle cell found in epithelia, e.g. In the iris of the eye and in glandular tissue.
Infection	The invasion and multiplication of microorganisms in body tissues is called an infection.
Hydrolyze	Hydrolyze refers to break a chemical bond, as in a peptide linkage, with the insertion of the components of water, -H and -OH, at the cleaved ends of a chain. The digestion of proteins is hydrolysis.
Cell wall	A cell wall is a more or less solid layer surrounding a cell. They are found in bacteria, archaea, fungi, plants, and algae.
Bacteria	The domain that contains procaryotic cells with primarily diacyl glycerol diesters in their membranes and with bacterial rRNA. Bacteria also is a general term for organisms that are composed of procaryotic cells and are not multicellular.
Lysozyme	Lysozyme is an enzyme (EC 3.2.1.17), commonly referred to as the "body's own antibiotic" since it kills bacteria. It is abundantly present in a number of secretions, such as tears (except bovine tears).
Middle ear	Middle ear refers to one of three main regions of the vertebrate ear; a chamber containing three small bones that convey vibrations from the eardrum to the inner ear.

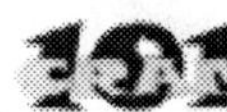

Cartilage	Cartilage is a type of dense connective tissue. Cartilage is composed of cells called chondrocytes which are dispersed in a firm gel-like ground substance, called the matrix. Cartilage is avascular (contains no blood vessels) and nutrients are diffused through the matrix.
Pinna	The pinna is the visible part of the ear that resides outside of the head. It acts as a funnel, amplifying the sound and directing it to the ear canal. While reflecting from the pinna, sound also goes through a filtering process which adds directional information to the sound.
Elastic cartilage	Elastic cartilage is a stiff yet elastic tissue found in the pinna of the ear and several tubes, such as the walls of the auditory and eustachian canals and larynx.
External auditory meatus	The external auditory meatus is a tube running from the outer ear to the middle ear. The net effect of the head, pinna, and ear canal is that sounds in the 2,000 to 4,000 Hz region are amplified by 10 to 15 dB.
Auditory	Pertaining to the ear or to the sense of hearing is called auditory.
Submucosa	The tissue layer just under the epithelial lining of the lumen of the digestive tract is referred to as the submucosa.
Hair follicle	A hair follicle is part of the skin that grows hair by packing old cells together. Attached to the follicle is a sebaceous gland, a tiny sebum-producing gland found everywhere except on the palms and soles of the feet.
Cerumen	Earwax, also known by the medical term cerumen, is a yellowish, waxy substance secreted in the ear canal of humans and many other mammals.
Ossicle	An ossicle is one of the small bones of the middle ear. They serve to transmit sounds from the air to the fluid filled labyrinth (cochlea). They are in order from the eardrum to the inner ear, the malleus, incus, and stapes.
Tympanic membrane	Tympanic membrane is a thin membrane that separates the outer ear from the middle ear. Its function is to transmit sound from the air to the ossicles inside the middle ear.
Pharynx	The pharynx is the part of the digestive system and respiratory system of many animals immediately behind the mouth and in front of the esophagus.
Mastoid process	The mastoid process is a conical bump of the posterior portion of the temporal bone that is situated behind the ear in humans and many other vertebrates and serves as a site of neck muscle attachment (the Sternocleidomastoid, Splenius capitis, and Longissimus capitis).
Eustachian tube	The Eustachian tube (or auditory tube) is a tube that links the pharynx to the middle ear. Normally the Eustachian tube is closed, but it can open to let a small amount of air through to equalize the pressure between the middle ear and the atmosphere.
Auditory tube	Extension from the middle ear to the nasopharynx which equalizes air pressure on the eardrum is called the auditory tube.
Periosteum	The periosteum is an envelope of fibrous connective tissue that is wrapped around the bone in all places except at joints.
Round window	Round window refers to membrane-covered opening between the inner ear and the middle ear.
Oval window	Oval window in the vertebrate ear is a membrane-covered gap in the skull bone, through which sound waves pass from the middle ear into the inner ear.
Malleus	The malleus is hammer-shaped small bone or ossicle of the middle ear which connects with the incus and is attached to the inner surface of the eardrum. It transmits the sound vibrations from the eardrum to the incus.

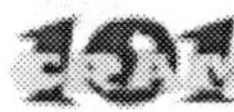

Stapes	The stapes is the stirrup-shaped small bone or ossicle in the middle ear which attaches the incus to the fenestra ovalis, the "oval window" which is adjacent to the vestibule of the inner ear. It is the smallest bone in the human body. The stapes transmits the sound vibrations from the incus to the membrane of the fenestra ovalis.
Incus	The incus is the anvil-shaped small bone or ossicle in the middle ear. It connects the malleus to the stapes. The incus only exists in mammals, and is derived from a reptilian upper jaw bone, the quadrate.
Subarachnoid space	Subarachnoid space is the interval between the arachnoid and pia mater. It is occupied by a spongy tissue consisting of trabeculæ of delicate connective tissue, and intercommunicating channels in which the subarachnoid fluid is contained.
Cochlea	The cochlea is a coiled, tapered tube containing the auditory branch of the mammalian inner ear. Its core component is the Organ of Corti, the sensory organ of hearing.
Labyrinth	The labyrinth is a system of fluid passages in the inner ear, comprising the vestibular system and the auditory system, which provides the sense of balance.
Utricle	A fluid-filled inner ear chamber containing hair cells that detect the position of the head relative to gravity is an utricle.
Vestibule	Vestibule refers to the cavity enclosed by the labia minora, it is the space into which the vagina and urethral opening empty.
Semicircular canals	The semicircular canals are three half-circular, interconnected tubes located inside each ear that are the equivalent of three gyroscopes located in three planes perpendicular (at right angles) to each other.
Cranial	In the limbs of most animals, the terms cranial and caudal are used in the regions proximal to the carpus (the wrist, in the forelimb) and the tarsus (the ankle in the hindlimb). Objects and surfaces closer to or facing towards the head are cranial; those facing away or further from the head are caudal.
Cranial nerve	A cranial nerve is a nerve that emerges from the brainstem instead of the spinal cord. Nerves I and II are named as such, but are technically not nerves, as they are continuations of the central nervous system.
Potassium	Potassium is a chemical element in the periodic table. It has the symbol K (L. kalium) and atomic number 19. Potassium is a soft silvery-white metallic alkali metal that occurs naturally bound to other elements in seawater and many minerals.
Endolymph	Endolymph is the fluid contained in the membranous labyrinth of the inner ear. It is similar in composition to Cerebrospinal Fluid, or the intracellular fluid in the cells of the air.
Macula	The macula is an oval yellow spot near the center of the retina of the human eye. Near its center is the fovea, a small pit that contains the largest concentration of cone cells in the eye and is responsible for central vision.
Microtubule	A hollow rod of the protein tubulin in the cytoplasm is referred to as the microtubule.
Hair cell	The hair cell is a sensory cell of both the auditory system and the vestibular system in all vertebrates. In mammals, the auditory hair cells are located within the organ of Corti on a thin basilar membrane in the cochlea of the inner ear.
Base	The common definition of a base is a chemical compound that absorbs hydronium ions when dissolved in water (a proton acceptor). An alkali is a special example of a base, where in an aqueous environment, hydroxide ions are donated.
Efferent nerve	An efferent nerve carries nerve impulses away from the central nervous system. A motor nerve is an efferent nerve involved in muscular control.

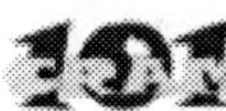

Crystal	Crystal is a solid in which the constituent atoms, molecules, or ions are packed in a regularly ordered, repeating pattern extending in all three spatial dimensions.
Cupula	The semicircular canals in the ears are filled with a fluid called endolymph and they contain a motion sensor with little hairs (cilia) whose ends are embedded in a gelatinous structure called the cupula. The cupula and the hairs move as the fluid moves inside the canal in response to an angular acceleration.
Basilar membrane	The basilar membrane within the cochlea of the inner ear separates two liquid filled tubes that run along the coil of the cochlea, the scala media and the scala tympani. This separation is the main function of the basilar membrane in the hearing organ of all land vertebrates.
Stereocilia	Stereocilia are mechanosensing organelles of hair cells, which respond to fluid motion or fluid pressure changes in numerous types of animals for numerous functions. As acoustic sensors in mammals, they are lined up in the Organ of Corti in the cochlea of the inner ear.
Tectorial membrane	Membrane that lies above and makes contact with the hair cells in the spiral organ is the tectorial membrane.
Diverticulum	A diverticulum is an outpouching of a hollow (or a fluid filled) structure in the body. Its use implies that the structure is not normally present, although embryologically, some normal structures begin development as a diverticulum arising off of another structure.
Scala media	Scala media is a endolymph filled cavity inside the cochlea, located in between the scala tympani and the scala vestibuli, separated by the basilar membrane and Reissner's membrane(the vestibular membrane) respectivly.
Scala vestibuli	Scala vestibuli is a perilymph filled cavity inside the cochlea of the inner ear. It is separated from the scala media by Reissner's membrane and extends from the oval window to the helicotrema where scala tympani continues.
Scala tympani	The purpose of the perilymph filled scala tympani and scala vestibuli is to transduce the movement of air that causes the tympanic membrane and the ossicles to vibrate, to movement of liquid which, depending of frequency, causes the basilar membrane to reach a peak amplitude at a specific site.
Helicotrema	The helicotrema is the part of the cochlear labyrinth where the scala tympani and the scala vestibuli meet. It is also known as the cochlear apex.
Perilymph	Perilymph is a fluid located within the cochlea in 2 of its 3 compartments; the scala typmani and scala vestibuli.
Organ of corti	The organ of Corti is the organ in the inner ear of mammals that contains the auditory sensory cells, the so-called hair cells. It is situated on the basilar membrane and protrudes into the scala media. It contains four rows of hair cells whose hair bundles stick out from its surface.
Ligament	A ligament is a short band of tough fibrous connective tissue composed mainly of long, stringy collagen fibres. They connect bones to other bones to form a joint. (They do not connect muscles to bones.)
Afferent neurons	In the nervous system, afferent neurons--otherwise known as sensory or receptor neurons--carry nerve impulses from receptors or sense organs toward the central nervous system. This term can also be used to describe relative connections between nervous structures.
Inhibition	The ability to prevent from making some cognitive or behavioral response is called inhibition.
Angular	The angular is a large bone in the lower jaw of amphibians, birds and reptiles, which is

connected to all other lower jaw bones: the dentary (which is the entire lower jaw in mammals), the splenial, the suprangular, and the articular.

Vestibular apparatus The vestibular apparatus is the sensory system that provides the dominant input about our movement and orientation in space. Together with the cochlea, the auditory organ, it is situated in the vestibulum in the inner ear.

Skeletal muscle Skeletal muscle is a type of striated muscle, attached to the skeleton. They are used to facilitate movement, by applying force to bones and joints; via contraction. They generally contract voluntarily (via nerve stimulation), although they can contract involuntarily.

Tensor tympani The tensor tympani muscle arises from the auditory tube and inserts onto the handle of the malleus, damping down vibration in the ossicles and so reducing the amplitude of sounds. It is supplied by the medial pterygoid nerve from the mandibular nerve.

Neurotransmitter A neurotransmitter is a chemical that is used to relay, amplify and modulate electrical signals between a neuron and another cell.

Etiology The apparent causation and developmental history of an illness is an etiology.

Concept A mental category used to class together objects, relations, events, abstractions, or qualities that have common properties is called concept.

CPSIA information can be obtained at www.ICGtesting.com
Printed in the USA
LVOW09s1516120214
373435LV00001B/78/A